Principles and Practice of Restorative Neurology

Butterworths International Medical Reviews

Neurology

Published titles

Principles and Practice of Restorative Neurology

Edited by

Robert R Young MD
Professor and Vice Chair, Department of Neurology, University of California at Irvine, California, USA; Chief, Neurology Service, Veterans Affairs Medical Center, Long Beach, California, USA

and

Paul J Delwaide MD, PhD
Chief, Departement Universitaire de Neurologie, Hopital de la Citadelle, Liege, Belgium

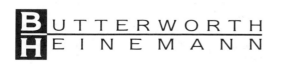

BUTTERWORTH
HEINEMANN

Butterworth-Heinemann Ltd
Linacre House, Jordan Hill, Oxford QX2 8DP

 PART OF REED INTERNATIONAL BOOKS

OXFORD LONDON BOSTON
MUNICH NEW DELHI SINGAPORE SYDNEY
TOKYO TORONTO WELLINGTON

First published 1992

British Library Cataloguing in Publication Data
A catalogue record for this book is available from the British Library

ISBN 0 7506 1172 3

Typeset in Great Britain by Latimer Trend & Company Ltd, Plymouth
Printed in Great Britain at the University Press, Cambridge

Contents

Contributors

Albert J. Aguayo
Neuroscience Unit, McGill University, Montreal General Hospital, Montreal, Canada

Paul Bach-y-Rita
Department of Rehabilitation Medicine, University of Wisconsin, Madison Medical School, Madison, USA

Michael H. Brooke
Division of Neurology, University of Alberta Medical School, Edmonton Alberta, Canada

Paul J. Delwaide
Departement Universitaire de Neurologie, Hopital de la Citadelle, Liege, Belgium

Rene Elkin
Medical Rehabilitation Research and Training Center, Albert Einstein College of Medicine, New York, USA

Alan I. Faden
Departments of Neurology and Pharmacology, Georgetown University Medical Center, Washington DC, USA

Theodore Friedmann
Department of Pediatrics, Center for Molecular Genetics, University of California at San Diego, School of Medicine, La Jolla, California, USA

Fred H. Gage
Department of Neurosciences, University of California at San Diego, School of Medicine, La Jolla, California, USA

Jeremy R. M. Haigh
Department of Clinical Neuroscience, Merck Sharp & Dohme Research Laboratories, Terlings Park, Harlow, UK

Richard Langton Hewer
Department of Neurology, Frenchay Hospital, Bristol, UK

Richard A. L. Macdonell
Department of Neurology, Austin Hospital, Heidelberg, Australia

Fletcher H. McDowell
Burke Rehabilitation Center; Professor of Neurology, Cornell University Medical College, New York, USA

D. Lindsay McLellan
University of Southampton Rehabilitation Unit, Southampton General Hospital, Southampton, UK

C. David Marsden
University Department of Clinical Neurology, Institute of Neurology, The National Hospital for Nervous Diseases, London, UK

Joseph B. Martin
School of Medicine, University of California at San Francisco, San Francisco, California, USA

Ronald G. Marteniuk
Faculty of Applied Sciences, Simon Fraser University, Burnaby, Canada

Hirotaro Narabayashi
Neurological Clinic, Nakameguro, Tokyo, Japan

John G. Nicholls
Department of Pharmacology, Biocenter of the University of Basel, Basel, Switzerland

John M. Oxbury
Neurology Department, Radcliffe Infirmary, Oxford, UK

S. Scott Panter
Letterman Army Institute of Research, Blood Research Division, Presidio of San Francisco, California, USA

Aftab E. Patla
Department of Kinesiology, University of Waterloo, Waterloo, Ontario, Canada

G. L. Pennisi
Department of Neurology, University of Catania, Sicily, Italy

Mehdi Sarkarati
Harvard Medical School, Spinal Cord Injury Service, West Roxbury Veterans
Administration Medical Center, Boston, Massachusetts, USA

Labe C. Scheinberg
Albert Einstein College of Medicine, New York, USA

Jean Siegfried
AMI Klinik im Park, Zurich, Switzerland

Marc Sindou
Department of Neurosurgery, Hopital Neurologique, Université de Lyon, Lyon,
France

Michael Swash
Department of Neurology, The London Hospital, London, UK

Michael Traub
Department of Clinical Neuroscience, Merck Sharp & Dohme Research
Laboratories, Terlings Park, Harlow, UK

Joe M. Watt
Glenrose Rehabilitation Hospital, Edmonton, Alberta, Canada

Robert R. Young
Department of Neurology, University of California at Irvine, California, USA;
Neurology Service, Veterans Affairs Medical Center, Long Beach, California, USA

Foreword

'Neurobiological research will provide the miracles of tomorrow', is the last sentence of the chapter by Young and Sarkarati (pages 125–35). For neurobiologists who study cellular and molecular mechanisms of repair, it is the work described in this volume that constitutes a miracle of today compared to say 10 or 15 years ago. At the technical level, the use of infrared or laser devices that enable quadriplegics to control a computer with their eyes, functional electrical stimulation that allows limbs to be moved effectively or respiration to proceed, orthopedic devices that make walking possible for paraplegics, all constitute extraordinary advances not even to be dreamed of when I studied medicine in the mid 1950s. Neither could one then have guessed at MRI and PET scanning, or the application of modern surgical, biochemical, pharmacological, genetic, and molecular biological techniques to restorative neurology, which has proceeded at such an astonishing pace.

In what way could experiments now being conducted on basic mechanisms in neurobiology provide 'miracles' for the future? Since I have never succeeded in prophesying any of the advances that actually did happen, attempts to make predictions must seem pretentious. What may however be possible is to emphasize certain avenues of research that define key problems. One major question concerns the ability of neurons in the adult mammalian CNS to grow, reform connections, and restore function after injury. Contrary to previous dogma, recent experiments (particularly those of A. Aguayo, M. Schwab, and their colleagues), show that CNS neurons have extensive powers of regeneration after their axons have been severed. It is now known that proteins expressed by oligodendrocytes can inhibit growth and can be blocked by specific antibodies, allowing impressive growth of neurons across a spinal cord lesion. Similarly, retinal ganglion cells grow new axons over several centimeters to end in superior colliculus where they form synapses after they have been provided with a favorable conduit of Schwann cells. The identification of specific molecules that enhance and inhibit nerve growth for specific types of neurons constitutes one major avenue of basic research for which one can foresee applications. Another is the use of optical recording techniques pioneered by L. Cohen, A. Grinvald, G. Blasdell, and others (see, for example, T'so DY, Frostig RD, Lieke EE, and Grinvald A (1990) Functional organization of primate visual cortex revealed by high resolution optical imaging, *Nature*, **249**, 417–20). By measuring changes in absorbance through a small opening in the skull, it is already possible to delineate ocular dominance columns, orientation columns, and the cytochrome oxidase color sensitive 'blobs' in the visual cortex of a living monkey without the use of electrodes. These detailed measurements of cortical activity in real time in response to precise visual stimuli, rich in form, depth, movement, and color, can at present be made through the dura mater, only after the skull has been opened. Nevertheless, in the last few years, resolution and the depth of tissue that can be investigated have improved so dramatically that one can perhaps foresee applications to neurology.

A further, fairly safe prediction, relates the development of better pharmacological agents, methods of delivery, and understanding of transmitter mechanisms. In this context, GABA provides an example of how basic research can contribute, with no hint of an application to clinical medicine at the time it was done. The role of GABA as an inhibitory transmitter and its mechanism of action were first considered to be interesting, not in mammalian brain but in peripheral axons of crustaceans.

A major problem for those of us studying basic mechanisms is the challenge of understanding how effectively the mammalian CNS can repair itself after injury. Axonal growth is not enough. For function to be restored, axons must not only regrow to their original destinations, they must branch and form connections on the right targets and not the wrong ones with appropriate synapses, excitatory or inhibitory, strong or weak. Specificity of reconnection is a prerequisite for recovery of function. The way in which neurons achieve the specificity during development or CNS regeneration (in lower animals) remains unknown. What molecules enable cells to recognize one another? How could a complex layered structure, such as the frontal lobe, rewire itself? Do pathways for pain regenerate better than those for movement control? Even in the best of all possible worlds, however, it is difficult to imagine that regeneration could be sufficient on its own without restorative neurology. Molecular and cellular biological mechanisms cannot be expected to solve all the problems that a physician has to handle treating patients with damage to the CNS. What seems so different now, compared to previous years, is that medical practitioners, as is so clearly demonstrated in this book, are not simply aware of the latest advances in basic science but are able to search for new ways of implementing them to the benefit of their patients. The collaboration of scientists working at the laboratory bench with practitioners of restorative neurology seems fruitful, timely, of mutual interest, and likely to grow in the future. The appeal of restorative neurology for a basic scientist like myself is the high interest of these problems, the immense challenge of helping the patients, and the hope of being able to contribute perhaps to the foundations from which the practical 'miracles' of the future could develop.

J. G. Nicholls MD, PhD, FRS
Biocenter, University of Basel, Basel, Switzerland

Series Preface

For almost a quarter of a century (1951–1975), subjects of topical interest were written about in the periodic volumes of our predecessor, *Modern Trends in Neurology*. Although both that series and its highly regarded editor, Dr Denis Williams, are no longer with us, the legacy continues in the present Butterworths series in Neurology. As was the case with *Modern Trends*, the current volumes are intended for use by physicians who grapple with the problems of neurological disorders on a daily basis, be they neurologists, neurologists in training, or those in related fields such as neurosurgery, internal medicine, psychiatry, and rehabilitation medicine.

Our purpose is to produce monographs on topics in clinical neurology in which progress through research has brought about new concepts of patient management. The subject of each monograph is selected by the Series Editors using two criteria: first, that there has been significant advance in knowledge in that area and, second, that such advances have been incorporated into new ways of managing patients with the disorders in question.

This has been the guiding spirit behind each volume, and we expect it to continue. In effect we emphasize research, both in the clinic and in the experimental laboratory, but principally to the extent that it changes our collective attitudes and practices in caring for those who are neurologically afflicted.

C. D. Marsden
A. K. Asbury
Series Editors

1
Introduction—why restorative neurology?

P. J. Delwaide and R. R. Young

Neurologic impairments and disabilities constitute important medical and socio-economic problems. Paradoxically, treatment of chronic neurologic diseases has been considered frustrating and of little value. Neurology has been viewed as a medical specialty more concerned with diagnosis than with therapy.

This opinion should now be changed. In the last 20 years, indisputable progress has been made in the discovery of techniques which reduce patients' disabilities and ameliorate their discomfort. However, to an extent unusual in other medical disciplines, these therapeutic modalities are not represented only by drugs but involve various procedures; surgical, psychological or rehabilitative in nature. Parkinson's disease provides a good example of the way in which different useful techniques have evolved. In the 1960s, before the advent of dopamine precursors and agonists, patients benefited from stereotactic surgery. In the 1980s, the major problem was to define optimal strategies of pharmacologic treatment. The 1990s promise neural grafting although it will certainly not replace drug therapy and has yet to establish its proper place in overall management. New approaches have been developed for the management of patients with spinal cord injuries which aim to reduce the extent of their lesions and make their lives longer and more productive. In neurology, disability is not only the consequence of dysfunctions in cell metabolism but often results from disruptions of neuronal circuits; These disconnections trigger compensatory and adaptive mechanisms which, when understood, may be improved by drugs or by alternative strategies such as training or correction of imbalance between excitatory and inhibitory processes.

There are many new therapeutic techniques to complement well established ones but they may appear disparate and clinicians are faced with confusing choices, sometimes in competition with one another, to improve their patients' function. Classically trained doctors may be reluctant to turn to new techniques but many clinicians are interested in the rationale, principles and achievements of these unusual or new procedures. They are anxious to identify those which are well-founded and derive directly from advances in the field of neuroscience and to discriminate them from other empirical ones which are advocated on the basis of anecdotal evidence. In addition, some clinicians are eager to learn about research techniques, such as neural grafting, which hold promise for the future.

2   *Principles and Practice of Restorative Neurology*

The above mentioned considerations have promoted the development of this book, *Principles and Practice of Restorative Neurology*. Each term in the title deserves comment.

The principles describe the rationale behind available therapeutic techniques as well as future ones which will derive from actual achievements in experimental neurology. They indicate, from a theoretical point of view, the promises and limitations of transposition to human pathology of advances being made in animal laboratories. This intellectual approach, however, is not sufficient for clinicians who have to make decisions for individual patients, choose the best treatment and learn to apply it. Practice is thus a complementary aspect which derives from principles or sends investigators back to the laboratory to discover new principles. Practice refers to the well established procedures that have proved useful including how and when to apply them.

Although all of us would welcome critical and quantitative analyses of techniques currently employed in the practice of restorative neurology, such data, for the most part, do not exist. Collecting such data is an important aspect of the future of restorative neurology.

Restorative neurology is a subspecialty of neurology; it deals with techniques and strategies used to restore a disordered nervous system to a state of optimal function. Restorative neurology is characterized by a pathophysiological approach to nervous system disease and, as such, differs from neurosurgery which is primarily an anatomical discipline and from pharmacology which relies essentially on neurochemistry. However, restorative neurology tries to integrate these modalities of treatment into a comprehensive approach to the patient's disability; it combines disparate disciplines, including new techniques derived from neurobiology, in a pragmatic attempt to improve neurologic functions. It is thus not surprising that restorative neurology encompasses a range of interests; some of these include pharmacology, plasticity, retraining, motivation, substitution, rehabilitation, functional surgery, neural grafting, and genetic engineering.

To be applied effectively, these various modalities of treatment require specialists so restorative neurology relies on a team of physicians, scientists and paramedical personnel assisting them. A coordinator experienced in many of the various aspects of care must define strategies of treatment and assess overall results. At this time, a neurologist seems best suited for that role.

In addition to being multidisciplinary, restorative neurology is uniquely dependent upon the following two endeavors. First is *quantitative evaluation of neurologic deficits* which is the cornerstone of restorative neurology. Proposed therapeutic efforts must prove their efficacy on an objective basis; quantitative assessment is mandatory if one is to be able to compare results and outcomes. This goal is difficult to achieve because tools of assessment are in development and rarely incorporated into the routine practice of most neurology departments. A continuous effort must be maintained to obtain reliable methods of assessment and, considering the interest raised in recent years by quantification of neurologic deficits, codification and generalization of these procedures which can be accepted worldwide may be expected. The second essential endeavor is *clinical neurophysiology*. In addition to providing objective data to contribute to assessment, clinical neurophysiology also permits pathophysiological analyses of the consequences of nervous system lesions. These results are useful to explain not only the general mechanisms involved in common syndromes such as spasticity but also to specify the unique functional particularities of individual patients. Clinical neurophysiology provides means to help understand defective function of the nervous system, develop strategies to correct abnormalities and assess the results. Finally, clinical neurophysiology has practical advantages because its equipment and techniques are widely available and not expensive; however, they are time-consuming.

One may, however, ask whether restorative neurology is a new field in neurology or is only a new name for an old practice, namely rehabilitation. Where does restorative neurology find its place and where are its borders with established medical specialities? We believe restorative neurology has a specific place in the treatment of individuals with neurologic disorders which can best be understood by considering schematically the sequence of events occurring immediately after a nervous system lesion. Similar considerations apply to patients following initial diagnosis of a chronic progressive disorder.

The first step is to make a correct diagnosis including a lesion's localization and extent. If possible, adequate measures are taken immediately to halt progression of the lesion and suppress its effects. This phase is that of diagnosis and acute treatment and may require an Intensive Care Unit. If acute management does not succeed completely, the patient is left with a permanent lesion and following that, biological processes such as plasticity and compensatory mechanisms enter into play to rearrange the nervous system and restore function. A pathophysiological approach to the patient combined with good knowledge of neurobiology may at that stage help one to enhance the recovery process. This is the role of restorative neurology. Many complementary techniques, and new ones appear regularly, are put in place to limit or compensate for disability.

This part of the treatment is the responsibility of a neurologist who knows nervous system semeiology and has the background to understand future developments in neurobiology. Neurologists are accustomed to interpreting results of sophisticated procedures such as brain mapping, MRI and CT scans. The role of the neurologist is not to apply all the therapeutic techniques but to act instead as a coordinator, defining the best strategy and the timing for specific specialists, such as speech therapists, to intervene.

When the lesion has reached a stable state, rehabilitation and retraining may commence. This aspect is more concerned with protheses, occupational therapy and readaptation to society. The burden of socio-economic factors is particularly obvious at this stage and social workers assist the rehabilitation team to reintegrate the patient into society.

This sequence of medical care delivery is only a scheme; in many instances, one or two steps may be missing and multiple interactions and overlapping efforts are needed between the various phases. However, such a sequence corresponds to the evolution of a neural lesion and identifies individual responsibilities throughout the course of a neurologic disease. If not yet clearly or officially formulated, this opinion appears to be shared by an increasing number of clinicians.

This book is not intended to be a treatise on therapy for chronic neurological diseases. It aims, instead, to underline critically the convergence of distinct techniques in some selective exemplary areas of neurology. The editors are aware that it does not cover all the interesting aspects and apologize for that. For example, adult rather than pediatric neurologic disorders are emphasized and retraining of cortical functions after a stroke or a head injury is not discussed. These related aspects are well covered in other textbooks to which we recommend the reader (Illis *et al.*, 1982; Kaplan and Ceullo, 1985; Maloney *et al.*, 1985; Leek *et al.*, 1986). We hope neurologists will find useful information here for understanding the rationale of standard as well as new therapeutic approaches and their application. However, our ultimate goal would be to stimulate young investigators to work on these problems to provide a firmer basis for an integrated therapy of neurological deficits.

References

Illis LS, Sedgwick EM and Glanville HJ (eds) (1982) *Rehabilitation of the Neurological Patient*, Oxford, Blackwell Scientific
Kaplan PE and Ceullo LS (eds) (1985) *Stroke Rehabilitation*, Boston, Butterworths
Leek JC, Gershwin ME and Fowler WW (eds) (1986) *Principles of Physical Medicine and Rehabilitation in Musculo-skeletal Diseases*, Orlando, Straton
Malony FP, Burk JS and Ringel SP (eds) (1985) *Interdisciplinary Rehabilitation of Multiple Sclerosis and Neuromuscular Disorders*, Philadelphia, Lippincott

2
Epidemiology of disability
D. L. McLellan

Discussion of this topic has become less complicated since the World Health Organization (WHO) formulated technical definitions for the terms disability, impairment, and handicap, which are described in the International Classification of Impairments, Disabilities, and Handicaps (WHO, 1980). The purpose for which epidemiological information is collected determines what information is sought (Wood and Badley, 1988).

From a health service perspective, knowing about the impairments and disabilities caused by different diseases helps in calculating the cost-effectiveness of their prevention and treatment. From the perspective of social services, or from the viewpoint of those responsible for housing and transport, the physical and social effects of disability are more immediately relevant than the impairments or the diseases (or trauma) that have caused them. Yet another perspective is that of the politician concerned to maximize the contribution to society by people with disadvantages. The effect of such disadvantages can often be reduced not by changing the people themselves, but by improving their physical environment, the resources available to them, and the willingness of the rest of society to recognize and encourage their contribution. These points are summarized in Table 2.1.

The relationship between disease and handicap is extremely complex, even when acute and transient conditions are excluded from discussion. Many diseases or injuries cause impairments, that is loss of a part or function. Some impairments lead to disability, that is any restriction or lack, resulting from an impairment, of ability to perform an activity in the manner or within the range considered normal for a human being (WHO, 1980). For example, someone with severe arthritis of both hips has impairment of hip movement and of the capacity to bear weight, causing the disabilities of being unable to walk upstairs or for distances of more than 300 metres outside the house. These disabilities would not cause dependency in someone who lived in a bungalow next to a supermarket, but would do so for someone living in a small two-storey house in a rural location.

The wider dimension, which most closely approaches the experience of the disabled person, is captured by the term handicap. Handicap is the restriction of the social role that would otherwise be normal for that person, taking into account their personal attributes, age, resources, environment, and appropriate cultural factors. If the person with arthritis was unable to continue at work, play tennis, or maintain social

Table 2.1 Summary of criteria that determine the collection of information for epidemiological studies

Perspective	Purpose of data collection	Data needed
Health and medical services	To determine impact of disease on costs and the quality of life	Disease-specific information relating mechanism of disease to disability and handicap
Social services or local authorities responsible for personal services	To determine the nature of the needs of disabled people whose independence is compromised	Prevalence and pattern of dependency (physical, social, or financial) caused by disability
Disabled people, politicians	To determine the nature and extent of the handicaps imposed: (a) by treatable or preventable conditions (b) by society	Pattern, prevalence, and causes of preventable handicap

contacts, there would be three handicaps, which could reduce the quality of life very significantly without necessarily leading to dependency.

A further degree of complexity that causes problems in surveys is the extraordinarily varied and unpredictable relationship between the operation of these factors in different individuals. It is often impossible to predict individual dependency from a list of disabilities, let alone from an inventory of their impairments or diseases. Dependency is crucially affected by the environment and resources of the disabled person. Handicap is even harder to predict because social attributes and objectives may be independent of impairment, but greatly constrained by the particular physical environment, and the attitudes and behaviour of other people.

For an individual, the cause or causes of impairment may themselves influence dependency and handicap. For example, multiple sclerosis may cause difficulty in walking, urgency of micturition, some impairment of judgement and decision making, and a tendency to unpredictable fatigue. These may seem modest impairments but they could translate in practice to daily incontinence (if the only toilet is upstairs), loss of employment (if the employer cannot accept unpredictable fluctuations in performance), and social isolation (if there is a breakdown in planning and consistency of making social contacts). Furthermore, this disabled person, his family and friends have to come to terms with the experience and prospect of a fluctuating and unpredictable decline in function over many years. The identity of the disease itself, multiple sclerosis in this example, has implications that contribute to the dependency and handicap experienced, which cannot be predicted by the impairments (or even the disabilities) alone.

People with disabilities have frequently expressed the view that advice provided through community services by people who are not familiar with their disease tends to miss the real target (Wood and Badley, 1988). It is equally clear that medical treatment given in the absence of any consideration of handicap may not only be wasteful but positively counter-productive.

These issues need to be kept clearly in mind when reading the data from surveys and considering their implications.

INSTRUMENTS FOR RECORDING IMPAIRMENT, DISABILITY, DEPENDENCY AND HANDICAP

One of the intentions of the WHO definitions (WHO, 1980) was to establish an agreed set of standards for the collection of data in the hope that all surveys would use them and therefore provide data that could be compared. However, this has not really succeeded, especially in relation to handicap where the necessary complexity of the inventories makes them impracticable for most surveys. By contrast, the concepts of impairment, disability, and handicap are now generally accepted and form part of most recent surveys of disability.

The most comprehensive survey yet undertaken in a developed country has been by the Office of Population Censuses and Surveys (OPCS) commissioned by the Department of Health and Social Security of the United Kingdom in 1984 (Green, 1988; Martin, Meltzer and Eliot, 1988; Martin and White, 1988; Bone and Meltzer, 1989; Martin and Meltzer, 1989; Meltzer, Smyth, and Robus, 1989; Smyth and Robus, 1989). The OPCS surveyed disabled people living in private households, disabled adults permanently resident in communal establishments, and 'carers', defined as people who are looking after, or providing some regular service for, a sick, handicapped, or elderly person, living in their own or another household.

For the survey of adults living in private households, a large sample of the general population (100 000 addresses) was screened to identify people with some form of disability. Subsequently, interviewers approached all disabled people under 60 years of age and half those 60 or more years of age. People with mental, intellectual, and sensory disabilities were surveyed as well as those with physical disabilities. Recognizing the hazards in attempting to predict overall disability from an inventory of impairments or disabilities, the survey team defined a set of scales of severity of disability. They are quite complex and the reader is referred to the illustrated cases given in the report (Martin, Meltzer, and Eliot, 1988).

The survey collected information about limitations in performing particular activities, but provided no direct measure of the overall, combined effect of all limitations. A criterion of overall severity was required in order to enable disabilities to be compared and to combine information about different disabilities into an overall measure. This was done by a panel of judges, which included professionals with expertise in disability, people carrying out research on disability including staff from the OPCS working on the surveys, people with disabilities, carers, and people from voluntary organizations concerned with disability. The panel performed a set of exercises designed to obtain an inventory of judgements in a systematic way. Scales were developed in 10 main areas of disability: locomotion, reaching and stretching, dexterity, sight, hearing, personal care, continence, communication, behaviour, and intellectual functioning.

The results showed that the average placement given by the panel could be predicted by taking into account only the three most severe disabilities, and considering only their level of severity, rather than which area of function they derive from. The three separate severity scores were then combined according to the formula:

worst + 0.4 (second worst) + 0.3 (third worst) = overall disability score

However, it became necessary to add three further categories of disability, which were consciousness (thus enabling epilepsy to be included), digestion, and disfigurement.

Table 2.2 Prevalence of disability in the UK in adults over 16 years of age, for 1000 people within each age group (Warren, 1989)

Age group	Prevalence	Age group	Prevalence
16–24	25	65–69	280
25–54	59	70–74	350
55–59	157	70 +	600
60–64	207	All (16+)	142

Table 2.3 Relationship between severity scores and age in the adult population of the UK (Martin, Meltzer, and Eliot, 1988)

Severity score	Prevalence per 1000 population of UK within age groups						Total all ages
	16–29	30–49	50–59	60–69	70–79	80 and over	
1–2	7	16	50	97	141	144	47
3–4	6	15	35	59	98	132	33
5–6	7	13	26	42	82	156	29
7–8	4	8	15	26	55	149	20
9–10	3	3	7	16	32	133	13

The experience of the panel of judges enabled the range of disabilities in each category to be divided into 10 and then, using the above formula, an overall severity score, also ranging from 1–10, was constructed. A series of 'pen pictures' was published to illustrate some of the exercises upon which this categorization was based. For example, someone with severity score one may be 59 years of age, deaf in one ear, and who had difficulty hearing someone talking in a normal voice in a quiet room; someone with severity score five may be 75 years of age with phlebitis, experiencing incontinence at least once every 24 hours, and unable to walk more than 50 yards or manage more than 12 steps. Severity score 10 included, for example, someone 86 years of age with severe dementia of the Alzheimer type, or severe impairments of motor, sensory, and communicating functions, and incontinence as a result of a stroke.

It was recognized that both the individual scales and the techniques used to arrive at an overall score introduced factors that reflected handicap as well as disability. Therefore, strictly speaking, they are not 'pure' disability scales. Nevertheless, these scales will be of great value in future epidemiological studies and in monitoring services, because they provide a basis for comparing severity of disabilities between studies, different services, or the same service at different times.

These surveys revealed a prevalence of disability in the UK population of 11%, or 14% of all those 16 years of age or more. Severity scores five to ten accounted for 44% of disabled adults.

The estimated prevalence of disabilities in the UK in adults over 16 years of age, for 1000 people within each age group, is shown in Table 2.2; the relationship between the severity scores and age is shown in Table 2.3. Disability of all categories increases

Table 2.4 Prevalence of disability in different fields estimated for adult UK population over 16 years of age (Martin, Meltzer, and Eliot, 1988)

Field of disability	Prevalence per 1000	Field of disability	Prevalence per 1000
Locomotion	99	Behaviour	31
Hearing	59	Reaching and stretching	28
Personal care	57	Communication	27
Dexterity	40	Continence	26
Sight	38	Eating, drinking, and digestion	6
Intellectual functioning	34	Consciousness	5

greatly in prevalence with increasing age. Furthermore, 58% of people with disabilities living in private households were 65 years of age or over, and 32% were 75 years of age or over. By contrast, of those living in communal establishments, 67% of adults with disabilities were 75 years of age or over.

PREVALENCE OF DIFFERENT FIELDS OF DISABILITY IN THE UK POPULATION

In descending order the prevalence of disability in the UK, according to fields of function, per 1000 adults 16 years of age and over is shown in Table 2.4.

Although these figures are of some value in indicating the frequency of different components of disability, an individual disabled person often has more than one disability. The very wide range of possible combinations emphasizes the need for a broad understanding of disability and for service delivery to be finely tuned to each individual situation.

DISEASES RESPONSIBLE FOR DISABILITY IN THE UK COMMUNITY

The prevalence of diseases causing chronic disability is usually greater than the prevalence of disabilities, because not all the people with a disease are disabled by it. In addition, methods and definitions used in epidemiological surveys are different from those used in disability surveys, and indeed the OPCS surveys did not collect precise information about the underlying diagnosis of the impairments.

Warren (1989) has compared the prevalence rates per 10 000 of the adult population investigated in these OPCS surveys with findings in a number of epidemiological studies of different diseases. Using this information, he has been able to estimate the proportion of people with a particular disease who are likely to be disabled by it; Table 2.5 is derived from Warren's analysis. Unfortunately, there is no direct survey data in which both sets of information were collected and so factors such as under-reporting caused by embarrassment, acceptance of a degree of disability as 'normal', and the under-reporting of mild cognitive impairments could all be contributing to the derived percentages in the third column of Table 2.5. However, these are the best current indications of the prevalence of disability in different diseases, as perceived by the people who have the disease.

Table 2.5 Prevalence, for 10 000 of the UK population, of diseases with disabilities and perceived disablement in OPCS surveys (Warren, 1989)

Disease or condition	Estimated prevalence of disease collated from epidemiological studies	Prevalence of disablement in OPCS surveys	Derived percentages of subjects likely to be disabled
Osteoarthritis and arthritis	2100	288	14
Deafness	1000	430	43
Impaired vision	520	250	48
Incontinence	500	210	42
Senile dementia	240	39	16
Coronary heart disease	200	86	43
Bronchitis and emphysema	180	69	38
Rheumatoid arthritis	175	43	25
Stroke	77	65	87
Epilepsy	50	30	60
Stomas	16	7	44
Parkinsonism	14	11	79
Multiple sclerosis	12	10	83

Table 2.6 Prevalence in adults of disabilities from the seven most common general causes (Martin and White, 1988)

Impairments	% of disabled adults in private households	% of disabled adults in communal establishments
Musculoskeletal	46	37
Hearing	38	13
Sight	22	17
Cardiovascular system	20	16
Nervous system	13	30
Respiratory system	13	6
Mental function	13	56

These data demonstrate that for an individual, the chances of becoming disabled are much greater with some diseases than others. Previous surveys, in which the thresholds for accepting the presence of disability were higher, tend to give rather lower percentages of disablement, although the rank order of the capacity of different diseases to cause severe disability is similar in all surveys in developed countries (Badley, Thompson, and Wood, 1978; Harris *et al.*, 1986). Therefore most people with stroke, parkinsonism, and multiple sclerosis have disability of some kind, whereas only one in every five people with arthritis is disabled at any point in time. Nevertheless, there will be 30 times more people with disabilities caused by arthritis than there are with disabilities caused by multiple sclerosis because arthritis is much more common.

Some indication of the propensity of different diseases to cause severe disability can be judged by comparing figures from disabled people living in private households with those living in communal establishments (Table 2.6). It is important to remember that those living in communal establishments tend to be older so that diseases affecting the elderly which do not reduce life expectancy, will be prominently represented. The figures shown in Table 2.6, and corroborated by previous surveys (Badley, Thompson, and Wood, 1978; Harris *et al.*, 1986), suggest that disorders of the nervous system are particularly likely to cause severe disability and dependency, especially when physical impairment co-exists with impairment of cognitive function or behaviour.

The OPCS surveys showed that elderly women are more likely to be disabled than elderly men, even when the greater life expectancy of women has been taken into account. The surveys also showed that once a correcting factor had been applied to the populations of different regions of the UK, in order to standardize differences in the distribution of ages, the North, Wales, Yorkshire, and Humberside had the highest prevalence of disabilities, whereas the southern regions of London, the South East, East Anglia, and the South West had lower than average disability rates. The reasons for these differences in prevalence between elderly men and elderly women, and between the populations in different parts of the UK, are not known.

DISABILITY IN CHILDREN

A concurrent OPCS survey of children under 16 years of age in the UK (Bone and Meltzer, 1989; Smyth and Robus, 1989) showed a 3% prevalence of disabilities. This is less than in previous surveys, which might reflect a more rigorous definition of disability despite the fact that the threshold for disability used in the OPCS surveys is lower than the threshold in most other surveys.

Commonly, children have more than one type of disability and the most prevalent had to do with behaviour. This contrasts with the findings in adults, which were dominated by the high frequency of locomotor disability in elderly people. This difference between children and adults could have been accentuated by a tendency to under-report disorders of mental function and behaviour by elderly people.

Additionally, 2% of disabled children lived in communal establishments, compared with 7% of disabled adults. Apart from disturbances of mental function and behaviour, disorders of the nervous system (especially epilepsy), the respiratory system (especially asthma), and ear complaints were reported relatively frequently. The number of children in each category of disability were similar, in contrast to adults in whom disability tended to become increasingly severe with advancing age. This probably reflects the fact that in childhood, most disabilities have a single cause in each case and many of these may be relatively stable. In contrast, the older adult tends to accumulate a number of unrelated and progressive disabilities with advancing age.

CATEGORIES OF DISEASE THAT COULD GIVE RISE TO DISABILITY IN DEVELOPED AND DEVELOPING COUNTRIES

Because of the different demography of disease in developing countries, it is likely that the range of disability in developing countries is very different from that recorded in the OPCS surveys of the UK. Another way of categorizing diseases, which is of particular value for planning medical services in developing countries, is to class them according to whether they are acute (resulting from injury or infection), developmental (resulting from congenital disorders or malnutrition), or chronic (the category that includes many of the diseases shown in Table 2.5, together with mental illness and abuse of drugs and alcohol). Wood (1983) estimated the contribution of these different classes of disorder to disability in the world population, taking as his base, the WHO estimate of the world population of disabled people, approximately 450–500 million at that time. Just over 25% of all cases were caused by acute conditions, especially infections, with 36% being caused by chronic disorders. Because most developmental and acute conditions are potentially preventable, by a combination of public health, immunization, improved nutrition, and the prevention of accidental injury, these figures indicate that appropriate public health and social measures can reduce the number of disabled people worldwide by almost 66% even in the absence of improvements in medical treatment or rehabilitation.

At a time when rehabilitation services worldwide are under severe resource pressure, it is clear that appropriate public health measures could release over-stretched rehabilitation resources. Therefore, those with unpreventable disabilities could have more resources to help them achieve rehabilitation.

However, such measures would not affect the circumstances of those with established disability whose personal rehabilitation had gone as far as it could. In both developed and developing countries, there continues to be a very great need to reduce the external physical, financial, and social constraints that exclude disabled people from the full range of social activities.

EXTERNAL CONSTRAINTS THAT CONTRIBUTE TO HANDICAP

Handicap is the result of disability and external constraints acting on the disabled person. One such constraint is lack of effective personal finance. The OPCS surveys in the UK (Martin and White, 1988; Smyth and Robus, 1989) provide for the first time systematic information about the financial consequences of disability. It is illuminating to observe the power of epidemiological techniques in detecting subtle influences operating in society, although the findings of such surveys cannot be extrapolated to countries with different social, political, medical, or physical environments.

Only 30% of disabled adults under pensionable age in the UK were working, ranging from 48% of those with severity score 1 (mildest) to 2% of those with severity score 10 (most severe). Unmarried disabled adults and those 50 years of age or over were less likely to be working than those who were married or under 50 years of age.

Disabled men and women in full-time employment earned less than non-disabled people, which was not accounted for by differences in the hours worked. Married disabled adults were less reliant on state benefits because many non-disabled spouses worked.

People who had acquired disabilities in adult life were usually better off than those whose disabilities dated from childhood. This was partly because of their access to training and experience before the onset of disability and partly to the fact that they had accumulated pensions and other assets before becoming disabled.

Disabled non-pensioner families had on average only 72% of the income of non-disabled families. The state benefits received by disabled adults and their families were greatest for married non-pensioners with children and least for unmarried pensioners. State benefits (including retirement benefit) were the main source of income for 75% of disabled adults in the UK.

Being disabled not only reduces income but carries its own costs. Altogether, 60% of disabled adults incurred regular extra expenditure because of their disability and 24% had unfulfilled needs for additional increased expenditure. Additional expenditure was lowest for disabilities of communication, and progressively higher for disabilities of intellectual function, hearing, sight, consciousness, dexterity, reaching and stretching, continence, behaviour, personal care, disfigurement (which included amputations), and locomotion.

This is not the same order of categories as the prevalence date itself (see Table 2.4). It is clear that the financial impact of disability, unlike the overall severity score, does vary according to the particular categories of disablement involved. Therefore, a person with a head injury, whose main disabilities are in the categories of locomotion, personal care, and behaviour, is likely to have higher costs than a person whose disabilities involve a combination lower down the list, such as sight, consciousness, and dexterity, despite registering the same overall severity score.

A further refinement of these surveys was to calculate the equivalent resources of disabled families, which is the income remaining after disability-related expenditure is taken into account. Families with lower incomes spent a greater proportion of their income on disability-related expenses. Those with disabilities with severity score one spent 4% of their income on such items, compared with 15% for those with severity score 10.

Finally, it was possible to establish that subjective experience of hardship of disabled families related more strongly to equivalent resources than to equivalent income. Results showed that 3% of pensioners, 23% of single adults, and 36% of single parents were in financial difficulties.

These findings may be of relatively little direct interest to those in countries other than the UK, but they are important in illustrating some of the mechanisms by which disability creates handicap; they also illustrate the potential power of such surveys in monitoring the effectiveness of general political and fiscal measures in the prevention of handicap. Survey work can also throw considerable light upon the identity and circumstances of those caring for disabled people (Green, 1988; McLellan *et al.*, 1989).

IMPACT OF REHABILITATION MEDICINE ON DISABILITY AND HANDICAP

Remarkably little epidemiological work has been done in evaluating the effectiveness of rehabilitation medicine. Useful insights can be gained into the impact of medicine not only by diagnostic categorizing of disease in survey work, but by detailed analysis of individual conditions.

For example, episodes of low back pain are extraordinarily frequent in developed countries. Frank and Hills (1988) estimated that one episode per year occurs for each 2.5 people of the population of the UK. However, only 9.6% of the 22.9 million episodes occurring each year lead to consultation with a general medical practitioner (personal physician), only 1.4% are referred to a hospital, only 0.3% result in hospital admission and only 0.04% lead to surgery. Such estimates place the role of the general medical practitioner, and the surgeon, in relieving the disability associated with low back pain, into different perspectives according to individual viewpoint along the cascades.

A major difficulty in defining the impact of a disease and its treatment is that single surveys can provide only a guide to the situation at a particular time. Even if a specific survey of the impact of a complex disease, such as multiple sclerosis, is performed and records not only the disability but associated handicaps, hardships, and effects upon the carer, it is not possible to extrapolate in a way that illuminates the actual process where impairments lead to handicaps as the disease progresses (McLellan *et al.*, 1989). For such work, repeated surveys using comparable methodology need to be performed at intervals appropriate to the pattern of the disease, and the physical and social changes expected in the survey population.

Although surveys of defined populations with particular diseases are becoming increasingly sophisticated, the resources needed for the repeated surveys necessary to establish how handicap is generated are beyond those of most charitable organizations. In most countries such repeated surveys, like large point prevalence surveys, inevitably depend upon a commitment of government funds.

CONCLUSION

The epidemiology of disability is a relatively young science and a great deal of work remains to be done, particularly in developing countries where the impact of public health measures is likely to be of crucial importance in reducing the number of disabled people and releasing resources for rehabilitation of people with disabilities and the support of their families. Data relating to attitudes and behaviour of non-disabled people towards those with disabilities could identify further fields for action in the search for ways to minimize handicap associated with disabling disease.

References

Badley EM, Thompson RP, and Wood PHN (1978) The prevalence and severity of major disabling conditions – a re-appraisal of the Government Social Survey of the handicapped and impaired in Great Britain, *Int J Epidemiol*, 7, 145–51

Bone M and Meltzer H (1989) *OPCS surveys of disability in Great Britain report 3: The prevalence of disability among children*, London, HMSO

Frank AO and Hills JE (1988) Spinal Pain, In Frank AO and Magurie GP, eds, *Disabling Diseases*, Oxford, Heinemann Medical

Green H (1988) *General Household Survey 1985 No. 15 Supplement A: Informal Carers*, London, HMSO

Harris, EA, Moore CI, Jack, A, and Fraser PR (1986) *Estimates of the population of disabled persons in New Zealand*, Accident Compensation Corporation, Wellington Business and Economic Research

Martin J, Meltzer H, and Eliot D (1988) *OPCS surveys of disability in Great Britain report 1: The prevalence of disability among adults*, London, HMSO

Martin J and White A (1988) *OPCS surveys of disability in Great Britain report 2: The financial circumstances of disabled adults living in private households*, London, HMSO

Martin J, White A, and Meltzer H (1989) *OPCS surveys of disability in Great Britain report 4: Disabled adults: services, transport and employment*, London, HMSO

McLellan DL, Martin JP, Roberts M, Spackman A, McIntosh-Michaelis S, Nichols S *et al.* (1989) *Multiple sclerosis in the Southampton District*, Southampton University Rehabilitation Research Unit

Meltzer H, Smyth M, and Robus N (1989) *OPCS surveys of disability in Great Britain report 6: Disabled children: services, transport and education*, London, HMSO

Smyth M and Robus N (1989) *OPCS surveys of disability in Great Britain report 5: The financial circumstances of families with disabled children living in private households*, London, HMSO

Warren M (1989) The prevalence of disability, *J Roy Coll Physicians Lond*, 23, 171–5

Wood PHN (1983) Prospects for control, In Wilson J, ed, *Disability prevention, the global challenge*, Leeds Castle Foundation and Oxford University Press, 87–97

Wood PHN and Badley EM (1988) The Epidemiology of Disablement, In Goodwill J and Chamberlain MA, eds, *Rehabilitation of the Physically Disabled Adult*, London, Croom Helm, 6–23
World Health Organization (1980) *The international classification of impairments, disabilities and handicaps – a manual of classification relating to the consequences of disease*, Geneva, WHO

3
Quantitative evaluation of the results of restorative neurology

P. J. Delwaide and G. Pennisi

For more than a century, neurologic semiology has defined typical clinical syndromes and succeeded in attributing them to localized lesions within the CNS. In recent years, these clinical efforts have been complemented by an impressive development of instrumental procedures which help one reach a precise diagnosis. In contrast with the wealth of means to recognize whether, where, and to what extent the nervous system is lesioned, advances have been uncertain in assessment of functional or social consequences of these lesions.

There are many reasons for this discrepancy. In diagnosis, the signs, irrespective of their intensity, often have full value in localising a lesion. If assessment is considered, every sign has to be graded and weighted, but semiology has not concentrated on this aspect. If combinations of signs lead easily to recognition of a syndrome, all its constituents contributing to disability are not necessarily mixed in fixed proportions and they don't evolve in parallel. Therefore, grading one sign is not enough to reflect the consequences of a neural lesion and there is often a problem to determine which are of functional interest. For example, Babinski's sign, so important in diagnosis, has a very limited role, if any, in disability imposed by the upper motorneuron syndrome. If, beyond the signs, functions are considered, the problem is not easier. Functions often deal with various aspects of relational life and, in that field, interpersonal variability is obviously great. Even the choice of adequate study parameters is largely open to debate and not yet standardized.

Although the need for reliable and well established methods of assessment had been less than urgent because few effective measures were able to modify the outcome of neural lesions, at least in their chronic stages, the situation has changed with therapeutic advances. With the development of more active treatments in many fields and the search for new ones, the necessity to appreciate and measure modifications in the neurological status is increasingly apparent and interest in objective methods of assessment is growing (Capildeo and Orgogozo, 1988; Munsat, 1989). Because of the very biology of the CNS, these methods should be sensitive because repair is incomplete and therapies usually of limited efficacy. The problems are therefore complex but deserve consideration and effort. Neurologists are aware that if a new drug were able to improve, for example, a chronic state like dementia, by 5–10%, they could easily overlook it in the absence of simple, reliable, and universally accepted methods to quantitate deficits.

Therefore, it is not surprising that intensive efforts are made around the world to elaborate, validate, and promote techniques, clinical or instrumental, which can objectively reflect impairments or disabilities caused by nervous system lesions. In fact, rather than a shortage of proposed methods there are, on the contrary, too many of them. The problem is that very few are validated and enjoy a large popularity. Each center, even each clinician, is developing personal rating scales depending on individual patient populations and the specific questions encountered. Unfortunately, few of these methods fulfill the requirements of a comprehensive assessment of neurological status. Concerning evaluation of consequences of a neural lesion, the present period is reminiscent of the early days of neurologic semiology. Many individual attempts are proposed but consensus on a battery of well codified and internationally acknowledged methods has not yet been reached.

GENERAL PRINCIPLES OF NEUROLOGIC ASSESSMENT

Before considering how to assess neurological function, it is worth considering what to assess. In fact, assessment can be performed at successive levels along a sequence going from neural lesion to handicap.

When a pathological process develops within the nervous system, it may cause a single or multiple lesions. The lesions may remain clinically silent but be detected by various paraclinical techniques such as MRI. For therapeutic purposes, it may be interesting to know the number and size of these lesions even if they have no clinical manifestations. It is therefore useful to have codified techniques able to specify the lesions; this represents the first level of assessment. Multiple sclerosis (MS) provides clear examples of lesions without clinical signs. MRI may reveal multiple large plaques of demyelination in a patient with a normal clinical examination. Visual evoked potentials may often document optic neuritis while ophthalmologic examination finds normal visual acuity.

Commonly, lesions within the CNS manifest themselves by neurologic signs and symptoms, which depend on the nature, location, and volume of the lesions. The signs reveal without doubt that CNS function is impaired. Impairment can be defined as any loss or abnormality of psychological, physiological or anatomical structure or function that reflects disturbances within the nervous system. A single lesion may lead to various impairments depending on many factors such as its precise localization and side, its nature, and the age of the patient. An identical lesion may result, especially in the chronic stage, in variable impairment, in absence of any therapeutic intervention, as a result of compensation and neuronal plasticity. Therefore, even if lesion and impairment are related, there is at the same time, no strict correlation between them. Consequently, assessment of impairment itself is necessary, which constitutes the second level of assessment. Impairment represented by neurologic signs and symptoms is influenced by many factors, which are related as follows:

$$\text{Impairment} = \frac{(\text{volume of the lesion} \times \text{location}) \times \text{number}}{\text{natural recovery} \times \text{plasticity} \times \text{therapeutic efficacy}}$$

Impairment(s) may or may not lead to functional consequences, which are called disabilities. Disability, according to the definition given by the World Health

Organization (WHO), is concerned with compound or integrated activities expected of a person, such as are represented by tasks and behaviours (e.g. walking and eating). A disability is any restriction or lack resulting from an impairment of ability to perform an activity in the manner or within the range considered normal. Disability may be temporary or permanent, reversible or irreversible, and progressive or regressive. It reflects disturbances at the level of the person. Theoretically, it depends on many factors:

$$\text{Disability} = \frac{\text{impairment(s)} \times \text{involved function} \times \text{evolution (complications)}}{\text{compensation/substitution} \times \text{therapy} \times \text{personal factors (motivation)}}$$

Neurologists are frequently faced with evaluation of disabilities; reduction of disability is the aim of all therapeutic measures. As shown by the two equations above, disability is not synonymous with impairment and not directly correlated with it. Disability has to be evaluated separately, which is the third level of assessment.

Disability may or may not be responsible for handicaps. Handicap is a disadvantage for a given individual, resulting from an impairment or disability that limits or prevents the fulfillment of a role that is normal (depending on age, sex, social, educational, and cultural factors) for that individual. Handicap therefore represents socialization of an impairment or disability, and is a phenomenon that deals with socio-economic consequences of disability. Handicap is estimated by the following formula:

$$\text{Handicap} = \text{disability(ies)} \times \text{socio-economic factors}$$

Evaluation of a handicap is in fact an administrative task, not a medical responsibility or function. However, non-medical factors have proved extremely difficult to measure and, for this reason, disability is a very important criterion for practical purposes. Determination of a handicap constitutes the fourth level of assessment.

The concepts of lesion, impairment, disability, and handicap appear to be linked in a simple linear progression, but in many instances, the situation is more complex. The sequence may be interrupted at any stage and, for example, a patient can be impaired without disability. We have already mentioned that in an MS patient, a residual Babinski's sign may be found at a neurological examination (impairment) but walking may not be affected (disability 0). Handicap may arise from impairment without the mediation of a disability. Sequelae of facial palsy, for example, may be a disadvantage in social life (handicap) but it would be difficult to identify any disability related to them.

The distinction between impairment, disability, and handicap has been promoted by the WHO (1980). An agreement between experts has been reached on definition and classification of consequences of diseases. However, it seems that these concepts encounter difficulties in becoming part of everyday language of neurologists and problems persist with terminology. For example, as quoted by Willoughby and Paty (1988), the 'Disability' Status Scale (DSS) introduced by Kurtzke (1961) concerns impairments more than disabilities.

The system proposed by the WHO is merely an international classification and is not intended for scoring neurologic deficits. To date, there is no unified coding system that has been patronized by an international organization but, if such a system is developed, there is little doubt that it will be adapted to the present WHO classification. That means that various levels of assessment will be considered and that specific methods will be proposed for each step of the sequence going from lesion to handicap. If scores are obtained for each level, it is important to clearly differentiate their meaning so as to have a precise idea of what is really being measured and the true significance of any observed change. The equations above make clear the differences between each level. Similarly, it would be unwise to extrapolate from one category of results to conclusions concerning other aspects.

If one of the major problems in assessment is to know precisely at what level evaluation has to be made, and to tailor techniques and methods according to the problem under study, there are other problems to solve. The tests employed have to fulfill general criteria; they must be valid, accurate, reliable, sensitive, reproducible, and easily practicable (Maurer and Commenges, 1988; Tourtellotte and Syndulko, 1989).

Validity means how well or how closely the test measures the true or actual value of what it is intended to measure. The problem has to be well defined and the techniques, well adapted. As symptomatology is most often multidimensional, the question of choice of judgement criteria or rating scales is still debated. Although useful in diagnosis, some signs are not necessarily good indicators of clinical changes. In any case, the selection should be adapted to the question under study. For example, if a drug is supposed to reduce parkinsonian tremor, it is not appropriate to evaluate its efficacy by selecting one of the general rating scales for Parkinson's disease which is made up of a large number of items. It is better to choose a scale designed to evaluate tremor exclusively. In this case, assessment has to be sign, rather than disease, specific.

Even an essentially valid criterion has also to be reliable, which means not blurred by large and random errors of measurement which can come from variations over time in a patient or inadequacy in scaling step width. Psychologists have studied the problems of validity and reliability for measurement of mental abilities and a vast literature exists on these topics (Levy, 1973; Shrout and Fleiss, 1979; Cho 1981).

Sensitivity is of special importance when measurement is used as a means to assess changes in the clinical picture. The number of possible scores may vary from two (present or absent) to a continuous scale with usually 3 to 10 steps for ordinal criteria. There is no general answer to the question of what choice is better. Sometimes, the sensitivity of a scale is greater when the number of possible scores is increased. But, if the error of observation is of the same size as the step width, that is not the case. One should choose only as many scores as can be described unequivocally by words.

Reproducibility applies whether the test is carried out repeatedly by the same observer or by multiple observers. Often the inter-rater reproducibility is estimated by taking into account the ratings of more than two raters and using measures of concordance or various coefficients of intraclass correlation.

Practicability is a limiting factor. The tests to be performed should be as simple as possible and the raters should clearly understand what is asked of them.

It is interesting to note that all the above mentioned properties are interrelated. For example, practicability is closely related to validity and reliability. Mathematical models have been used (Maurer and Commenges, 1988) to establish relationships between validity, reliability, and sensitivity. More practically, the various features of a test should be studied using proper methodology. For example, sensitivity could be estimated by the probability with which a true difference resulting from a treatment can be detected by an appropriate statistical test with a fixed number of patients or, conversely, by the number of patients that are needed to detect such a difference with a fixed, predetermined probability. Whenever possible, neurologic signs should be scored using physical units. However, that is not always possible so, often, ordinal scales must be used. The use of ordinal scales raises some theoretical problems. Guidelines for their construction and utilization as measures of outcome have not been clearly formalized. Nevertheless, McKenzie and Charlson (1986) have proposed standards for their use. The individual ranks should be clearly defined and mutually exclusive. They should be ordered in hierarchical progression, and concordance between scale scores and the other measures of outcome should be evaluated. As such scales are frequently used to quantify phenomena that are not truly dimensional, non-parametric statistics are preferred to parametric ones (Forrest and Andersen, 1986) but often, this requirement is not fulfilled in reported results of therapeutic trials.

Another problem concerns the validity of adding the various scores measured within a syndrome. Aggregate (Stewart, Ware, and Brook, 1981) or megascores are claimed to give a better and more comprehensive overview of a patient. In fact, although the advantages of such a method seem obvious, rules governing the combinations of the various items are not clear. Strong objections have been raised against the validity of performing simple additions, although this method is sometimes employed. A critical review of published results in clinical trials identifies many situations where ordinal scales are not used properly, indicating a need for further information and training in the field of quantification of neurologic deficits.

Assessment is an important aspect of restorative neurology and forms the basis for appreciating its achievements. Assessment concerns lesions, impairment, and disabilities equally. It is therefore not surprising that parallel evaluations must sometimes be conducted to reflect the situation at these various levels. In addition to the importance of assessing precisely, restorative neurology is also very much concerned with pathophysiological aspects resulting from lesions within the CNS. Most of the therapies it uses rely on that approach. Therefore, evaluation of the clinical picture is not operational enough and needs to be complemented by data coming from clinical neurophysiology. These data are objective and often quantitative and informative about residual activities within a lesioned part of the CNS. They constitute a complementary evaluation which, however, cannot be assigned a specific place in the sequence going from lesion to handicap, although they most often concern evaluation of lesion.

The field of restorative neurology begins immediately after the initial diagnostic procedures. Its first aim is to evaluate, as objectively as possible, lesions, impairment, and disabilities, and the functional consequences of a lesion in physiological terms. After that, restorative neurology mobilizes all possible therapeutic means, such as drug therapy, surgery, or physical therapies, to restore functions as much as possible. After that step, the patient is transferred to rehabilitation medicine where there are experts in physical medicine who should be more concerned with handicaps and socio-economic factors. Rehabilitation therapists are joined in their efforts by other professionals, such as social workers, to reintegrate the patient into society. There may thus be little overlap between restorative neurology and rehabilitation.

Evaluation of lesions

For a long time, simple biological indices reflecting the extent and severity of a brain lesion have been sought but the results of these searches are largely disappointing.

Technical refinements in brain imaging techniques, especially in computerized tomography and MRI, have made it possible to visualize neural lesions and define their volume and location (Young *et al.*, 1981; Lukes *et al.*, 1983). In addition, they are able to reveal silent lesions and, for that reason, are increasingly used in therapeutic trials in MS. As these examinations can be repeated many times over the course of the disease, they permit useful comparisons and may reflect the efficacy of therapies aimed at reducing the number and size of lesions.

With these techniques, it is sometimes difficult to distinguish between parts of the nervous system that are dead and those areas where cells are lesioned but nevertheless viable. This is an important problem when patients are seen in the acute phase after a nervous system lesion (Freund and Bauer, 1982; Wise *et al.*, 1983; Powers *et al.*, 1985). One solution is sometimes to use radioligands (Benavides *et al.*, 1988) but, when available, the best solution is offered by PET scans, which add useful metabolic information and assist in appreciating cell survival in damaged areas. Moreover, PET scans can also detect unexpected changes at some distance from a neural lesion. For example, hypometabolism in frontal lobes has been reported after cerebellar lesions. These distant abnormalities may help to explain some clinical peculiarities (Shimoyama *et al.*, 1988). Results from clinical neurophysiology examinations sometimes complement the data generated by imaging techniques, but they chiefly concern intensity of the dysfunctions brought about by a lesion rather than its volume.

If the advantages of directly evaluating a neural lesion are clear (objective and quantitative data on the volume, location, and evolution of a lesion), its limitations are also evident. The data concern only lesion characteristics and are not sign or disease specific. It is well known, for example, that a lesion may look very stable according to the presently available imaging methods while impairment and disability regress. Conversely, reduction of a lesion is only suggestive of possible improvement but certainly not evidence for it. Many biological factors that intervene in natural recovery, such as plasticity, compensation, and awakening of quiescent neurons, are not taken into account by these techniques. Finally, although non-invasive, the majority of these brain imaging techniques are expensive and not available everywhere, especially in hospitals for chronic patients. For research purpose, these limitations can sometimes be overcome, although not always in routine practice.

Evaluation of impairments

Physicians alone are competent to measure impairment. This assessment requires good clinical knowledge and is based on physical examination eventually assisted by laboratory investigations.

CLINICAL EXAMINATION
A precise description of the patient's status is the basis for impairment assessment. First, all abnormal signs and symptoms are listed. For diagnostic purposes, it suffices that a sign is present; its intensity acquires great importance for assessment. The 'all or none' law does not apply in restorative neurology. On the contrary, distinct degrees must be considered and examination should be maximally quantitative. Unfortunately, such measurements are not always possible or reliable for all signs. There are few well established methods for scoring common signs. For example, briskness of tendon jerks, one of the most common neurologic signs, is not yet scored in a uniform way by all neurologists. Some recognize three grades for tendon jerks (absent, normal, and increased), whereas others report four or five levels. When no physical

measurements can be obtained, ordinal scales are used, but they seem to vary from hospital to hospital. Fortunately, some signs can be evaluated with generally accepted scales such as the Ashworth scale for spasticity (Ashworth, 1964).

Whenever possible, direct measurements should be performed and expressed in physical units. A list of possible parameters would be too long, although some relevant parameters include range of voluntary motion at a joint (in degrees) and force of handgrip and wrist extensors; time during which a patient perceives vibration when a tuning fork is applied on the malleolus; and time needed to perform a well specified task (walking 10 meters or climbing five stairs). The problem with neurological examinations is that signs can be so many and varied that precise measurement of all of them would be practically impossible. A choice is arbitrarily made between them, often making comparisons impossible.

For practical purposes, only one sign out of a syndrome is sometimes considered, such as tremor in Parkinson's disease, or incontinence or spasms in the upper motorneuron syndrome. In these situations, limited clinical rating scales have been developed, which are sometimes weighted, assigning different values according to the various affected body areas (more points for arm tremor than for tongue tremor) and severity. Provided that the scale is valid and well adapted to the problem under study, such focused scales are useful and can be recommended.

To cope with the problem of inter-rater reliability, video recordings of patients are increasingly popular, especially in the field of abnormal movements. Many raters, therefore, have the possibility of rating a given patient and comparing the situation at various stages of the disease.

The advantages of assessing impairment by clinical examination are evident. Every clinician, in any circumstance, is able to collect relevant information and rate them numerically by making use of the various available scales. These procedures are inexpensive and easy. The time needed is in general compatible with the duration of a routine examination. However, subjectivity remains a problem, and inter-rater reliability may be poor. As a consequence, comparisons of results obtained by two neurologists may be hazardous even if those provided by the same observer for different patients are valid. Moreover, results refer necessarily to the patient's situation during the examination; diurnal fluctuations, for example, are not taken into account. It is often possible to increase precision and reliability of clinical assessment but to the detriment of the time needed to fill in the charts. When the procedure becomes more time consuming, it loses some of its specific advantages. The real problem with clinical assessment is that few methods have been carefully evaluated and recognized worldwide.

LABORATORY INVESTIGATIONS

Contrary to many general diseases, neurologic dysfunctions are generally not correlated with a simple biological parameter. Some muscular dystrophies may however represent an exception to that rule. As clinical examination is not entirely satisfactory in assessing impairment, many attempts have been made to complement it by objective, reproducible data about neurologic signs. Clinical neurophysiological techniques are often used with the sole aim of providing a permanent and quantifiable document. As will be discussed, this represents only one use of these techniques. For example, EMG recordings of tremor or clonus permit the measurement of exact frequency, the duration of the sign, or both. Triaxial accelerometry can assess tremor amplitude. As can be seen by these examples, one single sign out of a syndrome is recorded but the results are clearly not lesion or disease specific. Sometimes, a larger scope than a single sign is considered. For ataxia, force platforms are becoming popular; for gait disturbances, various techniques are available including polarized light recording, electromyography, and vector diagrams.

Cognitive functions can also be evaluated by a battery of psychometric tests. Often they are optimally utilized by psychologists who are trained in assessment of higher functions. In any given laboratory, techniques are usually well standardized and results reproducible. From laboratory to laboratory, however, there may be changes in the techniques making comparisons hazardous.

Therefore, laboratory investigations *can* provide objective quantifiable data; they are, however, limited for achieving a complete assessment. They concern, in general, one or few aspects of a whole syndrome. Moreover, they are instrumental, time-consuming, expensive, and not standardized enough to allow interlaboratory comparisons.

Evaluation of disability

Disability is the inability to perform a common human activity that usually results from impairments. Evaluation of disability is no longer the exclusive responsibility of the physician, and typically is made by health care professionals aided by members of the family. Disability represents objectification of impairments and, as such, reflects disturbances at the level of the whole person. Disability is not disease specific; the same degree of disability may arise following a CNS disease or trauma affecting the limbs.

Disability is appreciated by the way a patient performs composite activities or behaviors that are generally accepted as essential components of everyday life. Activities such as walking, eating, dressing, and speaking are ranked and the patient is assigned a specific score. These behaviours are often called activities of daily living (ADL). There are various scales for activities of daily living and new ones are regularly proposed. For MS, there is a long tradition of constructing and using disability rating scales, dating back to Alexander in 1951. The most popular is Kurtzke's method, which has been tested in a cooperative study on the effects of ACTH in acute exacerbations of MS (Kurtzke, 1970). However, many investigators found Kurtzke's scales insufficiently detailed; Kurtzke tried to overcome this problem by proposing his expanded disability status scale (Kurtzke, 1983). Alternative scales are available but not recognized worldwide. Moreover, many of them contain measures of impairment and of disability. For Parkinson's disease, as quoted by Lang and Fahn (1989), there were almost as many rating scales as there were groups of investigators performing clinical trials in that disorder. However, a consensus has recently been reached on a new and largely accepted scale, the unified Parkinson's disease rating scale (Fahn and Elton, 1987). It has been suggested that disability scales could serve to assess the results of treatment or disease progression by dividing the present grade of disability by the duration of the disease (in years or months). This method is however open to criticism and needs further evaluation. In fact, it would only be valid if modifications evolve linearly with time.

Another problem concerns scales based on combined scores because they record items cumulatively resulting from a single impairment. Caution is needed before expressing disease severity by a single index.

Once again, it is important to stress the difference between impairment and disability. A small degree of spasticity is clearly an impairment but its contribution to disability depends on its localization; in the lower limbs, it may help the patient to walk because it provides a firm support to the body.

CLINICAL NEUROPHYSIOLOGY

As already emphasized, clinical neurophysiology (Sedgwick, 1982) plays a special role in restorative neurology; it has various complementary aims. Some techniques are diagnostically oriented, others pathophysiologically. They provide objective, often quantitative, data which are of considerable interest for assessment. In that field, some general advantages may be underlined:

1) Quantitative results, when available, permit intra- and inter-individual comparisons.
2) Most of the techniques are standardized, distributed worldwide, and offer precise norms that can be used to match the results obtained in one given patient. Comparisons between various laboratories are therefore easier.
3) Often a battery of complementary tests (see Table 3.1) can be applied to one patient enabling the clinician to judge the coherence between the results.
4) The techniques are risk free, in general non-invasive, and require limited cooperation by the patient. In addition, they are cheap and may be easily repeated.

Clinical neurophysiology cannot however pretend to give a unique and comprehensive means of assessing the neurological picture. There are evident limitations including:

1. With some tests, the results may be difficult to quantify especially when they derive from a sampling technique. Needle electromyography or microneurography offer clear examples of such a limitation and routine EEG does not easily provide quantitative data.
2. Often, one limited aspect of complex and multiple functions is measured. For peripheral nerve function assessment, for example, nerve conduction velocities reflect only speed in the fastest conducting fibres. As stressed by Burke (1985), this constitutes only a small part of nerve physiological function and the results may not be closely linked to clinical complaints. In Charcot Marie-Tooth disease, for example, sensory symptoms are few and subtle despite dispersed low-amplitude sensory action potentials that have a maximal conduction velocity of $10-15\,\mathrm{ms}^{-1}$. On the other hand, somatosensory evoked potentials recorded after mixed nerve stimulation primarily provide information about proprioceptive fibers and do not necessarily reflect correctly abnormalities in cutaneous fibers and in skin sensitivity.
3. Results of clinical neurophysiology help in defining lesions and in evaluating their repercussions. The techniques are therefore valid for assessment of neural lesions and impairment, but they don't provide any idea about disability and, of course, cannot be used to measure it.
4. The techniques are not applicable in all circumstances.

In brief, clinical neurophysiology is a priviledged means to objectively assess lesions and impairments but it cannot be used alone to substitute for the clinical approach that it assists. However, in addition to its role in assessment, clinical neurophysiology is unique in being able to express results of lesions and impairments in physiological terms. Therefore, the results constitute a firm basis upon which to elaborate therapeutic strategies based on pathophysiological data. Clinical neurophysiology can point out functional difficulties and verify to what extent various types of therapy

Table 3.1 Partial list of neurophysiological investigations

Level of the nervous system	Test	Remarks
Cerebral cortex	– EEG	Qualitative
	– Spectral EEG	Quantitative
	– Mapping	Quantitative
	– Motor potentials	Qualitative
	– Cortical stimulation	Quantitative
Brain stem	– BAER	Quantiative
	– Blink Reflex	
Sensory pathways	– SSEP	Quantitative
(periphery to cortex)	– Dorsal column conduction velocity	but just one
	(direct or indirect techniques)	aspect
Motor pathways	– Cortical and spinal stimulation	Quantitative
(cortex to periphery)	– Needle EMG	Qualitative
Spinal cord	– Spinal conduction velocity:	
	see sensory and motor pathways, below	
	– H reflex/H/M ratio	Quantitative
	– F wave	Qualitative
	– Interneurons: Presynaptic inhibition	Quantitative
	IA inhibitory interneuron	
	IB interneuron	
	Renshaw cell	
	– Flexor reflexes	Qualitative
Nerve	– Sensory and motor conduction velocity	Quantitative but just one aspect
	– Somatosensory Evoked Potentials	Quantitative
	– Microneurography	Qualitative
Neuromuscular	– Stimulodetection	Quantitative
junction	– Jitter	Quantitative
Muscle	– Routine EMG	Qualitative

correct them (Delwaide, 1985). Moreover, it permits the pathophysiological study in man of many syndromes that are very imperfectly reproduced in animals. This pathophysiological aspect, chiefly research oriented, has recourse to standardized techniques but also to a large variety of protocols designed for one specific purpose and, therefore, restricted to few laboratories. Despite their interest, it is not possible to review these latter and we will limit ourselves to the most common.

Many techniques are available in almost all laboratories and can be applied to various levels of the nervous system, from the cerebral cortex to muscle. Table 3.1 lists some of them. This is not the place for an exhaustive discussion of methodology, intrinsic value, and limitations of each of them. The interested reader can consult the many specialized textbooks (Chiappa, 1990; Aminoff, 1986; Duffy, 1986; Kimura, 1987). In this chapter, only selected aspects will be considered.

Cerebral cortical activity can be evaluated by EEG, evoked potentials, and event-related evoked potentials, as well as by cortical stimulation.

Routine EEG gives a crude idea of the functioning of the cerebral cortex; its major limitation is related to a lack of possible quantification. For this reason, EEG is often regarded as disappointing from the point of view of assessment. Recent advances have however opened up new perspectives as a result of easy-to-operate, highly sophisticated recorders. Spectral analysis is now integrated into routine work in many laboratories of clinical neurophysiology and the results so far obtained renew interest in an old technique. Coherence of rhythms between the two cerebral hemispheres can be easily appreciated. EEG Brain Mapping, which computes the values of spectral analyses over many scalp derivations, is also promising but is still in a developmental phase and awaits controlled studies of larger series before being incorporated into the battery of essential tests for cortical function. Reservations about this technique, which have recently been made by a subcommittee of the American Academy of Neurology (Fahn *et al.*, 1989), apply more to its diagnostic uses than to its value for assessment. Long duration EEG recordings, often coupled with video monitoring, as used for diagnosing epilepsy, should be added in selected cases to the conventional techniques.

Evoked potentials, certainly the somatosensory but also the visual and auditory, are widely used to evaluate conduction in specific neural pathways. The main parameter recognized as useful is the latency; whereas amplitude and configuration are less reliable, they may nevertheless be indicative of asymmetries between the hemispheres. Here again, caution is necessary in assessing the value of evoked potentials; only one function of selected pathways is evaluated. This function can be quantified but it would be an error to equate the results of one single test with an exhaustive evaluation of impairment (even more, of a disability) of the sensory pathways. Cortical motor functions can be studied by the premotor and Bereitschaft-potentials. This approach is promising as exemplified by interesting data reported for Parkinson's disease (Dick *et al.*, 1989) but it remains more a research tool than a routine paraclinical test.

Various restricted parts of the cortex can be activated by transcranial stimulation, electric or more often magnetic, but the motor cortex has been investigated most often. With the exception of some papers on its value in predicting the outcome of stroke patients (McDonnell, Donnan, and Bladin, 1989), the usefulness of the technique has not been fully appreciated. Stimulation of the motor cortex is intended to test conduction velocity in fibers of the pyramidal tract. It would be an error to consider it an adequate and complete test of the function of this tract or of the motor cortex itself.

At the brainstem level, brainstem auditory evoked responses (BAER) have become classical because it has been shown that each peak corresponds to an anatomical relay in the acoustic pathway from ear to cerebrum. This technique is intensively used in comatose patients, and in those presenting with a permanent lesion in the brainstem. Before the generalized use of BAER, blink reflexes enjoyed great favor. Their methodology is well established and standardized; its two component response with potential for habituation offers many parameters to be studied, the significance of which is increasingly established. Consistent abnormalities have been described in many situations such as Parkinson's disease or the upper motorneuron syndrome and they may evolve in parallel with the clinical status (see Ongerboer de Visser, 1983; Kimura *et al.*, 1985). Other brainstem reflexes such as the masseteric reflex could perhaps be useful, but are less well established (Cruccu, Fornarelli, and Manfredi, 1988).

The functions of the spinal cord are multiple; it is a reflex center, organized on a segmental or plurisegmental basis, but it also has conduction functions, both ascending and descending. Descending fibers also control the reflex organization at spinal cord level (Baldissera, Hultborn, and Illert, 1981).

Conduction velocity in the dorsal column can be measured directly or indirectly using somatosensory evoked potentials, F wave, and reflex muscle potentials (Eisen, 1986). Normal values of spinal conduction velocities are available. When slowing is observed, it can be generalized over all tested segments. In other cases, a well defined travelling wave can be easily followed to a certain level and is then not recordable rostrally, indicating a localized conduction block (Delwaide and Delwaide, 1987). The study of conduction velocities in dorsal columns can be complemented by conduction velocity in the pyramidal tract activated at various levels by magnetic or electric stimulation. Conduction velocity in other spinal pathways can only be estimated by indirect and complex procedures.

There is at present a large battery of electrophysiological tests enabling the study of various neurons and interneurons within the spinal cord. The majority of techniques rely on conditioning a monosynaptic reflex, the Hoffmann reflex, by procedures that activate well defined afferent fibers. The Hoffmann reflex (H reflex) methodology is now well standardized and the response is stable enough to be used as a test. When sciatic nerve stimulation is kept constant, H reflex amplitude variations reflect excitability changes of the soleus alpha motorneurons (provided that presynaptic inhibition acting on IA afferents is not modified at the same time). Using correctly timed stimulation of various nerves, the inhibitory effects of Renshaw cells, IA inhibitory interneurons, and IB interneurons can be measured (Delwaide, 1985). Presynaptic inhibition can be measured by two methods. The first consists of measuring inhibition of the H reflex brought about by vibration of the soleus. Vibration activates muscle spindles and sets off continuous discharges in IA fibers, which trigger a mechanism of presynaptic inhibition acting on homonymous fibers. The second is based on measurement on the surface of a positive wave elicited in the dorsal horn when responses to sciatic nerve stimulation are recorded by percutaneous electrodes and averaged (Delwaide, Schoenen, and De Pasqua, 1985). The ratio between the negative (S) and positive (P2) waves gives a measure of presynaptic inhibition.

The majority of spinal electrophysiological tests produce quantitative results, enabling one to define normal values with standard deviations. Abnormalities can therefore be easily recognized and quantified. The techniques mentioned above have contributed greatly to pathophysiological knowledge of many motor syndromes. They have also been used for assessment but the results are less encouraging because signs and symptoms are often caused by many mechanisms, rather than a single disturbed mechanism. If a neurophysiological abnormality may be corrected, for example by a drug, it does not mean that the modification will result in reduced impairment or disability. The electrophysiological techniques of spinal cord testing therefore reveal neurophysiological disturbances and are unique in that respect. However, they are not sufficient to characterize and evaluate an impairment and should complement the use of quantified examinations and rating scales.

In addition to techniques based on H reflexes, flexor reflexes have attracted attention. They allow definition of the electrical threshold of motorneuron activation through cutaneous afferents. It is possible to specify the pattern of muscle activations (Young, 1973). More complex protocols include mixing extero- and proprioceptive influences.

For nerves, the most usual techniques rely on measurement of conduction velocities, either motor or sensory, and search for nerve segments where there is slowing. Whenever sensory conduction velocity is difficult to measure, somatosensory evoked potentials can sometimes overcome the technical problems. In other circumstances, H reflex latencies, or F wave dispersion, are used to reflect the slowing of conduction velocities. The value and limitations of these techniques have been reviewed by Burke (1985) who stressed the fact that routine studies examine only limited aspects of the functions of a peripheral nerve, that an electrical stimulus setting up a single impulse in each axon is unphysiological, that electrical stimulation of a cutaneous sensory nerve bypasses receptors, and most distal parts of the axon, and finally that all axons are activated simultaneously. Non-routine techniques are now in development, which investigate aspects of nerve function other than conduction velocity; they include microneurography, use of physiological stimuli, measurement of refractory and supernormal periods, and study of dispersion and distribution of conduction velocities. They are not yet incorporated into everyday practice and their exact usefulness has still to be evaluated because some, such as microneurography, are time consuming and provide qualitative results because they are based on a sample of fibers which happen to have been recorded.

Function of the neuromuscular junction is assessed by stimulodetection where standardized programs of stimulation are applied to a nerve and global muscle responses are recorded both electrically and mechanically. The jitter phenomenon, reflecting conduction block within the motor nerve terminals, can complement stimulodetection. The myasthenic nature of the neuromuscular block is characteristic and can be reduced or suppressed by prostigmine.

Routine EMG provides irreplaceable data because it indicates the degree, total or not, of denervation. Later on, it reflects the process of sprouting ('coherent' EMG) and contributes to decisions about the extent of reinnervation. However, such an examination is not quantitative because the needle explores only restricted parts of the muscle under study. The results depend on the care and expertise of the examiner.

The techniques mentioned above do not represent all the possibilities offered by clinical neurophysiology. Many more tests have been proposed and some are considered as classic. For example, the recovery curves of the H reflex, plotted after paired stimulation of the sciatic nerve, have been extensively employed. However, these curves depend on many variables such as intensity of the conditioning and conditioned stimuli, and definition of normal values appears difficult. The curves are complex and consist of various phases whose physiological meaning is far from established. Therefore, departures from normal cannot be interpreted at present in physiological terms, and only represent a crude and unreliable estimation of changes brought about by a pathological state. The same can be said for the silent period, which depends on at least four factors, both peripheral and central. Other currently used tests are still debated. Long latency reflexes, elicited by an abrupt stopping of an ongoing voluntary movement, have been studied in Parkinson's disease and the upper motorneuron syndrome. The M2 component of the response has been considered as reflecting reflex activities in long loop neural pathways relaying in the motor cortex. However, many researchers are reluctant to subscribe to that interpretation and have proposed various alternative explanations. The reported changes in pathology may perhaps contribute to assessment, particularly in Parkinson's disease, but they cannot be interpreted in simple pathophysiological terms.

New techniques are regularly proposed but it is not enough to have an opportunity to gather quantified data. Before being accepted into a useful battery of tests applicable on a worldwide basis, a new method should be critically examined. Is it quantifiable? Is it easy to employ and not so sophisticated that it would be restricted to only few centres? Is it more sensitive than simple clinical examination and do the results evolve in parallel with clinical signs? What kind of information does it really produce? Clinical neurophysiology describes clinical problems in physiological terms and is an irreplaceable tool for pathophysiologically oriented studies that are the basis for original attempts to improve treatment. It enables the validation of hypotheses for promoting recuperation and its role is not only limited to assessment. Once its dual role has been fully understood, it should become a corner stone of restorative neurology.

CONCLUSIONS

A neurological lesion leads as a rule to multiple difficulties distinct in nature. For example, even a limited nerve lesion may be responsible for motor and sensory deficits in addition to pain. Therefore, monitoring of recovery needs to be multifactorial. In addition, consequences of a lesion manifest themselves in different ways, including impairment, disability, and handicap. There are various methods permitting the assessment of consequences at these levels, from lesion to handicap, and the differences between them has to be well understood as each has its specific advantages and limitations. Finally, as recovery from CNS lesions is often incomplete because of absence of regeneration, the methods selected have to be sensitive enough to appreciate subtle and discrete changes. However, methods should not be too sophisticated and time consuming because they cannot demand too much from the patient or medical and paramedical staff.

Efforts are now developed to provide ways of assessment that fulfill these requirements. Unfortunately, they are not yet standardized and accepted worldwide. Even methodology for elaborating rating scales is still open to discussion. In fact, few are validated and further efforts are needed to obtain for assessment something equivalent to a textbook of semiology. Therefore, it is necessary to combine various approaches, clinical and instrumental. These latter are not necessarily redundant but can be complementary as they provide information about various aspects of a clinical picture. In general, clinical methods are qualitative but have a larger scope than instrumental techniques. Instrumental techniques provide quantitative data but this information often concerns a very limited aspect of a clinical picture.

Finally, measurement must be relevant to the problem under study. For example, to study the progression of amyotrophic lateral sclerosis, the investigator may decide to evaluate the strength of the first dorsal interosseous muscle as one measure of outcome. If the patient is rapidly declining because of swallowing difficulties, the measurement of muscle strength in the hand is not very relevant because it does not adequately reflect the clinical course. In other words, even if a list of all the possible clinical charts, rating scales, and instrumental methods were available for any given disease, it would be unwise to choose one indiscriminately from that battery without prior consideration of actual clinical problems.

References

Alexander L (1951) New concept of critical steps in course of chronic debilitating neurologic disease in evaluation of therapeutic response, *Arch Neurol Psychiatry*, **66**, 253–8

Aminoff MJ (1986) *Electrodiagnosis in Clinical Neurology*, 2nd Edn, Edinburgh, Churchill Livingstone

Ashworth B (1964) Preliminary trial of carisoprodol in multiple sclerosis, *Practitioner*, **192**, 540–2

Baldissera F, Hultborn H, and Illert M (1981) Integration in spinal neuronal system, In Brooks VB, ed, *Handbook of physiology, Sect I, The nervous system, vol II, Motor control*, Am Phys Soc Bethesda, 509–95

Benavides J, Cornu Ph., Dennis T, Dubois A, Hauw JJ, MacKenzie ET *et al.* (1988) Imaging of human brain lesions with a W3 site radioligand, *Ann Neurol*, **24**, 708–12

Burke D (1985) Value and limitations of nerve conduction studies, In Delwaide PJ and Gorio A, eds, *Clinical Neurophysiology in Peripheral Neuropathies. Restorative Neurology*, Vol 3, Amsterdam, Elsevier, 91–102

Capildeo R and Orgogozo JM (1988) *Methods in Clinical Trials in Neurology. Vascular and Degenerative Brain Disease*, London, Macmillan

Chiappa KH (1990) *Evoked Potentials in Clinical Medicine*, 2nd Edn, New York, Raven Press

Cho DW (1981) Inter-rater reliability: intraclass correlation coefficients, *Educ Psychol Meas*, **41**, 223–6

Cruccu G, Fornarelli M, and Manfredi M (1988) Impairment of masticatory function in hemiplegia, *Neurology*, **38**, 301–6

Delwaide PJ (1985) Electrophysiological testing of spastic patients: its potential usefulness and limitations, In Delwaide PJ and Young RR, eds, *Clinical Neurophysiology in Spasticity*, Amsterdam, Elsevier, 185–204

Delwaide PJ and Delwaide C (1987) Electrophysiological testing of human spinal cord, *Neuro-Orthopedics*, **3**, 76–81

Delwaide PJ, Schoenen J, and De Pasqua V (1985) Lumbo-sacral spinal evoked potentials in patients with multiple sclerosis, *Neurology*, **35**, 174–9

Dick JR, Rothwell JC, Day BL *et al.* (1989) The Bereitschaftspotential is abnormal in Parkinson's disease, *Brain*, **112**, 233–44

Duffy FH (1986) *Topographic Mapping of Brain Electrical Activity*, Boston, Butterworths

Eisen AA (1986) Non invasive measurement of spinal cord conduction: review of presently available methods, *Muscle Nerve*, **9**, 95–103

Fahn S, Elton RL, and Members of the UPDRS Development Committee (1987) Unified Parkinson's disease rating scale. In Fahn S, Marsden CD, Goldstein M *et al.*, eds, *Recent developments in Parkinson's disease. II.* New York, MacMillan, 153–63

Fahn S *et al.* (1989) Report of the American Academy of Neurology, Therapeutics and Technology Assessment Subcommittee: Assessment: EEG brain mapping, *Neurology*, **39**, 1100–1

Forrest M and Andersen B (1986) Ordinal scale and statistics in medical research, *Br Med J*, **292**, 537–8

Freund HJ and Bauer HJ (1982) Regeneration and repair of the nervous system: clinical aspects. In Nicholls JG, ed, *Repair and Regeneration of the Nervous System*, New York, Springer Verlag

Kimura J (1987) Electrodiagnosis in distress of nerve and muscle: Principles and Practice, Philadelphia, FA Davis

Kimura J, Wilkinson JT, Damasio H, Adams HR, Shivapour E, and Yamada T (1985) Blink reflex in patients with hemispheric cerebrovascular accident (CVA), *J Neurol Sci*, **67**, 15–28

Kurtzke JF (1961) On the evaluation of disability in multiple sclerosis, *Neurology*, **11**, 686–94

Kurtzke JF (1970) Neurologic impairment in multiple sclerosis and the disability status scale, *Acta Neurol Scand*, **46**, 493–512

Kurtzke JF (1983) Rating neurologic impairment in multiple sclerosis: an expanded disability status scale (EDSS), *Neurology*, **33**, 1444–52

Lang AET and Fahn S (1989) Assessment of Parkinson's disease, In Munsat T, ed, *Quantification of neurologic deficit*, Boston, Butterworths, 285–309

Levy P (1973) On the relation between test theory and psychology, In Kline P, ed, *New Approaches in Psychological Measurement*, New York, Wiley, 1–42

Lukes SA, Crooks LE, Aminoff MJ *et al.* (1983) Nuclear magnetic resonance imaging in multiple sclerosis, *Ann Neurol*, **13**, 592–601

Maurer W and Commenges D (1988) Choice and analysis of judgement criteria, In Capildeo R and Orgogozo JM, eds, *Methods in Clinical Trials in Neurology. Vascular and Degenerative Brain Disease*, London, MacMillan, 29–56

McDonnell RAL, Donnan GA, and Bladin PF (1989) A comparison of somatosensory evoked and motor evoked potentials in stroke, *Ann Neurol*, **25**, 68–73

McKenzie CR and Charlson ME (1986) Standards for the use of ordinal scales in clinical trials, *Br Med J*, **292**, 40–3

Munsat TL (1989) *Quantification of Neurologic deficit*, Boston, Butterworths

Ongerboer de Visser BW (1983) Anatomical and functional organization of reflexes involving the trigeminal system in man: jaw reflex, blink reflex, corneal reflex and exteroceptive suppression, *Adv Neurol*, **39**, 729–38

Powers WJ, Grubb RL, Darriet D, and Raichle ME (1985) Cerebral blood flow and cerebral metabolic rate of oxygen requirement for cerebral function and viability in humans, *J Cereb Blood Flow Metab*, **5**, 600–8

Sedgwick EM (1982) Clinical Neurophysiology in Rehabilitation, In Illis LS, Sedgwick EM, and Glanville HJ, eds, *Rehabilitation of the Neurological Patient*, London, Blackwell Scientific, 85–121

Shimoyama I, Dauth GW, Gilman S, Frey KA, and Penney JB (1988) Thalamic, brainstem and cerebellar glucose metabolism in the hemiplegic monkey, *Ann Neurol*, **24**, 718–26

Shrout PE and Fleiss JL (1979) Intraclass correlations: uses in assessing reliability, *Psychol Bull*, **86**, 420–8

Stewart AL, Ware JE, and Brook RH (1981) Advances in the measurement of functional status: construction of aggregate indexes, *Med Care*, **XIX**, 473–88

Tourtellotte WW and Syndulko K (1989) Quantifying the neurologic examination: principles, constraints, and opportunities, In Munsat TL, ed, *Quantification of Neurologic Deficit*, Boston, Butterworths, 7–16

World Health Organization (1980) *International classification of impairments, disabilities and handicaps*, Geneva, WHO

Willoughby EW and Paty DW (1988) Scales for rating impairment in multiple sclerosis: a critique, *Neurology*, **38**, 1793–8

Wise RSJ, Bernardis S, Frackowiak RSJ, Legg NJ and Jones T (1983) Serial observations on the pathophysiology of acute stroke: the transition from ischemia to infarction as reflected in regional oxygen extraction, *Brain*, **106**, 197 222

Young RR (1973) The clinical significance of exteroceptive reflexes, In Desmedt JE, ed, *New Developments in Electromyography and Clinical Neurophysiology*, vol. 3, Basel, S Karger AG, 697–712

Young IR, Hall AS, Pallis CA, Bydder GM, Legg NJ, and Steiner RE (1981) Nuclear magnetic resonance imaging of the brain in multiple sclerosis, *Lancet*, **2**, 1066

4
Biochemical changes and secondary injury from stroke and trauma

S. Scott Panter and Alan I. Faden

Ischemic and traumatic injuries to the brain or spinal cord initiate a cascade of cellular reactions that cause delayed tissue damage. This process involves a variety of physiological and biochemical events resulting in disruptions of cellular metabolism and alterations of membrane integrity that lead to progressive secondary injury. Among the more important secondary injury factors that have been identified are ion fluxes (Young and Flamm, 1982; Stokes, Hollinden, and Fox, 1983; Siesjo and Bengtsson, 1989), excitotoxin release (Benveniste *et al.*, 1984; Faden and Simon, 1988; Choi, 1988; Faden *et al.*, 1989; Panter, Yum, and Faden, 1990), generation of free radicals (Demopoulos *et al.*, 1980; Braughler and Hall, 1989; Watson and Ginsberg, 1989), phospholipid hydrolysis and formation of products of arachidonic acid metabolism (Demediuk *et al.*, 1985; Faden, Chan, and Longar, 1987; Demediuk and Faden, 1988b; Hsu *et al.*, 1989), and changes in tissue concentrations of neuropeptides (Faden, 1988a; 1988b). Identification of such factors and characterization of the injury cascade has led to development of interventional strategies to limit delayed tissue damage, thereby enhancing neurological recovery. Successful application of these concepts to experimental models has led to the initiation of a number of clinical trials that are now in progress.

ION FLUXES

The entry of calcium into cells plays an important role in normal cellular function and physiology. Calcium influences vesicular fusion, stimulates the synthesis and quantal release of neurotransmitters, affects cellular cytoskeletal assembly and breakdown, and alters arachidonic acid metabolism and protein phosphorylation through the activation of phospholipases (Blaustein, 1988a; Seisjo, 1988). Calcium is present in the extracellular milieu at concentrations 10^4 fold higher than intracellular levels. Consequently, an important cellular function is the maintenance of this steep concentration gradient (Blaustein, 1988a; Seisjo, 1988).

Calcium is thought to enter cells through two types of cation channels. One is a voltage sensitive calcium channel (VSCC) that is activated upon membrane depolarization. Based upon functional differences, VSCC's have been further divided into three categories: T (transient), L (long-lasting), and N (neither T nor L) (Tsien *et al.*,

1988). Activation of postsynaptic VSCC's by normal neurotransmitter activity causes a brief influx of calcium, which is probably rapidly sequestered by calcium binding proteins (Blaustein, 1988b). The activation of these channels may play a role in normal neuronal activity and cellular homeostasis but has also been implicated in secondary injury (Wauquier, Ashton and Clincke, 1988). The second type of calcium channel is an agonist operated calcium channel (AOCC). In CNS tissue, this channel is associated with neurons and has been demonstrated to play a role in memory acquisition or long-term potentiation (Collingridge and Bliss, 1987), but it also has been linked to secondary injury (Choi, 1988; Siesjo and Bengtsson, 1989). The endogenous agonists for this class of calcium channel are the excitatory amino acids, glutamate and aspartate, with magnesium serving as an endogenous antagonist (Wroblewski and Danysz, 1989).

During the course of normal metabolism, intracellular concentrations of calcium are finely controlled by a number of mechanisms. First, calcium is extruded from the cell through an energy-dependent process. Second, the neurotransmitters that cause transient openings of VSCC's or AOCC's do not remain in the synaptic cleft for prolonged time periods (Siesjo, 1988; Siesjo and Bengtsson, 1989). Instead, they are metabolized or actively taken up by the presynaptic membrane or, in the case of glutamate, by glial cells. Third, the number of intracellular binding sites for calcium are thought to be able to accommodate brief increases in calcium concentration (Blaustein, 1988a). Finally, the AOCC is naturally modulated by extracellular magnesium, which is present at a concentration of approximately 1 mmol in CNS tissue (Vink, McIntosh, and Faden, 1991).

In injured CNS tissue, extracellular calcium concentrations decrease rapidly with a presumed concomitant increase in intracellular levels (Young and Flamm, 1982; Stokes, Hollinden, and Fox, 1983; Siesjo, 1988) During global ischemia, intracellular ATP pools decrease to zero within 5–7 minutes, impairing the ability of cells to extrude calcium (Siesjo, 1981). In addition, CNS injury may alter calcium metabolism in a second manner, by affecting total tissue and intracellular levels of magnesium (Vink, McIntosh, and Faden, 1991). Because magnesium is thought to modulate calcium transport systems, alterations in magnesium will presumably affect both calcium and intracellular metabolism (Nahorski, 1988; Stanfield, 1988; Vink, McIntosh, and Faden, 1991). One of the consequences of CNS injury, therefore, is the decompartmentalization of calcium, which moves along its concentration gradient into cells.

It has been hypothesized that cellular damage during ischemia may be diminished by the vascular and/or biochemical effects of VSCC blockers (Wauquier, Ashton, and Clincke, 1988). The use of calcium channel blockade in cerebral resuscitation following cardiac arrest and in different models of ischemia has been reviewed (Wauquier, Ashton, and Clincke, 1988; Rolfsen and Davis, 1989). A variety of calcium-channel blockers (including nimodipine, nicardipine, flunarazine, lidoflazine, nifedipine, and verapamil) increase cerebral blood flow through vasodilation, improve survival, restore cellular metabolism, or improve electrical activity after ischemia (Wauquier, Ashton, and Clincke, 1988; Rolfsen and Davis, 1989). On the basis of these preclinical studies, a controlled clinical trial was conducted using nimodipine following acute ischemic stroke (Gelmers *et al.*, 1988). Using a modified Mathew scale of neurological evaluation, a significant improvement was noted in the nimodipine group. In addition, nimodipine significantly decreased mortality during the four-week treatment period, but this benefit was restricted to men. It has been suggested that the significant difference in mortality between treatment and placebo groups may be attributed to an unusually high rate of mortality in the placebo group (Earnest, 1988). Preliminary results from a subsequent multicenter clinical trial suggest that nimodipine may be beneficial only in patients treated within the first 12 hours following cerebral infarct (Mohr *et al.*, 1989).

A number of preclinical studies have used nimodipine or verapamil to treat spinal cord ischemia or trauma; no beneficial effects have been found (Cheng *et al.*, 1984; Faden, Jacobs, and Smith, 1984a; Ford and Malm, 1985). However, a beneficial effect has been reported when nimodipine was administered with adrenaline or dextran following spinal cord trauma in rats (Guha, Tator, and Piper, 1987; Fehlings, Tator, and Linden, 1989). Similar results have been achieved with hetastarch and phenylephrine (Dyste *et al.*, 1989). Co-treatment with these agents prevented the hypotension associated with dihydropyridines. Because hypotension may be expected to exacerbate post-traumatic ischemia in tissue that has lost autoregulation, this finding may explain the lack of protective action with dihydropyridines when agents are used alone.

Thus, VSCC-blockers may hold promise for the treatment of cerebral ischemia, although further controlled clinical studies are needed, preferably using analogs that do not affect the systemic vasculature. The effects of these agents in CNS trauma are controversial and warrant additional preclinical investigation.

Magnesium is another divalent cation that has been implicated in secondary CNS tissue injury. Magnesium is normally present in approximately millimolar concentrations in the CNS, and there appears to be no intracellular–extracellular concentration gradient (Veloso *et al.*, 1973; Vink *et al.*, 1988). Approximately 8–10% of intracellular magnesium is thought to be free. Because ATP can be bound only as an ATP-magnesium complex, all reactions that utilize ATP also require magnesium (Aikawa, 1981; Vink *et al.*, 1988). Therefore, normal glycolysis, Krebs cycle activity, and oxidative phosphorylation each require magnesium. A second, important role for magnesium in cellular homeostasis is that of a calcium antagonist (Wroblewski and Danysz, 1989; Vink, McIntosh and Faden, 1991). Magnesium is thought to modulate presynaptic release of excitatory amino acid transmitters, and other studies suggest that magnesium is an important natural modulator of postsynaptic AOCC's.

Magnetic resonance spectroscopy (MRS) and atomic absorption spectrophotometry have been used to monitor changes in free intracellular (Mgf) and total tissue (Mgt) levels of magnesium, respectively. Following traumatic brain or spinal cord injury, both Mgf and Mgt decrease significantly (Lemke *et al.*, 1987; Vink *et al.*, 1988; Vink *et al.*, 1989b). The degree of Mgf decrease after traumatic brain injury was related to the severity of tissue injury (Vink, Faden, and McIntosh, 1988; Vink *et al.*, 1988). Animals maintained on a magnesium-deficient diet suffered significantly greater neurological deficits following traumatic brain injury; whereas treatment with magnesium sulfate either before or following injury was protective (McIntosh *et al.*, 1988; McIntosh *et al.*, 1989b). Moreover, three classes of experimental compounds (kappa opiate receptor antagonists, thyrotropin-releasing hormone analogs, and excitatory amino acid antagonists), which have been demonstrated to have beneficial effects on the outcome from traumatic brain injury, also reduce the post-traumatic decline in Mgf (Vink, McIntosh, and Faden, 1988; Faden *et al.*, 1989a; McIntosh *et al.*, 1989a; Faden, personal communication). Similar observations have been made with regard to changes in Mgt after spinal cord trauma (Lemke *et al.*, 1987).

When administered following cerebral ischemia, magnesium treatment appears to be beneficial (White *et al.*, 1983). In a 'community hospital clinical trial', the combination of magnesium with a VSCC blocker seemed to improve neurological outcome following global cerebral ischemia (Schwartz, 1984). These data, in conjunction with the preclinical data on spinal cord and brain trauma, suggest that magnesium may have a therapeutic role, either separately or as co-therapy for the treatment of stroke or CNS trauma (Goldman and Finkbeiner, 1988).

EXCITATORY AMINO ACIDS

Excitatory amino acid (EAA) neurotransmission has been determined to be crucial to the process of long-term potentiation (LTP), which is thought to play an important role in learning, memory, and synaptic plasticity (Wroblewski and Danysz, 1989). Five classes of EAA receptors have been identified in CNS. Named according to agonist selectivity for that specific receptor, they are the receptors for N-methyl-D-aspartate (NMDA), quisqualate (or alpha-amino-3-hydroxy-5-methylisoxazole-4-propionic acid, AMPA), kainate, 2-amino-4-phosphonobutyrate (AP4), and the most recently described *trans*-1-aminocyclopentane-1,3-dicarboxylic acid (ACDP) (Monaghan, Bridges, and Cotman, 1989).

In general, the manner through which activation of the EAA receptor accomplishes intracellular changes is subdivided into two categories, ionotropic or metabolotropic (Wroblewski and Danysz, 1989). In the former instance, the receptor is directly coupled to an ion channel, which upon activation, opens to permit an influx of extracellular ions, including calcium, thereby affecting calcium-dependent processes. The metabolotropic effects of EAA's, however, are mediated through the formation of two types of second messenger molecules, inositol-1,4,5-triphosphate (IP3) and 1,2-diacylglycerol (DG). IP3 is thought to increase calcium concentrations from intracellular stores through receptors on the endoplasmic reticulum, and DG participates in the activation of protein kinase C (Wroblewski and Danysz, 1989).

Under normal circumstances, the presence of EAA in the synaptic cleft is thought to be very transient (Siesjo and Bengtsson, 1989). Following neural injury, however, neurons may be exposed to much higher concentrations of glutamate for longer periods of time. This possibility has been confirmed recently using the technique of intracerebral microdialysis, which permits the *in vivo* sampling of extracellular fluid in the spinal cord or brain. In animal models of injury, extracellular glutamate and aspartate are reported to be significantly elevated following head trauma in rats, following spinal cord trauma in rabbits, and during both global (Graham *et al.*, 1990) and focal ischemia in rats (Benveniste *et al.*, 1984; Katayama *et al.*, 1988; Korf *et al.*, 1988; Faden *et al.*, 1989a; Panter, Yum, and Faden, 1990). Furthermore, the absolute concentration of EAA's and the time interval during which they are elevated following impact trauma to rabbit spinal cord is related to the severity of trauma (Panter, Yum, and Faden, 1990).

Studies performed in cell culture suggest that the process of cell damage following exposure to EAA is comprised of two phases. An acute phase is thought to result from the activation of the kainate/quisqualate-operated channels that permit neuronal potassium efflux and sodium influx (Rothman and Olney, 1986; Choi, 1988). The increase in intracellular sodium is accompanied by an influx of chloride ions and an overall increase in the osmolarity of the cell. As a result, water enters the cell producing edema. A second phase of excitatory amino acid activity is mediated by the N-methyl-D-aspartate (NMDA) receptor, which permits the influx of both monovalent and divalent cations, especially calcium (Rothman and Olney, 1986; Choi, 1988). Excessive stimulation of the NMDA receptor has been demonstrated to cause a rapid rise in the concentration of intracellular calcium and activate a number of calcium-dependent processes that are normally carefully regulated, including calcium-dependent proteases, kinases, phospholipases, and transglutaminases (Blaustein, 1988a; Siesjo and Bengtsson, 1989). These intracellular changes produced by calcium may contribute to cell death.

A number of studies conducted in animal models provide support for the theory that excitotoxicity may be a general component of many different types of CNS injury. The administration of NMDA antagonists has been demonstrated to attenuate certain consequences of both global and focal ischemia (see Albers, Goldberg, and Choi, 1989, for review). The earliest studies utilizing NMDA antagonists *in vivo* were performed in models of global cerebral ischemia (Simon et al., 1984) and hypoglycemia (Weiloch, 1985). Each group demonstrated protection by pretreatment with the competitive NMDA antagonist 2-amino-7-phosphonoheptanoic acid. Subsequently, many antagonists have been examined in a variety of models of global and focal cerebral ischemia with mixed results. However, a recent critical review of this literature concludes that the preclinical data support the initiation of Phase I dose-escalation trials for potential use of NMDA antagonists in the treatment of focal ischemia or stroke (Albers, Goldberg, and Choi, 1989).

Data from several studies indicate that excitatory amino acids are released following spinal cord and brain trauma (Katayama et al., 1988; Faden et al., 1989a; Panter, Yum, and Faden, 1990), and it has been suggested that excitotoxicity is an important component of traumatic injury to CNS tissue. When administered after injury, NMDA significantly worsened outcome from spinal cord trauma; whereas its stereoisomer, N-methyl-L-aspartate, which has a much lower affinity for the NMDA receptor, had no effect (Faden and Simon, 1988). Moreover, the non-competitive NMDA antagonists, dextrorphan and MK-801, significantly improved outcome after traumatic spinal cord injury in rats (Faden et al., 1988; Faden, Ellison, and Noble, 1989). Similar results were obtained with the competitive antagonist 3-(2-carboxypiperazin-4-yl)propyl-1-phosphoric acid (CPP) (Faden, Ellison, and Noble, 1989).

Dextrorphan treatment significantly improved behavioral outcome and limited changes in cellular bioenergetics and intracellular free magnesium following traumatic brain injury (Faden et al., 1989a). Treatment with the non-competitive NMDA antagonist phencyclidine (PCP) prior to brain trauma has also been demonstrated to have a beneficial effect on recovery (Hayes et al., 1988). The non-competitive NMDA antagonist MK-801 attenuated cerebral edema and restored intracellular magnesium homeostasis when administered after traumatic brain injury (McIntosh et al., 1989a). The results of these experiments suggest that EAA receptor antagonists may also have therapeutic potential for the treatment of CNS trauma (Judge et al., 1991; Nellgård and Wieloch, 1992; Le Peillet et al., 1992; Sheardown et al., 1990).

OXYGEN RADICALS

Although the absence of oxygen is extremely detrimental to CNS tissue, oxygen itself can be very toxic. Molecular oxygen is actually an extremely unreactive compound, but under certain conditions, it can undergo a series of one electron reductions, eventually forming water. Two of the intermediates in this reductive sequence, superoxide and the hydroxyl radical, contain an unpaired electron and are called oxygen free radicals. Toxicity of oxygen free radicals is normally minimized by careful compartmentalization of their synthesis, normal cellular defense mechanisms, and containment of reactive iron, which is a potent catalyst of free radical reactions.

There are two categories of cellular defense mechanisms, enzymatic and non-enzymatic (Cotgreave, Moldeus, and Orrenius, 1988). Among the enzymatic are superoxide dismutase, which catalyzes the dismutation of superoxide to hydrogen peroxide; catalase, which metabolizes hydrogen peroxide to molecular oxygen and water; and a variety of peroxidases, the most important of which may be glutathione peroxidase, which metabolizes hydrogen peroxide to water. The non-enzymatic defense mechanisms are primarily antioxidants, which comprise two categories. One group includes molecules such as alpha-tocopherol and ubiquinone, which function in lipophilic compartments. The second category includes uric acid and reducing reagents such as ascorbate or glutathione, which are more active in aqueous environments (Cotgreave, Moldeus, and Orrenius, 1988).

Another important endogenous line of defense against free radical damage is the careful control of free, reactive iron, which is usually controlled by proteins that sequester iron or iron-containing molecules (Cotgreave, Moldeus, and Orrenius, 1988). The concentration of reactive iron in the body is limited by two factors. First, at a physiological pH, free ferric iron in solution in excess of 2.5×10^{-18} mol L^{-1} precipitates as ferric hydroxide, which has a solubility constant of 10^{-36} mol L^{-1}, and second, essentially all of the body's iron is normally well contained by cells, binding proteins, or enzymes and is not considered to be labile (Griffiths, 1987; Cotgreave, Moldeus, and Orrenius, 1988). Neurotrauma or cerebral ischemia, however, may cause increased availability of free or reactive iron that can greatly exacerbate free radical damage (Braughler and Hall, 1989; Panter, Braughler and Hall, 1992).

In injured CNS tissue, iron that is localized in transferrin, ferritin, or hemosiderin may be released by two different mechanisms. First, although these proteins avidly bind iron at a physiological pH, at an acidic pH, such as that existing during lactic acidosis, reductive mobilization of iron may occur (Braughler and Hall, 1989). In addition, the superoxide anion may also serve as a reducing agent and release bound iron. A second possible source of iron arises from erythrocytes that have been trapped by extravasation or cessation of blood flow. As these cells lyse, they release hemoglobin, which also readily gives up its iron in a reducing environment (Braughler and Hall, 1989; Panter *et al.*, 1990.

Perhaps the strongest evidence for free radical involvement in CNS injury comes from studies of the relationship between antioxidants, largely vitamin E, and trauma or ischemia. A number of preclinical experiments have demonstrated that vitamin E protects cell membranes from free radical damage (Liebler, Kling, and Reed, 1986), and tissue concentrations of vitamin E have been reported to decrease following spinal cord trauma and cerebral ischemia/reperfusion in rats (Yoshida *et al.*, 1984; Kinuta *et al.*, 1989; Lemke *et al.*, 1990). Preclinical studies in dogs have shown that pretreatment with vitamin E resulted in a significantly greater recovery of brain electrical activity following cerebral ischemia (Fujimoto *et al.*, 1984). In a rat model of cerebral ischemia, vitamin E pretreatment significantly reduced the concentration of indicators of free radical-dependent lipid damage (Yoshida *et al.*, 1985). Finally, dietary vitamin E supplementation significantly improved cerebral blood flow in a condition of cerebral hypoperfusion caused by subarachnoid hemorrhage (Travis and Hall, 1987).

A number of reports suggest that vitamin E also protects tissue from the effects of post-traumatic spinal cord ischemia. Four hours following spinal cord contusion, 100% of all animals (cats) developed hypoperfusion, but none of the animals pretreated for five days with oral vitamin E and selenium (a co-factor for glutathione peroxidase) manifested ischemia (Hall and Wolf, 1986). Following five minutes of compression trauma to cat spinal cord, elevated concentrations of tissue free fatty acids were detected 30 minutes post-trauma. Pretreatment with oral vitamin E and selenium significantly reversed this effect and improved behavioral recovery (Anderson et al., 1985).

Alpha-tocopherol plays a central role in the maintainence of normal CNS structure and function, and preclinical data strongly suggest that pretreatment with vitamin E significantly attenuates the effects of CNS injury (Sokol, 1989). Unfortunately, vitamin E itself may not be an effective therapeutic agent if administered following injury. In rats, vitamin E is accumulated by the CNS in a manner different to other body tissues. Brain and spinal cord require a longer period of time to sequester vitamin E, but tissue concentrations of vitamin E are maintained for a longer period of time in brain (four week half-life) and spinal cord (11 week half-life) than in other tissues (Burton and Ingold, 1986; Ingold et al., 1987). Therefore, a long time period is required to increase CNS concentrations of vitamin E, but once accumulated, vitamin E persists much longer. Consequently, preclinical data suggest that chronic dietary supplementation with modest doses of vitamin E may have a neuro-protective effect (Sokol, 1989). The potential of vitamin E as a therapeutic agent intended to be administered acutely is minimal because of the time necessary to elevate membrane concentrations in brain or spinal cord.

The ability of vitamin E to attenuate the effects of CNS injury has stimulated the development of a class of compounds that have antioxidant properties and which will be effective when administered acutely. These compounds are called 21-amino steroids and are all derivatives based on the structure of the glucocorticoid, methylprednisolone, but they have been modified to eliminate any glucocorticoid activity (McCall, Braughler, and Hall, 1987). Some of these compounds have excellent antioxidant activity, and others probably act as lipophilic iron chelators; regardless, they are very effective inhibitors of lipid peroxidation *in vitro* (Braughler *et al.*, 1987).

Extensive preclinical experiments have been performed with U74006F, which is one of the 21-amino steroids that is thought to have the greatest therapeutic potential when administered following injury (Hall and Braughler, 1989). Using a murine model of head injury, U74006F significantly improved survival and neurological recovery following moderate or severe trauma (Hall *et al.*, 1988). When administered after spinal cord trauma in cats, U74006F significantly increased spinal cord blood flow and promoted functional recovery (Anderson *et al.*, 1988; Hall, 1988).

In a rat model of regional cerebral ischemia, post-occlusion administration of U74006F significantly reduced regional ion and water shifts, but the effect was not observed in the area of infarct, only in the tissues surrounding the infarct (Young, Wojak and DeCrescito, 1988). U74006F was also studied in a gerbil model of global cerebral ischemia and was found to reduce cell damage and improve survival after three hours of ischemia (Hall, Pazara, and Braughler, 1988). Finally, in a primate model of subarachnoid hemorrhage (SAH) induced cerebral vasospasm, U74006F significantly reduced the degree of vasospasm when administered 20 hours following inducement of SAH (Steinke *et al.*, 1989). Recently, however, U74006F was reported to have no effect on neurological outcome in cats subjected to severe thoracic spinal cord contusion (Gruner *et al.*, 1989; Wrathall, personal communication). In conclusion, preclinical data suggest that U74006F may be an effective therapeutic for treatment of CNS trauma or ischemia. Clinical trials in head injury are about to begin.

EICOSANOIDS

Eicosanoids are a large group of compounds that originate from the oxidative metabolism of arachidonic acid, which is a 20 carbon, polyunsaturated fatty acid component of CNS phospholipids and plasmalogens (Wolfe, 1982). Among the enzymatically-generated eicosanoids are prostanoids (prostaglandins and thromboxane) synthesized via cyclo-oxygenase activity, and leukotrienes and hydroperoxy fatty acids, which are formed through the lipoxygenase pathway (Needleman *et al.*, 1986) Normally, eicosanoids play a role in cellular inflammation, vascular homeostasis, and neuronal communication (Bazan, 1989; Hertting and Seregi, 1989). With the exception of the prostaglandin PGI_2, thromboxanes and leukotrienes are all capable of potentiating hypoperfusion by vasoconstriction, platelet aggregation, or modifications of the blood–brain barrier (Wolfe, 1982). After ischemia or trauma, eicosanoids may significantly impair microcirculation, increase platelet microthrombi formation, produce vasogenic edema, and generally potentiate hypoperfusion (Hsu *et al.*, 1989; Galli *et al.*, 1989).

CNS trauma results in significant elevations of total tissue free fatty acids and arachidonic acid (Demediuk *et al.*, 1985; Faden, Chan, and Longar, 1987; Demediuk and Faden, 1988b). Elevated tissue levels of free arachidonic acid are thought to arise from increased phospholipase activity and elevated phosphoinositide turnover (Black and Hoff, 1990), and neural tissue may convert a portion of this free arachidonate to eicosanoids (Hertting and Seregi, 1989). In addition, eicosanoids are released by platelets, activated neutrophils, and other cell types that concentrate in areas of tissue injury. Furthermore, free fatty acids are re-integrated into phospholipids and membranes through the process of reacylation, which is highly energy dependent. Consequently, elevated levels of free fatty acids may reflect, in part, post-ischemic or post-traumatic hypometabolism (Siesjo, 1984; Vink, Faden, and McIntosh, 1988; Faden *et al.*, 1989a; Hsu *et al.*, 1989; Vink *et al.*, 1989a).

The metabolism of arachidonic acid in resting tissue is under tight control, and basal eicosanoid concentrations are very low (Needleman *et al.*, 1986). After trauma or ischemia, however, their concentrations increase significantly and rapidly, seemingly in direct proportion to the severity of injury. This response has been confirmed in a wide variety of experimental models (Chan, Longar, and Fishman, 1983; Siesjo, 1984; Hsu *et al.*, 1985; Demediuk and Faden, 1988b; Hsu *et al.*, 1989).

The metabolism of arachidonic acid is normally modulated at a number of different steps, and once formed, eicosanoid activity is mediated through specific cellular receptors, which are in the process of being identified and characterized (Needleman *et al.*, 1986; Halushka *et al.*, 1989; Snyder and Fleisch, 1989). Consequently, arachidonic metabolism may be amenable to therapeutic manipulation via enzyme inhibition or receptor antagonism (Faden, Lemke, and Demediuk, 1988; Snyder and Fleisch, 1989).

A number of preclinical studies have used animal models of CNS injury to assess the therapeutic potential of agents that affect arachidonic acid metabolism. Using a cat model of spinal cord contusion, spinal cord blood flow was measured following injury, and four different agents that might alter eicosanoid production were examined: ibuprofen or meclofenamate, cyclo-oxygenase inhibitors; furegrelate sodium, a thromboxane A_2 synthetase inhibitor; and ciprostene calcium, a stable analog of PGI_2, which can induce vasodilation and inhibit platelet aggregation (Hertting and Seregi, 1989). Both of the cyclo-oxygenase inhibitors significantly improved spinal cord blood flow at four hours after injury (Hall and Wolf, 1986). The thromboxane synthetase inhibitor and PGI_2 analog were ineffective when administered alone but were very effective when combined (Hall and Wolf, 1986). Another combination, including the cyclo-oxygenase inhibitor indomethacin, PGI_2, and heparin was found to have a beneficial effect on behavioral recovery following spinal cord impact injury in cats (Hallenbeck, Jacobs, and Faden, 1983). The same combination of drugs significantly improved cortical sensory evoked responses following focal cerebral ischemia in dogs (Hallenbeck *et al.*, 1982). More recently, a selective thromboxane synthetase inhibitor, 1-benzylimidazole, was administered during and after transient forebrain ischemia in rats and significantly improved cerebral blood flow and restored metabolic activity (Pettigrew *et al.*, 1989). In addition, indomethacin pretreatment administered 10–15 minutes before fluid percussion brain injury in rats significantly improved survival (Kim *et al.*, 1989).

The inhibition of cyclo-oxygenase following CNS injury is thought to be beneficial; however, decreasing the activity of this pathway may increase substrate availability for the lipoxygenase pathway (Demediuk and Faden, 1988b). Alternatively, selective inhibition of lipoxygenases may shunt arachidonic acid metabolism toward prostaglandins and thromboxanes. Accordingly, mixed cyclooxygenase-lipoxygenase inhibitors, such as nafazatrom and BW755C, may have advantages over selective cyclo-oxygenase or lipoxygenase inhibitors. Administration of BW755C following spinal cord injury in rats resulted in significant neurological improvement (Faden, Lemke, and Demediuk, 1988). This compound has also proved effective in the treatment of fluid-percussion-induced traumatic brain injury and transient spinal cord ischemia in rabbits (Graham, Demediuk, and Faden, 1989).

A number of clinical trials have been performed testing compounds affecting eicosanoid production for the prevention of CNS injury, and it is generally accepted that the administration of aspirin can significantly reduce the frequency of stroke in patients with transient ischemic attacks (Sze *et al.*, 1988). Aspirin has also been administered to prevent recurrent stroke following an initial infarction (Bousser *et al.*, 1983; Swedish Cooperative Study, 1986), but it has not been utilized to limit secondary tissue damage following stroke.

It has been suggested that the potent vasodilator, prostacyclin, may be effective in the treatment of acute ischemic strokes. Three open label studies demonstrated efficacy (Gryglewski *et al.*, 1983; Hakim, Pokrupa, and Wolfe, 1984; Miller *et al.*, 1984), but double-blind, placebo-controlled trials did not (Martin *et al.*, 1984; Hsu *et al.*, 1987). These studies have been criticized on the basis of dosage of prostacyclin used and the time at which therapy was initiated. Negative results may also have arisen because prostacyclin causes systemic hypotension, which may have particularly adverse effects on an infarct area that has lost autoregulation (Picone *et al.*, 1990). Synthetic analogs of prostacyclin that are less hypotensive may have more promise as therapy for acute ischemic stroke.

In conclusion, *in vitro* and animal model studies have generated information that may be useful for developing more specific and effective therapeutics based upon altering arachidonic acid metabolism. Data from the clinical trials suggest that this approach may eventually be successful.

OPIOID PEPTIDES

Numerous peptides with CNS neurotransmitter or neuromodulator activity have been identified and characterized (Kow and Pfaff, 1988), and several have been implicated as factors affecting secondary tissue injury following stroke or trauma (Faden, 1988a; Holaday *et al.*, 1989). Studies in experimental shock led to hypotheses regarding involvement of endogenous opioids in CNS trauma (Holaday and Faden, 1978). Increased β-endorphin-like immunoreactivity was noted in plasma one hour following spinal cord injury (Faden, Jacobs and Holaday, 1981b), and dynorphin immunoreactivity significantly increased in spinal cord following trauma (Faden *et al.*, 1985b).

The possible link between endogenous opioids and trauma led to a number of studies that were performed to determine the possible benefits of administering the non-specific opioid antagonist, naloxone. In a rabbit model of spinal cord ischemia, naloxone administration significantly reduced histopathological changes and improved motor recovery (Faden *et al.*, 1984). Improved neurological recovery following spinal cord injury was observed in rats (Arias, 1985; 1987) and cats (Faden *et al.*, 1981; Young *et al.*, 1981; Faden, Jacobs, and Holaday, 1982; Flamm *et al.*, 1982). Other studies, however, failed to detect a beneficial effect of naloxone in spinal cord injury (Black *et al.*, 1986; Wallace and Tator, 1986; Holtz, Nyström, and Gerdin, 1989). These discrepancies might have been caused by differences among the models, drug dosages, outcome measures, or the period of time over which recovery is evaluated. Naloxone has also been demonstrated to significantly improve a variety of physiological variables after traumatic brain injury in cats (Hayes *et al.*, 1983).

Naloxone treatment has been shown to improve recovery after acute cerebral ischemia in a variety of experimental animals, including rats (Wexler, 1984; Phillis, DeLong, and Towner, 1985; Capdeville *et al.*, 1986; Hariri *et al.*, 1986; Skarphedinsson and Thoren, 1986), gerbils (Hosobuchi, Baskin, and Woo, 1982; Avery, Crockard, and Russel, 1983), dogs (Faden, Hallenbeck, and Brown, 1982), cats (Baskin, Hosobuchi, and Grevel, 1982; Levy *et al.*, 1982), and baboons (Baskin, Kieck, and Hosobuchi, 1982; Zabramski *et al.*, 1984). In contrast, other studies were unable to detect a beneficial effect of naloxone in gerbils (Holaday and D'Amato, 1982; Kastin, Nissen, and Olson, 1982; Levy, Pike, and Rawlinson, 1982), rats (Shigeno *et al.*, 1983; Stokes, Hollinden, and Fox, 1984; Young *et al.*, 1984; Phillis, DeLong, and Towner, 1985), cats (Hubbard and Sundt, 1983), and monkeys (Gaines *et al.*, 1984). Part of this variability may relate to differences in models and outcome measures (Faden, 1988a). In addition, opioid antagonists exhibit an inverted-U-shaped dose-response curve, and many of the experiments that failed to detect a naloxone-dependent improvement of neurological function did not determine the optimal dose for their experimental model (Faden, 1988a).

Further support for a potential pathophysiological role for endogenous opioids in CNS injury have come from studies with intrathecal opioid administration. Dynorphin A, a κ-receptor agonist, causes flaccid hindlimb paralysis following intrathecal injection in rats (Faden and Jacobs, 1983; Herman and Goldstein, 1985; Smith and Lee, 1988). This effect of dynorphin is dose-dependent and is attenuated in a stereospecific fashion by treatment with nalmefene, which possesses increased κ-receptor activity (Bakshi and Faden, 1990), or nor-binalthophimine, which is a κ-selective antagonist (Faden, 1989a). Several other groups have also shown that dynorphin-induced paralysis is modified by κ-active opioid antagonists (Przewlocki, Shearman, and Herz, 1983; Przewlocki *et al.*, 1983; Spampinato and Candeletti,

1985), although one group has failed to observe antagonism of paralysis by nor-binaltorphimine (Long *et al.*, 1989b). More recent experiments have shown that dynorphin-induced hindlimb paralysis can be attenuated by the administration of competitive or non-competitive NMDA receptor antagonists (Caudle and Isaac, 1988; Bakshi and Faden, 1990). These results suggest that opioid-dependent tissue damage may be mediated, in part, through excitotoxic mechanisms.

Based upon these studies, a number of κ-receptor antagonists have been tested for efficacy in the treatment of spinal cord and brain injury. WIN44,441-3, an opioid antagonist with increased κ-receptor activity, improved neurological outcome and reduced histopathology following ischemic injury to the spinal cord (Faden *et al.*, 1985a; Faden and Jacobs, 1985b) or brain (Andrews *et al.*, 1988). WIN44,441-3 also improved cardiovascular, respiratory, and electrical physiological variables after head trauma in cats (McIntosh *et al.*, 1985). These drug effects were stereospecific, inferring an opioid receptor-mediated mechanism of action. Nalmefene treatment significantly improved behavioral outcome and reduced histopathological, electro-physiological, and biochemical changes following traumatic spinal cord injury (Faden, Sacksen and Noble, 1988b). Nalmefene is an exomethylene derivative of naltrexone with increased activity at κ receptors. It also attenuated injury-dependent changes in tissue free fatty acids and excitatory amino acids in a rat model of global cerebral ischemia/reperfusion (Faden *et al.*, 1990). In the latter study, nalmefene also substantially enhanced the speed and degree of recovery of cellular bioenergetic state, tissue acidosis, and lactate accumulation after cerebral ischemia as shown by magnetic resonance spectroscopy. Following fluid-percussion-induced brain injury in rats, nalmefene treatment improved free intracellular magnesium concentrations and cellular bioenergetic state as shown by magnetic resonance spectroscopy, as well as behavioral recovery (Vink *et al*, 1990). Following temporary spinal cord ischemia in rabbits, nalmefene significantly improved behavioral outcome and neuronal survival (Yum and Faden, 1990). Nor-binaltorphimine, a highly-selective antagonist, significantly improved neurological recovery after traumatic spinal cord and brain injury in rats (Faden, Takemori and Portoghese, 1987; Vink, Portoghese and Faden, 1991).

On the basis of results from preclinical studies, opioid antagonists have been tested in humans with strokes of varying etiologies. There are many methodological problems with these studies. Some of these reports are anecdotal, and others describe results from uncontrolled, non-randomized trials. The etiology of the stroke was often not specified, and the time elapsed between the occurrence of stroke and treatment was inconsistent. Moreover, the dosages of antagonists used was, in some cases, 1000-fold less than the dosage determined to be optimal in preclinical studies. Four studies found that administration of either naloxone or levellorphan improved neurological function, at least transiently (Baskin and Hosobuchi, 1981; Jabaily and Davis, 1984; Handa *et al.*, 1985; Namba *et al.*, 1986). Three other studies failed to show improved outcome (Cutler *et al.*, 1983; Fallis, Fisher, and Lobo, 1984; Perraro *et al.*, 1984). In a trial, attempts were made to control stroke etiology and time to treatment; naloxone was effective in acute or hyperacute ischemia, but not in patients with cerebral infarct or hemorrhage (Estanol, Aguilar, and Corona, 1985). In phase I trials of naloxone in stroke patients, improvement without toxicity was noted in 13 of 27 patients (Adams *et al.*, 1986). Despite the safety and possible efficacy of opioid receptor antagonists, a well-designed, randomized and controlled clinical trial has not yet been reported. Additional clinical experimentation seems warranted (Faden, 1990). For the past 4 years, the National Acute Spinal Cord Injury Study has been conducting a randomized trial involving 10 spinal cord centers that are comparing treatment with naloxone, methylprednisolone, or placebo. Results from this nearly-completed study are not yet available. A randomized-trial of naloxone treatment in acute head injury is also in progress at San Francisco General Hospital.

THYROTROPIN RELEASING HORMONE

Thyrotrophin-releasing hormone (TRH) has been demonstrated to have neuroprotective effects when administered after brain and spinal cord trauma. Administration of TRH at high doses (mg kg^{-1}) improved neurological outcome following spinal cord trauma produced in cats by the weight-drop method (Faden, Jacobs, and Holaday, 1981a; Faden *et al.*, 1983; Faden, Jacobs, and Smith, 1984b). Protection was dose related, and TRH was effective even if administered 24 hours after trauma (Faden, Jacobs, and Smith, 1984b). TRH treatment also improved neurological recovery following spinal cord injury produced with a vascular clip in rats (Arias, 1987), and reduced edema following traumatic spinal cord injury in rats (Salzman *et al.*, 1987). In addition, treatment with TRH has been shown to be protective in models of brainstem compression in cats (Fukuda, Yoshiaki, and Nagawa, 1979) and head injury in mice (Manaka and Sano, 1978).

In contrast, other groups have failed to detect a beneficial effect of TRH administered following spinal cord trauma (Hoerlein *et al.*, 1985; Hoovler *et al.*, 1987; Holtz, Nyström, and Gerdin, 1989). It is not clear, however, that any of these studies used experimental models capable of discriminating a pharmacological effect, because each of the groups has reported negative results with a series of agents shown to be effective in other laboratories and models. In addition, the latter study examined neurological recovery at four days after trauma. Previous reports have clearly shown that improvement in behavioral outcome is not observed until at least one week after trauma, possibly because of the consequences of spinal shock during the acute phase (Arias, 1987; Faden, 1988b; 1989b).

A number of modifications of the tripeptide comprising TRH have been synthesized and tested for efficacy in cat and rat models of impact-induced spinal cord injury. Two analogs with modifications at the N-terminal end of the peptide (CG3509 and CG3703) were beneficial, and two analogs with a modified C-terminal (MK771 and RX77368) were not (Faden and Jacobs, 1985a; Faden, Sacksen, and Noble, 1988a). CG7303 also attenuated the effects of traumatic brain injury on physiological variables, EEG, cellular bioenergetics, and behavioral outcome (McIntosh, Vink, and Faden, 1988). Effects of CG3703 in spinal cord injury appeared to be related to restoration of ionic homeostasis and associated improvement in bioenergetic state (Faden *et al.*, 1990). Another N-terminal substituted TRH analog, YM-14673, significantly improved physiological variables and neurological outcome following brain and spinal cord trauma in rats (Faden, 1989b).

Similar improvements were noted when an imidazole-substituted TRH analog was administered after traumatic brain injury (Faden, personal communication). These studies have clearly shown that integrity of the C-terminus is necessary for neuroprotective actions in CNS trauma; whereas, modifications of the N-terminus or imidazole moiety may significantly increase drug potency and improve pharmacokinetic profiles. The synthesis of additional N-substituted analogs may yield compounds with considerable therapeutic potential for the treatment of CNS trauma.

TRH has been administered following models of cerebral ischemia in dogs and gerbils, and spinal cord ischemia in rabbits; these studies were unable to demonstrate a beneficial effect (Faden, Hallenbeck, and Brown, 1982; Hannon and Garcia, 1982; Holaday and D'Amato, 1982; Faden, 1988a). However, beneficial effects have been reported by several investigators using TRH analogs in cerebral ischemia (O'Shaughnessy, Rothwell, and Shrewsbury-Gee, 1989; Yamamoto *et al.*, 1989). These preclinical studies generally support the potential clinical evaluation of TRH or TRH analogs in CNS trauma. However, further experimental work is necessary before these compounds can be assessed for the treatment of stroke.

OTHER FACTORS

Other peptide and non-peptide modulators have been implicated as secondary injury factors. Somatostatin injections caused dose-dependent loss of motor function that was blocked by pretreatment with a somatostatin receptor antagonist (Long, 1988). The antagonist, however, also produced paraparesis when injected at high doses, which suggests that it is a partial agonist at the somatostatin receptor or that the antagonist may be acting through non-somatostatin-receptor mediated pathways at high doses (Long, 1988). Peptide analogs of substance P (SP) antagonists also display neurotoxic effects. One such antagonist, Spantide, caused neuronal necrosis when injected intrathecally or directly into the brain or spinal cord (Post *et al.*, 1985; Post and Paulsson, 1985; Hokfelt *et al.*, 1989; Holaday *et al.*, 1989). Both somatostatin and substance P are significantly decreased one week after traumatic spinal cord injury (Faden, Jacobs, and Helke, 1985). The results of these studies provide further evidence that neuropeptide response may be related to injury. Intrathecal injection of arginine[8]-vasopressin was also neurotoxic, perhaps acting as a vasoconstrictor (Long *et al.*, 1989a). Interestingly, the neurotoxic effects of Spantide were blocked by pretreatment with the tripeptide TRH (Post *et al.*, 1985; Hokfelt *et al.*, 1989). However, another research group has been unable to detect a neuroprotective effect of TRH against Spantide toxicity (Holaday *et al.*, 1989).

Immunoreactivity to a variety of peptides has been associated either directly with capillary endothelial cells or with nerve cells terminating on pial arteries. Among the peptides that have been studied are substance P, neurokinin A, calcitonin gene-related peptide, vasoactive intestinal polypeptide, and arginine vasopressin (Pearlmutter *et al.*, 1988; McCulloch and Edvinsson, 1989). These molecules may be involved in coupling changes in local cerebral blood flow to local neuronal activity; potential therapeutic or pathophysiological roles for most of these peptides have not been evaluated.

Recent experiments suggest that the kallikrein-kinin system may participate in the arachidonic acid cascade pursuant to fluid percussion traumatic brain injury in rats (Ellis, Chao, and Heizer, 1989). Additional studies have reported that significant neurofilament degradation occurred within 15 minutes of the onset of either permanent global or transient cerebral ischemia (Ogata *et al.*, 1989). Therefore, inhibitors of kinin production or neuronal proteases may represent other classes of compounds that may have efficacy for the treatment of CNS lesions.

Platelet activating factor (PAF), an alkyl-phospholipid, may alter neutrophil or leukocyte responses, modulate thrombus formation, stimulate the release of interleukin-1, interleukin-2, and tumor necrosis factor from platelets, and control blood–brain barrier permeability by affecting the cytoskeleton of the vascular endothelium (Braquet *et al.*, 1988; Braquet *et al.*, 1989a). PAF is thought to participate in a positive-feedback loop with cytokines, generally inducing cellular chemotaxis, free radical production, and inflammation. PAF also causes paraparesis in rats and marked reduction in blood flow after intrathecal administration in rats through a specific reception mechanism (Faden and Halt, in press). Several chemically unrelated antagonists of PAF (BN-52021, WEB-2086, and kadsurenone) have a beneficial effect on neurological outcome and physiological variables when administered preventively or after experimental stroke in gerbils or dogs (Braquet, Palubert-Braquet, Koltai *et al.*, 1989b). BN-52021 also significantly improved behavioral outcome of rats following traumatic brain injury (Faden and Tzendzalian, in press). Another antagonist, BN-50739, significantly decreased progressive hypoperfusion following laser injury in rat brain (Frerichs *et al.*, 1989). PAF antagonists may have particular value for the treatment of pathologies involving microvascular damage and may possess considerable potential for treatment of stroke or trauma.

CONCLUSION

Secondary tissue injury in the CNS involves numerous biochemical and physiological changes that can lead to progressive tissue damage. Preclinical data generated through animal models of CNS injury suggest that excitotoxicity, ion fluxes, production of free radicals, generation of eicosanoids, or alterations of tissue concentrations of neuropeptides are all involved in secondary injury. Attempts to modify these processes pharmacologically have been successful in various experimental models.

Taken together, these findings suggest that neurological deficits following stroke or CNS trauma in humans may be limited by early pharmacological interventions that block or attenuate the effects of specific biochemical factors.

References

Adams HP, Olinger CP, Barsan WG, Butler MJ, Graff-Radford NR, Brott TG *et al.* (1986) A dose-escalation study of large doses of naloxone for treatment of patients with acute cerebral ischemia, *Stroke*, **17**, 404–9

Aikawa JK (1981) *Magnesium: its biological significance*, CRC, Boca Raton

Albers GW, Goldberg MP, and Choi DW (1989) N-methyl-D-aspartate antagonists: ready for clinical trial in brain ischemia?, *Ann Neurol*, **25**, 398–408

Anderson DK, Braughler JM, Hall ED, Waters TR, McCall JM, and Means ED (1988) Effects of treatment with U-74006F on neurological outcome following experimental spinal cord injury, *J Neurosurg*, **69**, 562–7

Anderson DK, Saunders RD, Demediuk P, Dugan LL, Braughler JM, Hall ED *et al.* (1985) Lipid hydrolysis and peroxidation in injured spinal cord: partial protection with methylprednisolone or vitamin E and selenium, *Central Nervous System Trauma*, **2**, 257–67

Andrews BT, McIntosh TK, Gonzales MF, Weinstein PR, and Faden AI (1988) Levels of endogenous opioids and effects of an opiate antagonist during regional cerebral ischemia in rats, *J Pharmacol Exp Ther*, **247**, 1248–54

Arias MJ (1985) Effect of naloxone on functional recovery after experimental spinal cord injury in the rat, *Surg Neurol*, **23**, 440–2

Arias MJ (1987) Treatment of experimental spinal cord injury with TRH, naloxone, and dexamethasone, *Surg Neurol*, **28**, 335–8

Avery MS, Crockard H, and Russel RW (1983) Improved survival following severe cerebral ischemia using naloxone, *J Cereb Blood Flow Metab*, **3**, S331–S332

Bakshi R and Faden AI (1990) Competitive and non-competitive NMDA antagonists limit dynorphin A-induced rat hindlimb paralysis, *Brain Res*, **507**, 1–5

Baskin DS and Hosobuchi Y (1981) Naloxone reversal of ischemic neurological deficits in man, *Lancet*, **1**, 272–5

Baskin DS, Hosobuchi Y, and Grevel JC (1986) Treatment of experimental stroke with opiate antagonists, *J Neurosurg*, **64**, 99–103

Baskin DS, Kieck CF, and Hosobuchi Y (1982) Naloxone reversal of ischemic neurologic deficits in baboons is not mediated by systemic effects, *Life Sci*, **31**, 2201–4

Bazan NG (1989) Arachidonic acid in the modulation of excitable membrane function and at the onset of brain damage, *Ann NY Acad Sci*, **559**, 1–16

Benveniste HJ, Drejer J, Schousboe A, and Diemer NH (1984) Elevation of the extracellular concentrations of glutamate and aspartate in rat hippocampus during transient cerebral ischemia monitored by intracerebral microdialysis, *J Neurochem*, **43**, 1369–74

Black KL and Hoff JT (1990) Arachidonic acid metabolism in ischemia, In Weinstein PR and Faden AI, eds, *Protection of the brain from ischemia*, Baltimore, Williams and Wilkins, in press

Black P, Markowitz RS, Keller S, Wachs K, Gillespie J, and Finkelstein SD (1986) Naloxone and experimental spinal cord injury: part 1, high dose administration in a static load compression model, *Neurosurgery*, **19**, 905–8

Blaustein MP (1988a) Calcium and synaptic function, *Handbook of Experimental Pharmacology*, **83**, 276–304

Blaustein MP (1988b) Calcium transport and buffering in neurons, *Trends Neurosci*, **11**, 438–43

Bousser MG, Eschwege E, Haguenau M, Lefaucconnier JM, Thimbult N, Touboul D et al. (1983) Controlled clinical trial of aspirin and dipyradamole in the secondary premention of athero-thrombotic cerebral ischemia, *Stroke*, **14**, 5–14

Braquet P, Spinnewyn B, Blavet N, Marcheselli V, Rossawska M, and Bazan NG (1988) Platelet activating factor as a mediator in cerebral ischemia and related disorders, *Biomed Biochim Acta*, **47**, S195–S218

Braquet P, Paulbert-Brequet M, Koltai M, Bougain R, Bussolino F, and Hosford D (1989a) Is there a case for PAF antagonists in the treatment of ischemic states, *Trends Pharmacol Sci*, **10**, 23–30

Braquet P, Spinnewyn B, Demerle C, Hosford D, Marcheselli V, Rossowska M et al. (1989b) The role of platelet activating factor in cerebral ischemia and related disorders, *Ann NY Acad Sci*, **559**, 296–312

Braughler JM and Hall ED (1989) Central nervous system trauma and stroke I: Biochemical consideration for oxygen radical formation and lipid peroxidation, *Free Radic Biol Med*, **6**, 289–301

Braughler JM, Pregenzer JF, Chase RL, Duncan LA, Jacobsen EJ, and McCall JM (1987) Novel 21-aminosteroids as potent inhibitors of iron-dependent lipid peroxidation, *J Biol Chem*, **262**, 10438–40

Burton GW and Ingold KU (1986) Vitamin E: application of the principles of physical organic chemistry to the exploration of its structure and function, *Accounts of Chemical Research*, **19**, 194–201

Capdeville C, Pruneau D, Allix M, Plotkine M, and Boulu RG (1986) Naloxone effect on the neurological deficit induced by forebrain ischemia in rats, *Life Sci*, **38**, 347–442

Caudle RM and Isaac L (1988) A novel interaction between dynorphin (1-13) and an N-methyl-D-aspartate site, *Brain Res*, **443**, 329–32

Cheng MK, Robertson C, Grossman RG, Foltz R, and Williams V (1984) Neurological outcome correlated with spinal evoked potentials in a spinal cord ischemia model, *J Neurosurg*, **60**, 786–95

Choi DW (1988) Calcium-mediated neurotoxicity: relationship to specific channel types and role in ischemic damage, *Trends Neurosci*, **11**, 465–9

Collingridge GL and Bliss TVP (1987) NMDA receptors – their role in long-term potentiation, *Trends Neurosci*, **10**, 288–93

Cotgreave IA, Moldeus P, and Orrenius S (1988) Host biochemical defense mechanisms against prooxidants, *Ann Rev Pharmacol Toxicol*, **28**, 189–212

Cutler JR, Bredesen DE, Edwards R, and Simon RP (1983) Failure of naloxone to reverse vascular neurologic deficits, *Neurology*, **33**, 1517–8

Demediuk P and Faden AI (1988a) Excitatory amino acids in experimental spinal cord trauma: injury-induced changes in total tissue levels and pharmacological intervention with the competitive antagonist CPP, *Society of Neuroscience Abstracts*, **14**, 419

Demediuk P and Faden AI (1988b) Traumatic spinal cord injury in rats causes increases in tissue thromboxane but not peptidoleukotrienes, *J Neurosci Res*, **20**, 115–21

Demediuk P, Saunders RD, Anderson DK, Means ED, and Horrocks LA (1985) Membrane lipid changes in laminectomized and traumatized cat spinal cord, *Proc Natl Acad Sci USA*, **82**, 7071–5

Demopoulos HB, Flamm ES, Pietronigro DD, and Seligman ML (1980) The free radical pathology and the microcirculation in the major central nervous system disorders, *Acta Physiol Scand Suppl*, **492**, 91–119

Dyste GN, Hitchon PW, Girton RA, and Chapman M (1989) Effect of hetastarch, mannitol, and phenylephrine on spinal cord blood flow following experimental spinal injury, *Neurosurgery*, **24**, 228–34

Earnest MP (1988) Nimodipine in acute achemic stroke, *N Engl J Med*, **319**, 203

Ellis EF, Chao J, and Heizer ML (1989) Brain kininogen following experimental brain injury: evidence for a secondary event, *J Neurosurg*, **71**, 437–42

Estanol B, Aguilar F, and Corona T (1985) Diagnosis of reversible versus irreversible cerebral ischemia by the intravenous administration of naloxone, *Stroke*, **16**, 1006–9

Faden AI (1988a) Neuropeptides and central nervous system injury, *Arch Neurol*, **43**, 501–4

Faden AI (1988b) Role of thyrotropin-releasing hormone and opiate receptor antagonists in limiting central nervous system injury, *Adv Neurol*, **47**, 531–45

Faden AI (1989a) Opioid and nonopioid mechanisms may contribute to dynorphin's pathophysiological actions in spinal cord injury, *Ann Neurol*, in press

Faden AI (1989b) TRH analog YM-14673 improves outcome following traumatic brain and spinal cord injury in rats: dose-response studies, *Brain Res*, **486**, 228–35

Faden AI (1990) Role of opiate antagonists in the treatment of stroke, In Weinstein PR and Faden AI, eds, *Protection of the brain from ischemia*, Baltimore, Williams and Wilkins, 265–71

Faden AI, Chan PH, and Longar S (1987) Alterations in lipid metabolism, Na$^+$, K$^+$-ATPase activity, and tissue water content of spinal cord injury following experimental traumatic injury, *J Neurochem*, **48**, 1809–16

Faden AI, Demediuk P, Panter SS, and Vink R (1989a) The role of excitatory amino acids and NMDA receptors in traumatic brain injury, *Science*, **244**, 798–800

Faden AI, Ellison JA, and Noble LJ (1989) Effects of competitive and non-competitive N-methyl-D-aspartate antagonists in experimental spinal cord injury, *Eur J Pharmacol*, **175**, 165–74

Faden AI, Hallenbeck JM, and Brown CQ (1982) Treatment of experimental stroke: comparison of naloxone and thyrotropin-releasing hormone, *Neurology*, **32**, 1083–7

Faden AI and Halt P (1992) Platelet-activating factor reduces spinal cord blood flow and causes behavioral deficits following intrathecal administration in rats through a specific receptor mechanism, *J Pharmacol Exp Ther* (in press)

Faden AI and Jacobs TP (1983) Dynorphin induces partially reversible paraplegia in the rat, *Eur J Pharmacol*, **91**, 321–4

Faden AI and Jacobs TP (1985a) Effect of TRH analogs on neurological recovery after experimental spinal trauma, *Neurology*, **35**, 1331–4

Faden AI and Jacobs TP (1985b) Opiate antagonist WIN44,441-3 stereospecifically improves neurologic recovery after ischemic spinal cord injury, *Neurology*, **35**, 1311–5

Faden AI, Jacobs TP, and Helke CJ (1985) Changes in substance P and somatostatin in the spinal cord after traumatic spinal injury in the rat, *Neuropeptides*, **6**, 215–25

Faden AI, Jacobs TP, and Holaday JW (1981a) Thyrotropin-releasing hormone improves neurologic recovery after spinal trauma in cats, *N Engl J Med*, **305**, 1063–7

Faden AI, Jacobs TP, and Holaday JW (1981b) Endorphins in experimental spinal injury: therapeutic effect of naloxone, *Ann Neurol*, **10**, 326–32

Faden AI, Jacobs TP, and Holaday JW (1982) Comparison of early and late naloxone treatment in experimental spinal injury, *Neurology*, **32**, 677–81

Faden AI, Jacobs TP, Mougey E, and Holaday JW (1981) Endorphins in experimental spinal injury. Therapeutic effect of naloxone, *Ann Neurol*, **10**, 326–32

Faden AI, Jacobs TP, and Smith MT (1984a) Evaluation of the calcium channel antagonist nimodipine in experimental spinal cord ischemia, *J Neurosurg*, **60**, 796–9

Faden AI, Jacobs TP, and Smith MT (1984b) Thyrotropin-releasing hormone in experimental spinal injury: dose response and late treatment, *Neurology*, **34**, 1280–4

Faden AI, Jacobs TP, Smith MT, and Holaday JW (1983) Comparison of thyrotropin-releasing hormone (TRH), naloxone, and dexamethasone treatments in experimental spinal injury, *Neurology*, **33**, 673–8

Faden AI, Jacobs TP, Smith MT, and Zivin JA (1984) Naloxone in experimental spinal cord ischemia: dose response studies, *Eur J Pharmacol*, **103**, 115–20

Faden AI, Knoblach S, Mays C, and Jacobs TP (1985a) Motor dysfunction after spinal cord injury is mediated by opiate receptors, *Peptides*, **6** (Suppl 1), 15–17

Faden AI, Lemke M, and Demediuk P (1988) Effects of BW755C, a mixed cyclo-oxygenase-lipoxygenase inhibitor, following traumatic spinal cord injury in rats, *Brain Res*, **463**, 63–78

Faden AI, Lemke M, Simon RP, and Noble LJ (1988) N-methyl-D-aspartate antagonist MK801 improves outcome following traumatic spinal cord injury in rats: behavioral, anatomical, and neurochemical studies, *J Neurotrauma*, **5**, 27–37

Faden AI, Molineaux CJ, Rosenberger JG, Jacobs TP, and Cox BM (1985b) Endogenous opioid immunoreactivity in rat spinal cord following traumatic injury, *Ann Neurol*, **17**, 386–90

Faden AI, Sacksen I, and Noble LJ (1988a) Structure activity relationships of TRH analogs in experimental spinal injury, *Brain Res*, **448**, 287–93

Faden AI, Shirane R, Chang L-H, James TL, Lemke M, and Weinstein PR (1990) Opiate receptor antagonist improves metabolic recovery and limits neurochemical alterations associated with reperfusion and global brain ischemia in rats, *J Pharmacol Exp Ther* **255**, 451–8

Faden AI, Sacksen I, and Noble LJ (1988b) Opiate-receptor antagonist nalmefene improves neurological recovery after traumatic spinal cord injury in rats, *J Pharmacol Exp Ther*, **245**, 742–8

Faden AI and Simon RP (1988) A potential role for excitotoxins in the pathophysiology of spinal cord injury, *Ann Neurol*, **23**, 623–6

Faden AI, Takemori AE, and Portoghese PS (1987) κ-selective opiate antagonist nor-binaltorphimine improves outcome after traumatic spinal cord injury in rats, *Central Nervous System Trauma*, **4**, 227–237

Faden AI and Tzendzalian PA (1992) Platelet activating factor antagonists limit glycine changes and behavioral deficits after brain trauma, *Am J Physiol* (in press)

Faden AI, Tzendzalian P, Lemke M, and Valone F (1989b) Role of platelet-activating factor (PAF) in the pathophysiology of traumatic brain injury, *Society for Neuroscience Abstracts*, **15**, 1112

Fallis RJ, Fisher M, and Lobo R (1984) A double-blind trial of naloxone in the treatment of acute stroke, *Stroke*, **15**, 627–9

Fehlings MG, Tator CH, and Linden RD (1989) The effect of nimodopine and dextran on axonal function and blood flow following experimental spinal cord injury, *J Neurosurg*, **71**, 403–16

Flamm ES, Young W, Demopoulos HB, De Crescito V, and Tomasula JJ (1982) Experimental spinal cord injury: treatment with naloxone, *Neurosurgery*, **10**, 227–31

Ford WJ and Malm DN (1985) Failure of nimodipine to reverse acute experimental spinal cord injury, *Central Nervous System Trauma*, **2**, 9–17

Frerichs KU, Lindsberg PJ, Hallenbeck JM, and Feuerstein GZ (1989) Beneficial effect of platelet activating factor (PAF) antagonist in experimental neuroinjury in rats, *Society for Neuroscience Abstracts*, **15**, 1112

Fujimoto S, Mizoi D, Yoshimoto T, and Suzuki J (1984) The protective effect of vitamin E on cerebral ischemia, *Surg Neurol*, **22**, 449–54

Fukuda N, Yoshiaki S, and Nagawa Y (1979) Behavioral and EEG alterations with brainstem compression and effect of thyrotropin-releasing hormone (TRH) in chronic cats, *Nippon Yakurigaku Zasshi*, **75**, 321–31

Gaines C, Nehls DG, Suess DM, Waggener JD, and Crowell RM (1984) Effect of naloxone on experimental stroke in awake monkeys, *Neurosurgery*, **14**, 308–14

Galli C, Petroni A, Bertazzo A, and Sarti S (1989) Arachidonic acid and its metabolites during cerebral ischemia and recirculation, *Ann NY Acad Sci*, **559**, 352–64

Gelmers HJ, Gorter K, de Weerdt CJ, and Wiezer HJA (1988) A controlled trial of nimodipine in acute ischemic stroke, *N Engl J Med*, **318**, 203–7

Goldman RS and Finkbeiner SM (1988) Therapeutic use of magnesium sulfate in selected cases of cerebral ischemia and seizure, *N Engl J Med*, **319**, 1224–5

Graham SH, Demediuk P, and Faden AI (1989) Pretreatment with a mixed cyclo-oxygenase-lipoxygenase inhibitor improves behavioral and histological outcome following spinal cord ischemia-reperfusion, *Society for Neuroscience Abstracts*, **15**, 42

Graham SH, Shiraishi K, Panter SS, Simon RP, and Faden AI (1990) Changes in extracellular amino acid neurotransmitters produced by focal cerebral ischemia, *Neurosci Lett*, **110**, 124–30

Griffiths E (1987) Iron in biological systems, In Bullen JJ and Griffiths E, eds, *Iron and Infection*, New York, Wiley and Sons, 1–25

Gruner JA, Young W, Blight AR, and DeCrescito V (1989) Effect of 21-aminosteroid U74006F on sensory and motor recovery after severe thoracic spinal cord contusion injury in cats, *J Neurotrauma*, **6**, 197

Gryglewski RJ, Nowak S, Kostka-Trabka E, Kusmiderski J, Dembinska-Kiec A, Bieron K *et al.* (1983) Treatment of ischaemic stroke with prostacyclin, *Stroke*, **14**, 197–202

Guha A, Tator CH, and Piper I (1987) Effect of a calcium channel blocker on post-traumatic spinal cord blood flow, *J Neurosurg*, **66**, 423–30

Hakim A, Pokrupa RP, and Wolfe LS (1984) Preliminary report on the effectiveness of prostacyclin in stroke, *Can J Neurol*, **11**, 409

Hall ED (1988) Effects of the 21-aminosteroid U74006F on posttraumatic spinal cord ischemia in cats, *J Neurosurg*, **68**, 462–5

Hall ED and Braughler JM (1989) Central nervous system trauma and stroke II: Physiological and pharmacological evidence for involvement of oxygen radicals and lipid peroxidation, *Free Radic Biol Med*, **6**, 303–13

Hall ED, Pazara BA, and Braughler JM (1988) 21-aminosteroid lipid peroxidation inhibitor U74006F protects against cerebral ischemia in gerbils, *Stroke*, **19**, 997–1002

Hall ED and Wolf DL (1986) A pharmacological analysis of the pathophysiological mechanisms of posttraumatic spinal cord ischemia, *J Neurosurg*, **64**, 951–61

Hall ED, Yonkers PA, McCall JM, and Braughler JM (1988) Effects of the 21-aminosteroid U74006F on experimental head injury in mice, *J Neurosurg*, **68**, 456–61

Hallenbeck JM, Jacobs TP, and Faden AI (1983) Combined PGI$_2$, indomethacin, and heparin improves neurological recovery after spinal trauma in cats, *J Neurosurg*, **58**, 749–54

Hallenbeck JM, Leitch DR, Dutka AJ, Greenbaum LJ, and McKee AE (1982) Prostacyclin I$_2$, indomethacin, and heparin promote post-ischemic neuronal recovery in dogs, *Ann Neurol*, **12**, 145–56

Halushka PV, Mais DE, Mayeux PR, and Morinelli TA (1989) Thromboxane, prostaglandin and leukotriene receptors, *Ann Rev Pharmacol Toxicol*, **29**, 213–39

Handa N, Matsumoto M, Nakamura M, Yoneda S, Kimura K, Sugitani Y *et al.* (1985) Reversal of neurological deficits by levallorphan in patients with acute ischemic stroke, *J Cereb Blood Flow Met*, **5**, 469–72

Hannon CJ and Garcia AR (1982) Thyrotropin-releasing hormone (TRH) increases morbidity and mortality in the gerbil stroke model, *Neurosci Lett*, **33**, 299–303

Hariri RJ, Supra EL, Roberts JP, and Lavyne MH (1986) Effect of naloxone in cerebral perfusion and cardiac performance during experimental cerebral ischemia, *J Neurosurg*, **64**, 780–6

Hass WK and Kamm B (1984) The North American ticlopidine aspirin stroke study: structure, stratification variables, and patient characteristics, *Agents and Actions*, (Suppl), 273–8

Hayes RL, Galinet BJ, Kulkarne P, and Becker DP (1983) Effects of naloxone in systemic and cerebral responses to experimental concussive brain injury in cats, *J Neurosurg*, **58**, 720–8

Hayes RL, Jenkins LW, Lyeth BG, Balster RL, Robinson SE, Clifton GL *et al.* (1988) Pretreatment with phencyclidine, an N-methyl-D-aspartate antagonist, attenuates long-term behavioral deficits in the rat produced by traumatic brain injury, *J Neurotrauma*, **5**, 259–75

Herman BH and Goldstein A (1985) Antinociception and paralysis induced by intrathecal dynorphin A, *J Pharmacol Exp Ther*, **232**, 27–32

Hertting G and Seregi A (1989) Formation and function of eicosanoids in the central nervous system, *Ann NY Acad Sci*, **559**, 84–99

Hoerlein BF, Redding RW, Hoff EJ, and McGuire JA (1985) Evaluation of naloxone, crocetin, thyrotropin releasing hormone, methylprednisolone, partial myelotomy, and hemilaminectomy in the treatment of acute spinal cord trauma, *J Am Anim Hosp Assoc*, **2**, 67–77

Holaday JW and D'Amato RJ (1982) Naloxone or TRH fail to improve neurological deficits in gerbil models of 'stroke', *Life Sci*, **31**, 385–92

Holaday JW, Long JB, Martinez-Arizala A, Chen H-S, Reynolds DG, and Gurll NJ (1989) Effects of TRH in circulatory shock and central nervous system ischemia, *Ann NY Acad Sci*, **553**, 370–9

Hökfelt T, Tsuruo Y, Ulfhake B, Cullheim S, Arvidsson U, Foster GA *et al.* (1989) Distribution of TRH-like immunoreactivity with special reference to coexistence with other neuroactive compounds, *Ann NY Acad Sci*, **553**, 76–105

Holtz A, Nyström, and Gerdin B (1989) Blocking weight-induced spinal cord injury in rats: effects of TRH or naloxone on motor function recovery and spinal cord blood flow, *Acta Neurol Scand*, **80**, 215–20

Hoovler DW, Fujii E, Sheckowitz E, and Wrathall JR (1987) Lack of effect of naloxone or TRH on functional deficit in rats with contusive spinal cord injuries, *Society of Neuroscience Abstracts*, **13**, 1500

Hosobuchi Y, Baskin DS, and Woo SK (1982) Reversal of induced ischemic neurological deficits in gerbils by the opiate antagonist naloxone, *Science*, **215**, 69–71

Hsu CY, Faught RE, Furlan AJ, Coull BM, Huang DC, Hogan EL *et al.* (1987) Intravenous prostacyclin in acute nonhemorrhagic stroke: a placebo-controlled double-blind trial, *Stroke*, **18**, 352–8

Hsu CY, Halushka PV, Xu J, Hogan EL, Banik NL, Lee WA, and Perot PL (1985) Alteration of thromboxane and prostacyclin levels in experimental spinal cord injury, *Neurology*, **35**, 1003–9

Hsu CY, Liu TH, Hogan EL, Chao J, Sun G, Tai HH *et al.* (1989) Arachidonic acid and its metabolites in cerebral ischemia, *Ann NY Acad Sci*, **559**, 282–95

Hubbard JL and Sundt TM (1983) Failure of naloxone to affect focal incomplete cerebral ischemia and collateral blood flow in cats, *J Neurosurg*, **59**, 237–44

Huczynski J, Kostka-Trabka E, Sotowska W, Bieron K, Grodzinska L, Dembinska-Kiec A *et al.* (1985) Double-blind controlled trial of the therapeutic effects of prostacyclin in patients with completed ischaemic stroke, *Stroke*, **16**, 810–4

Ingold KU, Burton GW, Foster DO, Hughes L, Lindsay DA, and Webb A (1987) Biokinetics of and discrimination between dietary nRRR- and SRR-alpha-tocopherols in the male rat, *Lipids*, **22**, 163–72

Jabaily J and Davis JN (1984) Naloxone administration of patients with acute stroke, *Stroke*, **15**, 36–9

Judge ME, Sheardown MJ, Jacobsen P, and Honoré T (1991) Protection against post-ischemic behavioral pathology by the a-amino-3 hydroxy-5-methyl-4-isoxazolepropionic acid (AMPA) antagonist 2,3 dihydroxy-6-nitro-7 sulfamoyl-benzo(f)quinoxaline (NBQX) in the gerbil, *Neurosci Lett*, **133**, 291–4

Kastin AJ, Nissen C, and Olson RD (1982) Failure of MIF or naloxone to reverse ischemic-induced neurologic deficits in gerbils, *Pharmacol Biochem Behav*, **17**, 1083–5

Katayama Y, Cheung MK, Gorman L, Tamura T, and Becker DP (1988) Increase in extracellular glutamate and associated massive ionic fluxes following concussive brain injury, *Society of Neuroscience Abstracts*, **14**, 1154

Kim HJ, Levasseur JE, Patterson JL, Jackson GF, Madge GE, Povlishock JT *et al.* (1989) Effect of indomethacin pretreatment on acute mortality in experimental brain injury, *J Neurosurg*, **71**, 565–72

Kinuta Y, Kikuchi H, Ishikawa M, Kimura M, and Itokawa I (1989) Lipid peroxidation in focal ischemia, *J Neurosurg*, **71**, 421–9

Korf J, Klein HC, Venema K, and Postema F (1988) Increases in striatal and hippocampal impedance and extracellular levels of amino acids by cardiac arrest in freely moving rats, *J Neurochem*, **50**, 1087–96

Kow L-M and Pfaff DW (1988) Neuromodulatory actions of peptides, *Ann Rev Pharmacol Toxicol*, **28**, 163–88

Le Peillet E, Arvin B, Moncada C, and Meldrum BS (1992) The non-NMDA antagonists, NBQX and GYK1 52466, protect against cortical and striatal cell loss following transient global ischaemia in the rat, *Brain Res* **571**, 115–20

Lemke M, Demediuk P, McIntosh TK, Vink R, and Faden AI (1987) Alterations in tissue Mg^{++}, Na^+ and spinal cord edema following impact trauma in rats, *Biochem Biophys Res Commun*, **147**, 1170–5

Lemke M, Frei B, Ames BN, and Faden AI (1990) Decreases in tissue levels of ubiquinol-9 and -10, ascorbate, and alpha-tocopherol following spinal cord impact trauma in rats, *Neurosci Lett*, **108**, 201–6

Levy R, Feustel P, Severinghaus J, and Hosobuchi Y (1982) Effect of naloxone on neurologic deficit and blood flow during focal cerebral ischemia in cats, *Life Sci*, **31**, 2205–8

Levy DE, Pike CL, and Rawlinson DG (1982) Failure of naloxone to limit clinical or morphological brain damage in gerbils with unilateral carotid artery occlusion, *Society of Neuroscience Abstracts*, **8**, 248

Liebler DC, Kling DS, and Reed DJ (1986) Antioxidant protection of phospholipid bilayers by alpha-tocopherol, *J Biol Chem* **261**, 12114–9

Long JB (1988) Spinal subarachnoid injection of somatostatin causes neurological deficits and neuronal injury in rats, *Eur J Pharmacol*, **149**, 287–96

Long JB, Martinez-Arizala A, Johnson SH, and Holaday JW (1989a) Arginine[8]-Vasopressin reduces spinal cord blood flow after spinal subarachnoid injection in rats, *J Pharmacol Exp Ther*, **249**, 499–506

Long JB, Rigamonti DD, de Costa B, Rice KC, and Martinez-Arizala A (1989b) Dynorphin A-induced rat hindlimb paralysis and spinal cord injury are not altered by the kappa opioid antagonist nor-binaltorphimine, *Brain Res*, **497**, 155–62

Manaka S and Sano K (1978) Thyrotropin-releasing hormone tartrate (TRH-t) shortens concussion effects following head impact in mice, *Neurosci Lett*, **8**, 255–8

Martin JF, Hamdy N, Nicholl J, Lewtas N, Bergvall U, Owen P *et al.* (1985) Double-blind controlled trial of prostacyclin in cerebral infarction, *Stroke*, **16**, 386–90

McCall JM, Braughler JM, and Hall ED (1987) A new class of compounds for stroke and trauma: effects of 21-aminosteroids on lipid peroxidation, *Acta Anaesthesiol Belg*, **38**, 417–20

McCulloch J and Edvinsson L (1989) Peptidergic innervation of the cerebral vasculature and its functional significance, In Battaini F, Govoni S, Magnoni MS, and Trabucchi M, eds, *Regulatory mechanisms of neuron to vessel communication in the brain*, Berlin, Springer Verlag, 97–108

McIntosh TK, Agura VM, Hellgeth M, Rittner H, Faden AI, and Hayes RL (1985) Stereospecific efficacy of the opiate antagonist WIN44,441-3 in the treatment of head injury in the cat, *Society of Neuroscience Abstracts*, **11**, 1200

McIntosh TK, Faden AI, Yamakami I, and Vink R (1988) Magnesium deficiency exacerbates and pretreatment improves outcome following traumatic brain injury in rats: 31P magnetic resonance spectroscopy and behavioral studies, *J Neurotrauma*, **5**, 17–31

McIntosh TK, Soares HL, Hayes RL, and Simon RP (1989a) The N-methyl-D-aspartate antagonist MK-801 prevents edema and restores magnesium homeostasis following traumatic brain injury in rats. In Leahman J, ed, *Recent advances in excitatory amino acid research*, New York, AR Liss, 653–6

McIntosh TK, Vink R, and Faden AI (1988) An analogue of thyrotropin-releasing hormone improves outcome after brain injury: 31P-NMR studies, *Am J Physiol*, **254**, R785–R792

McIntosh TK, Vink R, Yamakami I, and Faden AI (1989b) Magnesium protects against neurological deficit after brain injury, *Brain Res*, **482**, 252–60

Miller VT, Coull BM, Yatsu FM, Shah AB, and Beamer NB (1984) Prostacyclin infusion in acute cerebral infarction, *Neurology*, **34**, 1431–5

Mohr JP, Dilanni M, Muschett JL, Riccio RV, and GH Besselaar Associates and the Nimodipine Study Group (1989). Nimodipine in acute ischemic stroke, *Ann Neurol*, **26**, 124

Monaghan DT, Bridges RJ, and Cotman CW (1989) The excitatory amino acid receptors, *Ann Rev Pharmacol Toxicol*, **29**, 365–402

Nahorski SR (1988) Inositol polyphosphates and neuronal calcium homeostasis, *Trends Neurosci*, **10**, 444–8

Namba S, Nishigake S, Fujiwara N, Wani T, Namba Y, and Masaoka T (1986) Opiate-antagonist reversal of neurological deficits – experimental and clinical studies, *Jpn J Psychiatry Neurol*, **40**, 61–79

Needleman P, Turk J, Jakschik BA, Morrison AR, and Lefkowith JB (1986) Arachidonic acid metabolism, *Annu Rev Biochem*, **55**, 69–102

Nellgard B, Wieloch T (1992) Postischemia blockade of AMPA but not NMDA receptors mitigates neuronal damage in the rat brain following transient severe cerebral ischemia, *J Cereb Blood Flow and Metab*, **12**, 2–11

Ogata N, Yonekawa Y, Taki W, Kannagi R, Murachi T, Hamakubo T *et al.* (1989) Degradation of neurofilament protein in cerebral ischemia, *J Neurosurg*, **70**, 103–7

O'Shaughnessy CT, Rothwell NJ, and Shrewsbury-Gee J (1989) Differential effects of two analogs of thyrotropin-releasing hormone (TRH) on cerebral infarction and blood flow following ischemia in the rat, *J Physiol (Lond)*, in press

Panter SS, Braughler JM, and Hall ED (1992) Dextran-coupled deferoxamine improves outcome in a marine model of head injury, *J Neurotrauma*, **9**, 47–53

Panter SS, England LJ, Hellard DM, and Winslow RM (1990) Factors affecting the stability of hemoglobin-bound iron, *Blood*, **76**, 72A

Panter SS, Yum SW, and Faden AI (1990) Alteration in extracellular amino acids after traumatic spinal cord injury, *Ann Neurol*, **27**, 96–9

Perraro F, Tosolini G, Pertoldi F, Sbrojavacca R, Beorchia A, Bulfoni A *et al.* (1984) Double-blind placebo-controlled trial of naloxone on motor deficits in acute cerebrovascular disease (letter), *Lancet*, 915

Pearlmutter AF, Szkrybalo M, Kim Yl, and Harik SI (1988) Arginine vasopressin receptors in pig cerebral microvessels, cerebral cortex and hippocampus, *Neurosci Lett*, **87**, 121–6

Pettigrew LC, Misra LK, Grotta JC, Narayana PA, and Wu KK (1989) Selective inhibition of thromboxane synthase enhances reperfusion and metabolism of the ischemic brain, *Ann NY Acad Sci*, **559**, 478–9

Phillis JW, DeLong RE, and Towner PT (1985) Naloxone enhances cerebral reactive hyperemia in the rat, *Neurosurgery*, **17**, 596–9

Picone CM, Rosenbaum DM, Pettigrew LC, and Yatsu FM (1990) Anticoagulants and antiplatelet aggregation agents, In Weinstein PR and Faden AI, eds, *Protection of the brain from ischemia*, Baltimore, Williams and Wilkins, 219–30

Post C, Freedman J, Hokfelt T, Jonsson J, Paulsson I, Arwestrom E *et al.* (1985) Neuronal damage induced by a substance P-antagonist is counteracted by thyrotropin releasing hormone, In Hokanson R and Sundler F, eds, *Tachykinin antagonists*, New York, Elsevier, 383–91

Post C and Paulsson I (1985) Antinociceptive and neurotoxic actions of substance P analogues in the rat's spinal cord after intrathecal administration, *Neurosci Lett*, **57**, 159–64

Przewlocki R, Shearman GT, and Herz A (1985) Mixed opioid/nonopioid effects of dynorphin and dynorphin-related peptides after their intrathecal injection in rats, *Neuropeptides*, **3**, 233–40

Przewlocki R, Stala L, Greczek M, Shearman GT, Przewlocki B, and Herz A (1983) Analgesic effect of μ-, δ-, and κ-opiate agonists and, in particular, dynorphin at the spinal level, *Life Sci*, **33** (Suppl 1), 649

Reuther R and Dorndorf W (1978) Aspirin in patients with cerebral ischemia and normal angiograms of non-surgical lesions, In Bredding K, Dorndorf W, Loew D, Marxd R, eds, *Acetylsalicylic acid in cerebral ischemia and coronary heart disease*, Stuttgart, FK Schaltauer, 97–106

Rolfsen JL and Davis WR (1989) Cerebral function and preservation during cardiac arrest, *Crit Care Med*, **17**, 283–92

Rothman SM and Olney JW (1986) Glutamate and the pathophysiology of hypoxic-ischemic brain damage, *Ann Neurol*, **19**, 105–11

Salzman SK, Hirofugi E, Knight PB, Llados, Eckman C, Beckman AL *et al.* (1987) Treatment of experimental spinal trauma with thyrotropin-releasing hormone: central serotonergic and vascular mechanism of action, *Central Nervous System Trauma*, **4**, 181–96

Schwartz AC (1984) Cerebral resuscitation in the community hospital, *Ann Emerg Med*, **13**, 872–3

Sheardown MJ, Nielsen EØ, Hansen AJ, Jacobsen P, Honoré T (1990) 2,3-Dihydroxy-6 nitro-7 sulfamoyl-benzo(F)quinoxaline: a neuroprotectant for cerebral ischemia, *Science*, **247**, 571–4

Shigeno T, Teasdale GM, Kirkham D, Mendelow D, Graham DI and McCulloch J (1983) Effect of naloxone on cerebral glucose metabolism in normal rats and rats with focal cerebral ischemia, *J Cereb Blood Flow Metab*, **3**, S528–S529

Siesjo BK (1981) Cell damage in the brain: a speculative synthesis, *J Cereb Blood Flow Metab*, **1**, 155–85

Siesjo BK (1984) Cerebral circulation and metabolism, *J Neurosurg*, **60**, 883–908

Siesjo BK (1988) Historical overview: calcium, ischemia, and death of brain cells, *Ann NY Acad Sci*, **522**, 638–61

Siesjo BK and Bengtsson F (1989) Calcium fluxes, calcium antagonists, and calcium-related pathology in brain ischemia, hypoglycemia, and spreading depression: a unifying hypothesis, *J Cereb Blood Flow Metab*, **9**, 127–40

Simon RP, Swan JH, Griffiths T, and Meldrum BS (1984) Blockage of N-methyl-D-aspartate receptors may protect against ischemic damage in the brain, *Science*, **226**, 850–2

Skarphedinsson JO and Thoren P (1986) The effects of naloxone on cerebral function in spontaneously hypertensive rats during hypotensive haemorrhage, *Acta Physiol Scand*, **128**, 597–604

Smith AP and Lee NM (1988) Pharmacology of dynorphin, *Annu Rev Pharmacol Toxicol*, **28**, 123–40

Snyder DW and Fleisch JH (1989) Leukotriene receptor antagonists as potential therapeutic agents, *Annu Rev Pharmacol Toxicol*, **29**, 123–43

Sokol RJ (1989) Vitamin E and neurologic function in man, *Free Radic Biol Med*, **6**, 189–207

Spampinato S and Candeletti SU (1985) Characterization of dynorphin A-induced antinociception at spinal levels, *Eur J Pharmacol*, **110**, 21–30

Stanfield PR (1988) Intracellular MG^{2+} may act as a co-factor in ion channel function, *Trends Neurosci*, **11**, 475–7

Steinke DE, Weir BKA, Findlay JM, Tanabe T, Grace M, and Krushelnycky BW (1989) A trial of the 21-aminosteroid U74006F in a primate model of chronic cerebral vasospasm, *Neurosurgery*, **24**, 179–86

Stokes BT, Fox P, and Hollinden G (1983) Extracellular calcium activity in the injured spinal cord, *Exp Neurol*, **80**, 561–72

Stokes BT, Hollinden G, and Fox P (1984) Improvement of injury-induced hypocalcia by high-dose naloxone intervention, *Brain Res*, **290**, 187–90

Swedish Cooperative Study (1986) High dose acetylsalicylic acid after cerebral infarction, *Stroke*, **18**, 325–34

Travis MA and Hall ED (1987) The effects of chronic two-fold dietary vitamin E supplementation on subarachnoid hemorrhage-induced brain hypoperfusion, *Brain Res*, **418**, 366–70

Tsien RW, Lipscombe D, Madison DV, Bley DR, and Fox AP (1988) Multiple types of neuronal calcium channels and their selective modulation, *Trends Neurosci*, **11**, 431–8

Veloso D, Guynn RO, Oskarsson M, and Veech RL (1973) The concentration of free and bound magnesium in rat tissues, *J Biol Chem*, **248**, 4811–9

Vink R, Faden AI, and McIntosh TK (1988) Changes in cellular bioenergetic state following graded traumatic brain injury in rats: determination by phosphorus 31 magnetic resonance spectroscopy, *J Neurotrauma*, **5**, 315–30

Vink R, Knoblach SM, and Faden AI (1987) 31P Magnetic resonance spectroscopy of traumatic spinal cord injury, *Magn Reson Med*, **5**, 390–4

Vink R, McIntosh TK, Demediuk P, Weiner MW, and Faden AI (1988) Decline in intracellular free Mg^{2+} is associated with irreversible tissue injury after brain trauma, *J Biol Chem*, **263**, 757–61

Vink R, McIntosh TK, and Faden AI (1988) Treatment with the thyrotropin-releasing hormone analog CG3703 restores magnesium homeostasis following traumatic brain injury in rats, *Brain Res*, **460**, 184–8

Vink R, McIntosh TK, and Faden AI (1991) Magnesium in neurotrauma: its role and therapeutic implications. In Searpa P and Carbone E, eds, *Magnesium and Excitable Membranes*, Berlin, Springer-Verlag, 125–45

Vink R, Portoghese PS, and Faden AI (1991) K-Opoid antagonist improves cellular bioenergetics and recovery after traumatic brain injury, *Am J Physiol*, **261** R1527–32

Vink R, McIntosh TK, Rombanyi R, and Faden AI (1990) Opiate antagonist nalmefene improves intracellular free Mg^{2+} bioenergetic state and neurologic outcome following brain injury in rats, *J Neurosci*, **10**, 3524–30

Vink R, Noble LJ, Knoblach SM, Bendall MR, and Faden AI (1989a) Metabolic changes in rabbit spinal cord after trauma: magnetic resonance spectroscopy studies, *Ann Neurol*, **25**, 26–31

Vink R, Yum SW, Lemke M, Demediuk P, and Faden AI (1989b) Traumatic spinal cord injury in rabbits decreases intracellular free magnesium concentrations as measured by 31P MRS, *Brain Res*, **490**, 144–7

Wallace MC and Tator CH (1986) Failure of blood transfusion or naloxone to improve clinical recovery after experimental spinal cord injury, *Neurosurgery*, **19**, 489–94

Watson BD and Ginsberg MD (1989) Ischemic injury in the brain, *Ann NY Acad Sci*, **559**, 269–81

Wauquier A, Ashton D, and Clincke GH (1988) Brain ischemia as a target for Ca^{2+} entry blockers, *Ann NY Acad Sci*, **522**, 478–90

Wieloch T (1985) Hypoglycemia-induced neuronal damage prevented by an N-methyl-D-aspartate antagonist, *Science*, **230**, 681–3

Wexler BC (1984) Naloxone ameliorates the pathophysiologic changes which lead to and attend an acute stroke in stroke-prone/SHR, *Stroke*, **15**, 630–4

White BC, Winegar CD, Wilson RF, and Krause GS (1983) Calcium blockers in cerebral resuscitation, *J Trauma*, **23**, 788–94

Wolfe LS (1982) Eicosanoids: prostaglandins, thromboxane, leukotrienes, and other derivatives of carbon-20 unsaturated fatty acids, *J Neurochem*, **38**, 1–14

Wroblewski JT and Danysz W (1989) Modulation of glutamate receptors: Molecular mechanisms and functional implications, *Annu Rev Pharmacol Toxicol*, **29**, 441–72

Yamamoto M, Shimizu M, Okada M, Terai M, Tamura A, Kirino T *et al.* (1989) Effects of YM-14673, a new TRH derivative, on behavioral changes after focal ischemia, *Ann NY Acad Sci*, **553**, 622–3

Yoshida S, Busto R, Santiso M, and Ginsberg MD (1984) Brain lipid peroxidation induced by postischemic reoxygenation in vitro: Effect of vitamin E, *J Cereb Blood Flow Metab*, **4**, 466–9

Yoshida S, Busto R, Watson BD, Santiso M, and Ginsberg MD (1985) Postischemic cerebral lipid peroxidation in vitro: modification by dietary vitamin E, *J Neurochem*, **44**, 1593–601

Young W and Flamm ES (1982) Effect of high-dose corticosteroid therapy on blood flow evoked potentials and extracellular calcium in experimental spinal injury, *J Neurosurg*, **57**, 667–73

Young W, Flamm ES, Demopoulos HB, Tomasula JJ, and De Crescito V (1981) Effect of naloxone on posttraumatic ischemia in experimental spinal contusion, *J Neurosurg*, **55**, 209–19

Young RSK, Hessert TR, Pritchard GA, and Yagel SK (1984) Naloxone exacerbates hypoxic-ischemic brain injury in the neonatal rat, *Am J Obstet Gynecol*, **150**, 52–6

Young W, Wojak JC, and DeCrescito V (1988) 21-aminosteroid reduces ion shifts and edema in the rat middle cerebral artery occlusion model of regional ischemia, *Stroke*, **19**, 1013–9

Yum SW and Faden AI (1990) Comparison of the protective effects of the N-methyl D-aspartate receptor antagonist, MK-801, and the opiate receptor antagonist, nalmefene, in spinal cord ischemia in rabbits, *Arch Neurol*, **47**, 277–81

Zabramski JM, Spetzler RF, Selman WR, Hershey LA, and Roessman U (1984) Naloxone improves neurologic function during and outcome after temporary focal cerebral ischemia, *Stroke*, **15**, 621–7

5
Applications of principles of brain plasticity and training to restore function

Paul Bach-y-Rita

Brain damaged patients improve with rehabilitation (Lehmann *et al.*, 1975a). However, knowledge of the most efficient rehabilitation procedures is limited at this time due to the lack of well planned, scientifically validated, controlled studies. Therefore, this chapter will discuss the present state of neurorehabilitation, relevant knowledge of neural mechanisms of recovery, and some of the interesting research areas that should lead to more scientific rehabilitation in the future.

There are a number of reasons why scientific neurorehabilitation studies have been scarce. One is that rehabilitation cannot be administered or injected, but must have the active cooperation of the patient and the therapist is often a facilitator. In addition to administering specific procedures, the therapist must teach the patient and the patient must do the work. In fact, education plays a key role in rehabilitation (this is reflected by the fact that in the USA the National Institute of Disability and Rehabilitation Research is in the Department of Education). Many factors in addition to medical treatment influence the outcome. Environmental, psychosocial, and motivational factors must also be considered (Bach-y-Rita, 1980; 1981; 1990a; Bach-y-Rita and Wicab Bach-y-Rita, 1990a, 1990b), and the pre-morbid educational level may also be a factor (Lehmann *et al.*, 1975b). It is particularly important to note that expectations of outcome may influence the results; two recent studies have shown that little or no recovery occurs after three months following a stroke (Lindmark, 1988; Kelley-Hayes *et al.*, 1989), although studies discussed below have shown that significant recovery can be obtained many years after the brain damage, with an appropriate rehabilitation program. This aspect is discussed elsewhere (Bach-y-Rita and Wicab Bach-y-Rita, 1990a, 1990b).

Other important barriers to scientific rehabilitation research exist. These include the long time-course of recovery; the difficulty of locating the precise site of the brain lesion and the problems of accurately matching groups; the high cost of extended programs; the lack of precise, sensitive measures of outcome; and the fact that efficacy evaluation is complicated by 'spontaneous' recovery, which occurs during the time that rehabilitation services are being delivered. However, these are not the principal barriers to scientific rehabilitation. The most important barriers are the absence of a tradition of scientific rehabilitation, the absence of role models, and the lack of an understanding of the need for theory as a basis of practice.

Rehabilitation practitioners are by nature service oriented. Their aim is to determine and deliver clinical services that may lead to improvement in their patients. Because thoroughly tested, theory-based rehabilitation methodologies are lacking, personal experience and anecdotal reports influence the choice of therapy. Rehabilitation methodologies, many of which bear the name of their major proponents, often acquire a semblance of scientific validation from pseudoscientific studies and post-hoc application of theoretical findings (Bach-y-Rita, 1989).

Historical factors also play a role in the present primitive state of neurorehabilitation. The importance of the brain's ability to modify functions and compensate for damage has only recently been appreciated. This includes factors related to the absence of interest in brain plasticity (Bach-y-Rita, 1988, 1990). The identification in the middle of the last century, of a specific area in the left temporal lobe related to speech (Broca, 1861), led to the determination of a concept of strict localization in the neurosciences. The great complexity of the brain may have contributed to the conceptual rigidity that developed; to organize all that was known into a cohesive, understandable form, anatomists had to compartmentalize, such as division of the cortex into 52 regions (Brodmann, 1909). The descriptions and illustrations of those components, each clearly separated from the others, gave rise to a concept of a rigid, sharply compartmentalized brain. Furthermore, the absence of significant regeneration in the brain (in contrast to organs such as the liver that have the capacity of mitotic division) combined to create an impression of a rigidly divided, non-plastic organ with little capacity to recover from damage. Therefore, significant recovery was rarely expected, and seldom sought.

During the 100 years following Broca's finding, occasional reports appeared revealing a significant potential for recovery with adequate rehabilitation. In 1915, Franz, Sheetz, and Wilson described the role of rehabilitation in obtaining functional recovery in long-standing hemiplegia. Their studies were inspired by laboratory observations, which suggested that conclusions regarding the permanency of paralysis from cerebral accidents were neither accurate nor scientifically based. Their studies showed that improvement can be rapid when the patient's active cooperation is obtained, and that elaborate apparatus is not needed. 'The principal requirement is a knowledge of the structures involved and their functional relations, with some ingenuity in the devising of means of bringing about movements of certain characters which should be practiced, and also different means which may help to stimulate the patient's interest and to show plainly to him the course of his improvement. . . . We should probably not speak of permanent paralysis, or of residual paralysis, but of uncared for paralysis.' (Franz, Sheetz, and Wilson, 1915).

Animal models are of great importance in the development of clinical procedures. Few good animal models have been described in neurorehabilitation. However, even these have been ignored. For example, in 1917, Ogden and Franz presented convincing evidence for the role of neurorehabilitation in the functional recovery of hemiplegic monkeys. Later, Travis and Woolsey (1956) demonstrated the importance of physical therapy in the functional recovery of brain-damaged monkeys. One of the best animal neurorehabilitation studies has been virtually uncited. Chow and Steward (1972) reported morphological, physiological, and behavioral correlates of a successful cat visual rehabilitation program. Hubel and Wiesel (1970) had previously demonstrated that if the eyelids of one eye of a kitten are sutured closed during the few months of the critical period of normal visual development, that eye will be permanently amblyopic following the removal of the sutures, even if the cat lives for five or more years with the eyelids functioning normally. Chow and Steward (1972) then explored whether recovery of vision can be obtained with an appropriate training (rehabilitation) program. They demonstrated some return of function (vision), as well as concomitant physiological (increased numbers of binocular cells in the visual cortex) and morphological (changes in the lateral geniculate) effects. They noted that the usual rewards were insufficient; the cats required periods of 'gentling' and petting to establish an affective bond with the experimenters.

NEURAL MECHANISMS OF RECOVERY

Now that evidence of the capacity to recover function following brain damage exists, there is great interest in elucidating neural mechanisms as well as the appropriate therapeutic approaches. In addition to physical rehabilitation, specific pharmaco-logical interventions (primarily related to neurotransmitters) and psychosocial issues are being actively studied. The degree of functional improvement is dependent on many factors including age, area damaged, amount of tissue damaged, rapidity of the damage, the rehabilitation program, and environmental and psychosocial factors. These and other aspects have been extensively examined elsewhere (e.g. Bach-y-Rita, 1980, 1981, 1990b, in press; Bach-y-Rita and Balliet, 1987; Bach-y-Rita and Bjelke, 1991; Bach-y-Rita and de Pedro-Cuesta, 1991; Bjelke *et al.*, in press; Boyeson and Bach-y-Rita, 1989; Bach-y-Rita and Wicab Bach-y-Rita, 1990a, 1990b) and will be briefly reviewed here.

Reorganization of function can occur even after the loss of hundreds of grams of brain mass, as studies of hemispherectomized patients revealed (Glees, 1980). While individual neurons do not appear to regenerate, there are a number of potential mechanisms of reorganization. For example, the neuronal processes 'axons and dendrites' appear to respond to functional demand (see also Bach-y-Rita, 1980), and in fact these processes constitute the major portion of the brain mass. Cragg (1968) demonstrated that only 3% of the volume of rat visual cortex is composed of cell bodies, and the rest (97%) is made up of axons, dendrites, glia, and blood vessels. The malleability of neuronal processes appears to extend into advanced old age. Buell and Coleman (1979) have shown in a study of brain plasticity that the length of the terminal dendritic segment of cortical pyramidal neurons is 25% longer in non-senile humans of 80 years of age than in normal persons of 50 years of age. They suggested that this might represent growth to compensate for normal cell loss.

There are many potential mechanisms of brain reorganization. Some frequently mentioned include the following (from Bach-y-Rita, 1988):

1. Sprouting, which is the growth from a cell body to another cell as a consequence of normal growth, a vacancy at a particular site, or a return to a particular site. Collateral sprouts are new axonal processes that have budded off an uninjured axon and grown to a vacated synaptic site. Collateral sprouting has been shown to occur in the CNS. However, sprouting can be adaptive or maladaptive, and its role in recovery from brain damage is still uncertain.

2. Denervation supersensitivity results in a permanent increase in neuronal respons-ivity to diminished input. The receptor site may become more sensitive to a neurotransmitter, or the receptors may increase in number. This may be a factor in CNS reorganization.

3. Behavior compensation following brain damage can result in new combinations of behaviors. For example, a patient may use different groups of muscles or cognitive strategies.

4. Unmasking, which is quiescent neuronal connections that are inhibited in the normal state, being unmasked following brain damage. This may be an important mechanism of recovery of function. Negative effects of unmasking may also occur. For example, the appearance of 'pathological' reflexes, such as a Babinski reflex, following brain injury may be caused by the unmasking of reflexes that were normal in infancy but had become inhibited during development.

Diaschisis has been mentioned as a basis for functional recovery since von Monakow (see Boyeson and Bach-y-Rita, 1989) suggested that functional disturbances that would spontaneously recover were primarily caused by depressions in tissues remote from, but connected to, the primary injury site; as the depressions (thought by him to be caused by loss of excitation) diminished in the remote structures, functional recovery occurred. Head (see Boyeson and Bach-y-Rita, 1989) discussed 'suspension of activity', a concept comparable to diaschisis. Head, as well as von Monakow, spoke against contemporary concepts of a rigid brain, since they noted significant recovery of function after brain damage. However, as diaschisis is a concept not yet explained by specific mechanisms, Feeney (in Boyeson and Bach-y-Rita, 1989) considers it a description of events that lacks strong explanatory power.

Boyeson and Bach-y-Rita (1989) have summarized a three-day conference in which a number of determinants of brain plasticity were evaluated including the following. Remote metabolic changes had been noted by Varon, who reported that, following frontal cortex damage, the contralateral cerebellum shows reduced activity, which was confirmed in PET scan studies of persons with long-standing post-traumatic hemiparesis (Perlman *et al.*, 1988). Boyeson noted that, if the rat contralateral cerebellum is made supersensitive by a unilateral ceruleus lesion two weeks before a sensorimotor cortex injury, total permanent recovery from hemiplegia is noted as little as one hour post infusion (24 hours after the cortical lesion); he suggested that the anatomical basis for the effect is the simultaneous projection of individual locus ceruleus cells to both contralateral cerebellum and ipsilateral sensorimotor cortex.

Glial cells are now considered to determine the micro-chemical environment that the neuron sees, including trophic factors such as those relating to cellular outgrowth and mechanisms of functional recovery.

Davis pointed out that four factors are of particular importance in regard to recovery of function after brain damage: location of the damage; the brain's response to injury, such as bleeding; the ability of the brain to respond to an injury by having an area that is uninjured perform a function that had previously been performed by the injured area; and neuronal rearrangement, demonstrable by anatomic methods (some of these rearrangements may be maladaptive).

In regard to the therapeutic roles of pharmacological agents, Fuxe considered that many of the effects of exogenous gangliosides are via the lipid part of the membrane. Animal studies revealed that if gangliosides are administered during the first 48 hours, there seems to be an increase in TH-immunoreactive cell bodies and increased cell survival, with increased functional recovery. Leon stated that gangliosides may in some way positively modulate neuronal trophic influences capable of antagonizing potential neurotoxic agents. They can change a number of membrane functional properties. When cells are pretreated for one hour with gangliosides, there is total protection from glutamate neurotoxicity *in vitro*; protection occurs even if they are given concurrently with the glutamate. The addition of sphingolipids (including gangliosides) to cerebellar granular cells *in vitro* can antagonize the protein kinase translocation. GM1 post-treatment of lesioned animals very soon after an ischemic episode results in less damage than in controls.

Agnati discussed gangliosides in relation to interactions between neurons and glia. Gangliosides, by modulating polyamine biosynthesis, can in some way increase the efficacy of the transformation of putrescine into GABA. In a rat model, gangliosides protected 40–50% of the striatal neurons and produced a large activation of astroglia, noted seven days later.

Stein noted that ganglioside treatment prevented loss of body weight following large cortical transections in rats, and produced early positive behavioral responses. However, 39 days after injury, the treated and untreated animals were not distinguishable. Combining ganglioside and amphetamine treatment was not beneficial. Stein noted that both beneficial and disruptive effects of ganglioside treatment can be noted. Convulsive activity can be increased. A frontal cortex transplant model revealed that successfully ganglioside-treated rats are actually worse one year later. He cautioned that, when clinical trials are planned, a number of factors must be taken into consideration (Boyeson and Bach-y-Rita, 1989).

The possible role of extra-synaptic receptor activation (volume transmission) in the brain during reorganization following brain damage has been discussed elsewhere (Bach-y-Rita, 1990a, b; Bach-y-Rita and Wicab Bach-y-Rita, 1990a).

PHYSICAL REHABILITATION

Procedures and techniques for the rehabilitation of individuals with brain damage have been extensively described elsewhere (e.g. DeLisa, 1988; Goodgold, 1986) and will not be detailed here. The techniques have developed out of practical experience rather than evolving from experimental evidence. At present, rehabilitation services are commenced as soon as possible after the neural damage, with initial interventions being primarily preventive. Rehabilitation can prevent: contractures by means of passive range of motion; bed sores by means of appropriate bed positioning and changing of position as well as special purpose mattresses and covers; dehydration and nutritional imbalances; and depression by appropriate psychosocial and environmental interventions.

As soon as possible after injury, often within the first few days, physical rehabilitation is commenced. The term is used here to include the various therapeutic approaches undertaken by members of the interdisciplinary rehabilitation team, such as physical therapy, occupational therapy, speech therapy, and recreational therapy. Rehabilitation nurses, psychologists, vocational rehabilitators, and others are included in the team in addition to the clinician trained in rehabilitation who is the team leader.

Multi-therapy rehabilitation begins as soon as possible and is as intense as possible. In fact, if there are not sufficient hours per day of therapy, reimbursement for the rehabilitation services may be withheld. Therapy usually involves having the patient taken to each therapist on a regular daily schedule. This program is sustained during the hospitalization period and is often continued when the patient is discharged.

It should be pointed out that there is little or no demonstrated scientific basis for most of the procedures, and few of the procedures have been validated by controlled studies. The importance of the intervention of the various therapies (e.g. speech, occupational, physical, and recreational therapy) has not been demonstrated. The requirements of neurorehabilitation are great, and the heavy demand for services has led to a considerable growth of neurorehabilitation facilities and professional groups.

Each group is firmly convinced of the need for, and value of, its services; both profit making and non-profit making facilities, units, and multi-site corporations have proliferated. Patients do improve and the services are reimbursed, and as a result new service units continue to appear. Yet there is a dearth of evaluation data. Not only is the relative contribution of each program and separately named therapy not firmly established, but the required level of participation by each of the medical specialties involved in rehabilitation has not been determined.

The early application of intensive rehabilitation may lead to the greatest level of recovery (e.g. monkey study by Black, Markowitz, and Cianci, 1975). However, there are negative issues to consider. The recently brain-damaged patient may have medical complications, and can be easily exhausted. The patient may not be psychologically ready; this and psychosocial issues may create barriers to full participation. The multi-therapy approach may be the most efficient way to deliver services, but may also give rise to problems. A great deal of the patient's limited energy may be squandered by delays in transportation of the patient from the hospital room to each therapy. Berenson (personal communication) followed patients, stopwatch in hand, from the hospital room to the various therapies. He compared the time the patient actually received therapy to the lost time in waiting for patient escort transportation within the hospital, and waiting for the therapist to finish with the previous patient. Although his untimely death prevented completion of the study, Professor Berenson's preliminary findings were that a large percentage of the 'therapy time' was expended in these extraneous activities.

Environmental factors must also be considered when evaluating neurorehabilitation. Patients kept in a rehabilitation ward are in an unfamiliar, often hostile environment, deprived of family and home. Rehabilitation facilities are often located in the basement or in other harsh settings. These and other environmental factors may influence rehabilitation outcome. In fact, evidence has shown that the view through the window may influence recovery from surgery. Ulrich (1984) showed that surgical patients assigned to rooms with windows looking out on a natural scene had shorter postoperative hospital stays, received fewer negative evaluative comments in nursing notes, and took fewer potent analgesics compared to matched patients in similar rooms with windows facing a brick wall of a building.

The appropriate environment for therapy is a subject of clinical importance. Whereas group activities and peer interactions may be appropriate for certain groups of patients, others, and in particular for certain therapeutic interventions, require complete concentration and a quiet environment. For example, electromyographic sensory feedback for developing neuromuscular control ideally requires quiet individual rooms because a high level of concentration is required (Bach-y-Rita and Balliet, 1987).

The therapeutic environment also includes the home and social environments. This has been well recognized and incorporated into most long-term inpatient rehabilitation programs by means of the judicious use of home leaves and weekend passes. In fact, a supportive family member may be able to undertake rehabilitation interventions that, although less technically developed than professional therapy, may be able to achieve significant functional gains in the familiar and supportive environment of the home; specific therapeutic activities may be more closely related to the patient's particular interests (Bach-y-Rita, 1980). Research into the effects of the various therapy environments may lead to the most appropriate use, at different stages of evolution of the brain-damaged patient, of acute hospital bedside rehabilitation, rehabilitation units in acute hospitals, late (chronic) rehabilitation units, specific rehabilitation hospitals, community rehabilitation facilities, nursing homes, and home programs.

In addition to appropriate studies on the efficacy of rehabilitation procedures, other models should be explored. Questions to be studied might include the following: 1. What is the most appropriate composition of the rehabilitation team? Is it necessary to have many individual therapists involved, or would a single rehabilitation therapist be more efficient and economical in certain circumstances? 2. When should rehabilitation services be emphasized? What is most appropriate in the acute stage, post-acute hospital stage, early outpatient stage, and late post-acute stage?

Questions of efficacy can best be explored using a model in which most of the variables can be controlled. In Sweden, a home rehabilitation program that allows control of many of the variables that are difficult to control in acute neurorehabilitation was developed (Bach-y-Rita and de Pedro-Cuesta, 1991).

LATE REHABILITATION

In the absence of rehabilitation, some recovery of function occurs in most brain-damaged people. It is assumed (e.g. Lehmann *et al.*, 1975a) that appropriate rehabilitation significantly increases the functional return. For the purpose of controlled studies, the 'spontaneous' recovery, which usually occurs through the first year or two after damage, makes it difficult to evaluate the specific effect of the rehabilitation. Such factors as increased attention from staff during rehabilitation, psychosocial factors, and motivation may play a role. In view of the clinical success of our late rehabilitation program, its suitability as a research model of neurorehabilitation is being explored.

One successful model of late rehabilitation involves facial paralysis. For example, an acoustic neuroma can lead to the loss of control of the facial musculature on one side as a result of destruction of the facial nerve. Patients who undergo an anastomosis between the facial and hypoglossal nerves provide a particularly interesting model of brain plasticity, because there is direct surgical evidence of a complete section of the facial nerve and the attachment of its peripheral portion to the central portion of the XIIth nerve. In these cases, reinnervation of facial muscles by nerves genetically programmed to control tongue muscles often leads to excellent muscle tone (and thus a relatively symmetrical face at rest), although dysfunction is apparent on movement. With such patients, we have evaluated rehabilitation programs specifically designed to obtain reorganization of function by reprogramming the motorneurons of the XIIth nerve on the operated side to become included in the facial motor programs (Balliet, 1985; Balliet, Shinn, and Bach-y-Rita, 1982).

As part of the late rehabilitation program, electromyographic (EMG) sensory feedback is often introduced. Much of the following section has been adapted from Bach-y-Rita and Balliet, 1987. The use of EMG sensory feedback in the neuromuscular retraining of stroke patients typically consists of five over-lapping steps (Balliet, 1985):

1) General relaxation, including the uninvolved extremity. Once a low-noise baseline is established.

2) Slow, reciprocal motor control of the uninvolved extremity is acquired.

3) This relatively slow motor control pattern is used as a model to suppress unnecessary muscle activity, facilitate voluntary contractions of the involved extremity, or both.

4) Voluntary reciprocal sequencing of the involved side is then partially established.

5) Voluntary reciprocal sequencing is used to generalize appropriate proprioceptive and kinesthetic sensibility of muscles and joints to functional tasks requiring more integrative motor control sequences.

This sequence is repeated in the clinic, and simple (usually non-EMG) exercises followed at home usually lead to the return of some amount of function.

EMG is used to provide 'sensory feedback' required for neuromuscular retraining, although effective neuromuscular retraining is not device dependent. The therapist should not only know how to use the EMG, but also to apply manual facilitation techniques (such as quick stretching) and many other modalities. The EMG acts as a sensory facilitator or substitution device. The therapist should verbally and manually help the patient to initiate the correct motor commands and to inhibit the incorrect motor commands through modalities that normally might have been insufficient to produce any apparent response. A very experienced therapist may often not require such a high-tech device, if sufficient sensory feedback information concerning the patient's ongoing neuromuscular status can be provided with some other method of facilitation, such as active assist, range of motion, and mirror exercises.

Participation by the patient and therapist

The active involvement of the patient may enhance the signal to noise ratio by increasing attention to the retraining information (signal) while decreasing attention to other information that is not related to actual retraining and proper functional motor control (noise). Learning is a conscious and cortically organized process (Finger and Stein, 1982); passive 'participation' relative to learning may not be possible, although passive treatment techniques should be used to promote range of motion and decrease the risk of contractures. Automatic and functional movement patterns may also be used to promote proprioception and kinesthetic sensibility and to facilitate active participation. It is the patient who really trains the patient; the therapist determines the specific program and delivers services, but is also a guide. Therefore, patients may be trained to be their own best therapists. Friends and family can be trained to perform facilitation, to give verbal reminders of correct behaviors, to help keep track of progress on goal attainment sheets, and provide positive moral support. The patient can also be taught related basic anatomy, physiology, and kinesiology in order to decrease dependency on the rehabilitation team (Bach-y-Rita and Balliet, 1987).

Home training of the post-acute patient results in cost-free therapy and extends resources. A 20:1 ratio of home to clinic training has been demonstrated to be successful (Balliet, Shinn, and Bach-y-Rita, 1982; Balliet, Levy, and Blood, 1986). Successful treatment cannot occur without a positive attitude and resulting encouragement from the therapist, which has been demonstrated in an animal model (Chow and Steward, 1972). Psychosocial issues may be the cause of apparent physiological plateaus, and can act as shields that are impenetrable to even the most effective therapy (Bach-y-Rita and Balliet, 1987).

The therapy environment

Most therapy is conducted in a 'gym' where numerous patients are being treated by many therapists. Although noisy conditions might be satisfactory for developing muscle strength or maintaining passive range of motion, they are not optimal for neuromuscular rehabilitation. A child learns to play the piano in isolation, who can concentrate, receive positive and negative feedback, and repeatedly modify neuromuscular programs. The child may benefit from occasional meetings with others who are practicing but usually does not practice with them. Similarly, a patient who is trying to re-establish neuromuscular control should be involved in support groups, but should 'practice' in a quiet individual room where concentration can be maximized. The velocity of movements appears to be an important consideration. Compensatory or uncoordinated movements appear to be perpetuated when the patient is allowed to move relatively fast or imprecisely, and therefore we use slow movements in our late rehabilitation programs. Uninteresting or non-functional tasks will result in fast, imprecise and improper motor control (Kottke, 1982).

Alertness and motivation appear to favor progress. Volitional motor control sequences will ultimately have to be practiced thousands of times to store a new motor program that is relatively fast, automatic, coordinated, effortless, functional, and generalizable; therefore, the motor sequences should be as interesting as possible (Bach-y-Rita and Balliet, 1987). Rehabilitation procedures individually designed in response to the patient's particular interests ('functional rehabilitation') fulfill many of these criteria; some fortunate patients have family members with a natural ability to develop such programs at home, and they may have very successful rehabilitation outcomes (Bach-y-Rita, 1980).

Muscle recruitment

There is usually an orderly and additive recruitment in size of motorneurons and their corresponding muscle fibers in normal animals and man. The smaller, slower, and weaker motor units are recruited before larger, faster, and stronger motor units (Henneman, Somjen, and Carpenter, 1965a, 1965b). In limbs as well as eye movements (Yamanaka and Bach-y-Rita, 1968), larger units are usually recruited at relatively high recruitment thresholds in a slow ramp contraction, but are not selectively recruited under rapid movement conditions (for review see Desmedt, 1983).

Patients with some neurological disorders such as complete nerve transection with surgical reunion, post-acute polymyositis (Milner-Brown *et al.*, 1981), and parkinsonism (Milner-Brown, Fisher, and Weiner, 1979) demonstrate recruitment disorders, which occur even when the number of motor units is within normal limits (compare Milner-Brown *et al.*, 1981). Muscle recruitment patterns in many of the common causes of brain dysfunction are not known. Recruitment order data for stroke and brain trauma patients would be helpful in developing appropriate rehabilitation procedures. The data may be relevant to the clinical observation that slow movements are more effective than fast movements.

ADAPTATION TO ABILITY

Work with late rehabilitation patients has revealed a psychological barrier to increased function. Patients with long-standing disability who show significant recovery are confronted with the need to adapt to increasing function. Studies on how physically disabled persons perceive their disability (Campbell, Cull, and Hardy, 1986; Weinberg and Williams, 1978) and how they assess the quality of their lives and the possibility of gaining abilities (Weinberg, 1984) revealed that stages of adjustment to disability, learned helplessness, and perceived interference of disability with the attainment of goals may influence the perception and the desirability of partial or complete recovery of abilities. The role of the family system and the cultural milieu can also be considered key influences on the outcome of rehabilitation, the desirability of recovery, or both (Bach-y-Rita and Wicab Bach-y-Rita, 1990a, 1990b). A suggested theoretical framework for studies in this area is that, following an illness or accident that produces an impairment, there is a process of adaptation to the disability. However, a rehabilitation program that produces an increase in ability also requires adaptation to a relatively non-disabled status. The adaptation to loss will include a process of mourning, including shock, denial, anger, sadness, and depression (Hughes, 1984), which will trigger individual coping mechanisms such as denial and compensation that will contribute to the nature of the adaptation to an impairment and consequent disability. Psychological processes such as cognitive appraisal and coping (Lazarus and Folkman, 1984) and social dimensions such as roles, status, support networks, and institutional and cultural definitions of disability should be considered mediating variables that contribute to the outcome of the rehabilitation process.

Patterson has recently discussed an aspect of the rehabilitation process that is usually overlooked, although it is relevant to the environmental factors discussed above. Patients in hospitals, but particularly those at home, may have great difficulty in adjusting to idleness and loss of the customary 40 to 60 hours of work per week. This is especially true of particular personality types, such as those whose lives revolve around physical activities in their vocations and avocations, and who have poor coping skills with little interest in other activities such as listening to music or reading. After an intense rehabilitation program in the hospital, they may be virtually inactive while waiting for something to heal. During that time much that is healthy and therapeutic could be introduced. Patterson discusses the use of taped material, exercises, and even yoga or meditation if the patient is receptive, in order to avoid the psychological damage that may occur with the absence of activity (Patterson, personal communication).

CONCLUSION

Significant recovery of function is possible following brain damage, and patients recover better with neurorehabilitation than without it. The brain is a plastic, malleable organ; appropriate physical rehabilitation, drug therapy to influence specific neurotransmitter systems, and psychosocial interventions are of considerable importance in obtaining maximum return of function. Potential for functional recovery persists for many years after the brain damage occurs, and specific late rehabilitation procedures have been developed to take advantage of that potential.

Although neurorehabilitation is effective, much remains to be determined in regard to the neural mechanisms involved in the recovery, which specific procedures are most effective, the optimal timing of the delivery of rehabilitation services, and the most efficient and cost-effective rehabilitation team structure. Well validated, scientifically based studies are required in the field.

Acknowledgment

Preparation of this report was supported in part by NIDRR Grant #G0087C2008.

References

Bach-y-Rita P (1980), ed, *Recovery of Function: Theoretical Considerations for Brain Injury Rehabilitation*, Bern SW, Hans Huber

Bach-y-Rita P (1981) Brain plasticity as a basis for the development of rehabilitation procedures for hemiplegia, *Scand J Rehabil Med*, **13**, 73–83

Bach-y-Rita P (1988) Brain plasticity, In Goodchild J, ed, *Rehabilitation Medicine*, St Louis, Mosby, 113–8

Bach-y-Rita P (1989) Theory-based neurorehabilitation, *Arch Phys Med Rehabil*, **70**, 162

Bach-y-Rita P (1990) Paul Broca: aphasia and cerebral localization; Citation Classic, *Current Contents: Institute for Scientific Information*, **22**, 18

Bach-y-Rita P (1990a) Thoughts on the role of the mind in recovery from brain damage. In John ER, Harmony T, Prichep L, Valdez-Soza M, and Valdez-Soza P, eds, *Machinery of the Mind*, Boston, Birkhauser, 353–9

Bach-y-Rita P (1991) Thoughts on the role of volume transmission in normal and abnormal mass sustained functions, In Fuxe K and Agnati LF, eds, *Volume Transmission in the Brain*, New York, Raven, 489–96

Bach-y-Rita P (1990b) Receptor plasticity and volume transmission in the brain: emerging concepts with relevance to neurologic rehabilitation, *J Neurol Rehabil*, **4**, 121–8

Bach-y-Rita P (in press) Volume (Extrasynaptic) Transmission. In Adelman G and Smith B, eds, *Neuroscience Year: Supplement 3 to the Encyclopedia of Neuroscience*, Boston, Birkhauser

Bach-y-Rita P and Balliet R (1987) Recovery from stroke, In Duncan PW and Badke MB, eds, *Motor Deficits following Stroke*, New York, Year Book, 79–107

Bach-y-Rita P and Bjelke B (1991) Lasting recovery of motor function, following brain damage, with a single dose of amphetamine combined with physical therapy; changes in gene expression? *Scand J Rehabil Med* **23**, 219–20

Bach-y-Rita and de Pedro-Cuesta J (1991) Neuroplasticity in the aging brain: development of conceptually based neurologic rehabilitation. In Molina A, Parreño J, Martin JS, Robles E and Moret A, eds, *Rehabilitation Medicine*, Amsterdam, Exerpta Medica, 5–12.

Bach-y-Rita P and Wicab Bach-y-Rita E (1990a) Biological and psychological factors in recovery from brain damage in humans, *Can J Psychol*, **44**, 148–65

Bach-y-Rita P and Wicab Bach-y-Rita E (1990b) Hope and active patient participation in the rehabilitation environment, *Arch Phys Med Rehabil*, **71**, 1082

Balliet R (1985) Motor control strategies in the retraining of facial paralysis, In Portman M, ed, *Proceedings of the Fifth International Symposium on the Facial Nerve* (Bordeaux, 1984), Paris, Masson, 465–9

Balliet R, Levy B, and Blood KMT (1986) Upper extremity sensory feedback therapy, *Arch Phys Med Rehabil*, **67**, 304–10

Balliet R, Shinn JB, and Bach-y-Rita P (1982) Facial paralysis rehabilitation: retraining selective muscle control, *Int J Rehabil Med*, **4**, 67–74

Bjelke B, Bach-y-Rita P, Anderson C, and Fuxe K (in press). Changes in patterns of c-fos immunoreactive neurons in the rat tel- and di-encephalon following d-amphetamine treatment combined with motor training following unilateral lesion of the sensory-motor cortex. *Neurosci Abstr*

Black P, Markowitz RS, and Cianca SN (1975) Recovery of motor function after lesions in motor cortex of monkey, In *Outcome of Severe Damage to the Central Nervous System*, CIBA Foundation, Amsterdam, Elsevier, 65–83

Boyeson MG and Bach-y-Rita P (1989) Determinants of brain plasticity, *J Neurol Rehabil*, **3**, 35–57

Broca P (1861) Remarques sur le siege de la faculte du language articule; suivies d'une observation d'a phemie (perte de la parole), *Bulletin Societe Anatomie de Paris*, **6**, 330–57

Brodmann K (1909) *Vergleichende Lokalisationslehre der Groshirnrinde*, Leipzig, Barth

Buell S and Coleman P (1979) Dendritic growth in aged human brain and failure of growth in senile dementia, *Science*, **206**, 854–6

Campbell ME, Cull JG, and Hardy RE (1986) Disabled persons' attitudes toward disability, *Psychology: A Quarterly Journal of Human Behavior*, **23**(2–3), 16–20

Chow KL and Steward DL (1972) Reversal of structural and functional effects of long-term visual deprivation in cats, *Exp Neurol*, **34**, 409

Cragg BG (1968) Are there structural alterations in synapses related to functioning? *Proc R Soc*, Ser. **B**, **171**, 319–23

DeLisa JA (1988), ed, *Rehabilitation Medicine: Principles and Practice*, Philadelphia, J. B. Lippincott

Desmedt JE (1983) Size principle of motorneuron recruitment and the calibration of muscle force and speed in man, In Desmedt JE, ed, *Motor Control Mechanisms in Health and Disease*, New York, Raven, 227–51

Finger S and Stein DG (1982) *Brain Damage and Recovery: Research and Clinical Perspectives*, Orlando, Academic Press

Franz IS, Sheetz ME, and Wilson AA (1915) The possibility of recovery of motor function in long-standing hemiplegia, *JAMA*, **LXV**, 2150–4

Glees P (1980) Functional reorganization following hemispherectomy in man and after small experimental lesions in primates. In Bach-y-Rita, ed, *Recovery of Function: Theoretical Considerations for Brain Injury Rehabilitation*, Bern SW, Hans Huber, 106–26

Goodgold J (1986), ed, *Rehabilitation Medicine*, St Louis, Mosby

Henneman E, Somjen G, and Carpenter DD (1965a) Functional significance of cell size in spinal motorneurons, *J Neurophysiol* **28**, 560–80

Henneman E, Somjen G, and Carpenter DD (1965b) Excitability and inhibitibility of motorneurons of different sizes, *J Neurophysiol*, **28**, 599–620

Hubel DH and Wiesel TN (1970) The period of susceptibility to the physiological effects of unilateral eye closure in kittens, *J Physiol (Lond)*, **206**, 419

Hughes F (1984) Reaction to loss: coping with disability and death. In Marinelli PR and Dell Orto EA, eds, *Psychological and Social Impact of Physical Disability*, New York, Springer, 131–6

Kelley-Hayes M, Wolf PA, Kase CS, Gresham GE, Kannel WB, and D'Agostino RB (1989) Time course of functional recovery after stroke: the Framingham study, *J Neurol Rehabil*, **3**, 65–70

Kottke F (1982) The neurophysiology of motor function, In Kottke F, Stillwell GK, and Lehmann JF, eds, *Krusen's Handbook of Physical Medicine and Rehabilitation*, Philadelphia, W. B. Saunders, 218–53

Lazarus SR and Folkman S (1984) *Stress, Appraisal, and Coping*, New York, Springer

Lehmann JF, DeLateur BJ, Fowler RS, Warren CG, Arnhold R, Schertzer G *et al.* (1975a) Stroke: does rehabilitation affect outcome?, *Arch Phys Med Rehabil*, **56**, 375–82

Lehmann JF, DeLateur BJ, Fowler RS, Warren CG, Arnhold R, Schertzer G *et al.* (1975b) Stroke rehabilitation: outcome and prediction, *Arch Phys Med Rehabil*, **56**, 383–9

Lindmark B (1988) Evaluation of functional capacity after stroke, with special emphasis on motor function and activities of daily living. *Scand J Rehabil Med Suppl*, **21**, 1–40

Milner-Brown HS, Fisher MA, and Weiner WJ (1979) Electrical properties of motor units in Parkinsonism and a possible relationship with bradykinesia, *J Neurol Neurosurg Psychiatry*, **42**, 35–41

Milner-Brown HS, Stein RB, Lee RG *et al.* (1981) Motor unit recruitment in patients with neuromuscular disorders, In Desmedt JE, ed, *Motor Unit Types. Recruitment and Plasticity in Health and Disease: Progress in Clinical Neurophysiology*, Basel, Karger, 305–18

Ogden R and Franz SI (1917) On cerebral motor control: the recovery from experimentally produced hemiplegia, *Psychobiology*, **1**, 33–49

Perlman S, Wilson MA, Blood K, Balliet R, Turski PA, Sunderland JJ, Rowe B, and Sackett JF (1988) Cerebellar metabolism of FDG in patients with brain damage, *J Nucl Med*, **29**, 822

Travis AM and Woolsey CN (1956) Motor performance of monkeys after bilateral partial and total cerebral decortication. *Am J Phys Med*, **35**, 273–310

Ulrich R (1984) View through a window may influence recovery from surgery, *Science*, **224**, 420–1

Weinberg N (1984) Physically disabled people assess the quality of their lives, *Rehabilitation Literature*, **45**(1–2), 12–15

Weinberg N and Williams J (1978) How the physically disabled perceive their disabilities, *J Rehabil*, **44**, 31–3

Yamanaka Y and Bach-y-Rita P (1968) Conduction velocities in the abducens nerve correlated with vestibular nystagmus in cats, *Exp Neurol*, **20**, 143–55

6
Recent developments in the pharmacotherapy of major neurological dysfunction

M. Traub, J. R. M. Haigh and C. D. Marsden

Before the introduction of levodopa for the management of Parkinson's disease, treatment of neurological disorders was largely based upon empirical observations. Since then, significant advances in therapy have frequently been limited by an ignorance of the underlying pathophysiological mechanisms, resulting in treatments that are usually symptomatic and often disappointing. An increasing knowledge of the pathophysiology of neurological disease has enabled the development of a number of pharmacotherapeutic strategies; concepts of neurotransmitter replacement and modulation of intrinsic neurotransmitter function by exogenous agents are well established, whereas the use of trophic factors and protection against putative toxic processes (such as the generation of free radicals) remain speculative.

This review will not attempt to encompass the whole range of pharmacological interventions for restoration of function in neurological disease; in particular, the drug treatment of pain is too large a topic to be covered here (refer to Volume 10 in this Series). We will examine current approaches to the pharmacotherapy of some major neurological disorders (Parkinson's disease, spasticity, dementia, epilepsy, and stroke), with particular reference to differences in the mechanisms of drug action.

PARKINSON'S DISEASE

In the early years of levodopa therapy for Parkinson's disease, the benefits of chronic, symptomatic treatment were clearly demonstrated by studies of patient morbidity (Hunt *et al.*, 1973) and mortality (Lees, 1986). However, subsequent long-term surveys have confirmed that within 10 to 12 years the majority of patients develop dyskinesias and troublesome fluctuations of mobility and that by this time mortality ratios begin to rise towards those reported in the pre-levodopa era (Curtis *et al.*, 1984).

The major challenge for novel, symptomatic treatments of Parkinson's disease is the prevention and adequate management of treatment-related fluctuations, but at present there is no consensus of aetiology. At one extreme, a commonly held view is that the development of late complications is caused in part by the adverse effects of chronic levodopa administration (Fahn and Bressman, 1984); in contrast, others have implicated progress of the underlying disease and argued in favour of early initiation of levodopa treatment (Markham and Diamond, 1981). Based on the hypothesis that chronic levodopa administration is, to some extent, responsible for the development of abnormal movements and fluctuations in motor performance, there have been a number of trials of early treatment with dopamine agonists, including bromocriptine, lisuride, and pergolide. In general, these studies indicate that such therapy results in a lower incidence of dose-related fluctuations, but that this is confounded by the very high drop-out rate (> 50% in one year) caused by a lack of efficacy when these agonists are used as monotherapy (Kurlan, 1988). Subsequent trials, in which bromocriptine has been administered with low doses of levodopa, have suggested that such early combination therapy produces an excellent clinical response with a lower incidence of late complications than observed when levodopa is used alone (Rinne, 1987). Such reports await confirmation in large, well controlled trials.

The finding that continuous intravenous infusions of levodopa (Quinn, Parkes, and Marsden, 1984) or a subcutaneous bolus of apomorphine (Hardie, Lees, and Stern, 1984) can reverse akinesia, even in patients suffering from severe 'on-off' fluctuations, indicates that striatal efferent mechanisms are relatively preserved even in the late stages of Parkinson's disease. Therefore, it should be possible to reduce fluctuations in performance by the maintenance of stable plasma levels of levodopa or a dopamine agonist. The promise of such treatments is probably best exemplified by studies employing chronic infusions of dopamine agonists. For example, Stibe *et al.* (1988) reported that chronic subcutaneous administration of apomorphine over 15 months reduced 'off' time from 10.1 to 3.8 hours per day and that, importantly, the theoretical risk of tachyphylaxis was not encountered.

Although parenteral or intraduodenal administration of anti-parkinsonian medication may be an appropriate last resort in patients with severe 'on-off' syndrome, there is clearly a need for a more acceptable method for maintaining stable plasma levels of levodopa or dopamine agonists. Controlled-release formulations of levodopa plus a peripheral dopa decarboxylase inhibitor (Madopar CR, Sinemet CR) have been developed and shown to confer significant benefit in terms of motor fluctuations (Lees, 1989). However, this improvement is modest by comparison with that achieved using apomorphine infusions. This limitation reflects the difficulty in maintaining stable plasma levels with oral levodopa, a drug possessing a short half-life and a narrow absorption window (mainly from the proximal duodenum). Hopefully this difficulty can be overcome by the development of either suitable pro-drugs of levodopa, or dopamine agonists that possess physicochemical characteristics appropriate for a controlled delivery system such as a transdermal patch.

The limitations of conventional anti-parkinsonian therapy have led a number of investigators to treat severely ill patients by transplanting autologous adrenal medulla or foetal ventral mesencephalic tissue within the striatum. The groundwork for this approach was laid in 1979 by studies showing that dopamine-rich grafts of foetal mesencephalon could partially reverse behavioural abnormalities in rats with lesions of the nigro-striatal system (Bjorklund and Stenevi, 1979; Perlow *et al.*, 1979). These reports have subsequently been extended to other models, including MPTP-induced parkinsonism in non-human primates (Sladek *et al.*, 1988). Adrenal medulla has been suggested to be an alternative source of dopaminergic tissue. There are practical and ethical advantages in using adult adrenal tissue as the donor material, but the majority of preclinical studies favour the use of foetal mesencephalic grafts. Transplanted foetal neurones are capable of long-term survival and form synaptic connections with the host striatum, whilst releasing dopamine under host afferent control (Lindvall, 1989). On the other hand, the benefit derived from adrenal grafts appears limited and transitory, unless nerve growth factor (NGF) is continuously infused into the host striatum (Stromberg *et al.*, 1985).

In 1987, Madrazo and coworkers claimed remarkable benefit from adrenal autografts in two young parkinsonian patients, using a technique in which adrenal tissue was implanted into a cavity at the head of the caudate nucleus. In a subsequent report the same group extended their trial to 22 patients and although four died post-operatively, 17 of the remaining 18 were reported to have good to moderate results (Madrazo, Drucker-Colin, and Torres, 1988). Unfortunately other investigators from the USA and Europe have been unable to confirm these dramatic claims and the majority have noticed only modest benefits from adrenal autografts with a significant morbidity from the procedure (Goetz *et al.*, 1989). Although the preclinical basis for transplantation of foetal material would appear stronger than that for adrenal autografts, the limited data from clinical studies remains controversial; certain preliminary reports have been highly enthusiastic (Madrazo *et al.*, 1988) whereas others have demonstrated only modest improvements at best (Lindvall *et al.*, 1989). In conclusion, there is ample preclinical evidence to suggest that transplantation may become important in the treatment of severe Parkinson's disease, but currently it must be regarded as a form of experimental therapy in the early stages of development.

The advances that have been made in the treatment of Parkinson's disease are largely based on replacement therapy; however, attempts at slowing the progress of cell death are now being investigated. At present, such trials of 'neuroprotective' treatment are based on somewhat speculative hypotheses. Therefore, on the assumption that Parkinson's disease is caused or exacerbated by free radical damage, a trial (DATATOP) has been undertaken to determine the possible benefit of chronic administration of the free radical scavenger, vitamin E. Furthermore, the potential role of deprenyl is being examined in the same study following the observation that inhibiting monoamine oxidase B protects against the development of MPTP-induced parkinsonism. Preliminary studies have demonstrated that deprenyl may slow the progress of Parkinson's disease (Parkinson Study Group, 1989; Tetrud and Langston, 1989). It is hoped that further preventive treatment will be developed once the mechanisms of cell death in Parkinson's disease are understood.

SPASTICITY

Central nervous system damage elicits two fundamental types of symptoms; those that are negative, such as weakness, paralysis, and lack of dexterity, and positive symptoms including excessive involuntary motor activity, commonly referred to as spasticity. The precise manifestations of spasticity (increased muscle tone, hyper-reflexia, and muscle spasms) depend upon the site and extent of the injury, but by definition always result from a lesion of the descending motor pathways. Combinations of positive and negative symptoms produce a variety of clinical profiles known collectively as spastic paresis (upper motorneuron syndrome); as a result, spasticity cannot be regarded as a single disorder and consequently should not be expected to respond consistently to single pharmacotherapy. Interestingly, patient disability in such cases arises predominantly from negative symptoms, yet positive signs are more obvious and, at present, the only ones responsive to pharmacological intervention. This anomaly underlies one of the principal inadequacies of current drug treatment. However, it should be remembered that a patient with flexor spasms and pain (generated by nerve impulses from nocioceptors) will often derive major benefit from a drug-induced reduction in such symptoms, even without a concomitant increase in strength and dexterity.

A comprehensive review of myorelaxant pharmacotherapy for spasticity would undoubtedly include medications such as opioids and botulinum toxin or curare-like neuromuscular blockers, which although effective at reducing muscle tone, flexor spasms, or both are, for various reasons, of little practical value in the treatment of spastic patients. In addition, numerous pharmacological agents (e.g. phenothiazines and propranolol) have been rendered virtually obsolete by the discovery of more effective alternatives. It is to three such alternatives that the following discussion is directed, forming as they do the mainstay of current antispastic therapy. All three, dantrolene, diazepam, and baclofen, evolved serendipitously before a greater understanding of the neurophysiology and neuropharmacology of motor control enabled the elucidation of their respective mechanisms of action. All three can cause potentially serious adverse effects but, as with other pharmacotherapy for chronic neurological disorders, it is the balance between safety and efficacy during long-term administration that is of paramount importance.

In contrast to both baclofen and diazepam, the principal site of action of dantrolene is peripheral, although some of its side-effects (drowsiness and confusion) are centrally mediated. Dantrolene acts directly on contractile mechanisms within muscle but has no specific effect on reflex pathways. By reducing the depolarisation-induced calcium efflux from sarcoplasmic reticulum, which is elicited by conducted muscle action potentials, dantrolene impairs 'excitation–contraction coupling' and thus the force produced by a muscle in response to electrical activation (Van Winkle, 1976). The result is a drug that causes mild to moderate generalized muscle weakness and has considerable antispastic/myorelaxant efficacy; for reasons that remain unclear, it has no effects on either cardiac or smooth muscle at antispastic doses. Thus, dantrolene is of particular use in patients with severe, prolonged muscle contraction who would not be incapacitated by the concurrent reduction in voluntary power. Patients who rely on their hemiplegic dystonia as an 'endogenous crutch' do not benefit from such therapy (Young and Delwaide, 1981). It is not usually possible to predict which patients will experience worthwhile benefit, but dantrolene can be useful irrespective of the spasticity type or lesion site; hence it has a role in cerebral spasticity, which is characteristically unresponsive to diazepam or baclofen. Unfortunately, a potential for hepatotoxicity has resulted in the more frequent use of baclofen (or diazepam) when the spasticity is of spinal origin.

Although little is known about the pathophysiology of spinal spasticity, oral baclofen (beta-4-chlorophenyl-gamma aminobutyric acid) has been used successfully for over 20 years in the treatment of flexor spasms. Like diazepam it appears to exert an antispastic effect directly on the spinal cord because efficacy is retained even in cases of complete cord transection. However, despite other similarities, these two compounds do not share a common mechanism of action: whereas diazepam appears to act primarily by facilitating $GABA_A$ receptor mediated presynaptic inhibition (see under Epilepsy, below, for more detailed explanation of benzodiazepine/GABA interactions), baclofen is an agonist at the $GABA_B$ (bicuculline-insensitive) receptor subtype (Price *et al.*, 1984). Here it functions both presynaptically to reduce excitatory amino acid release and also, at higher concentrations, postsynaptically to antagonise excitatory amino acid actions (Blaxter and Carlen, 1985). Both mechanisms serve to reduce activity in flexor reflex and pain pathways. Baclofen has now become the drug of choice for spinal spasticity, producing fewer alterations in cerebral function than diazepam or morphine, and avoiding the generalized muscle weakness characteristic of dantrolene. However, at high enough doses even baclofen can induce dose-limiting sedation when taken orally, a problem that has led to the development of intrathecal administration.

Despite being designed to penetrate the blood–brain barrier, baclofen, when infused into the subarachnoid space, produces levels in the CNS that are some orders of magnitude higher than can be achieved after oral administration (Penn, 1988). This may explain the increased antispastic effect of baclofen when given by this route, especially as the target $GABA_B$ receptors are located in the superficial layers (laminae I–IV) of dorsal grey matter where they are easily accessible to cerebrospinal fluid (CSF) (Price *et al.*, 1984). Double blind studies of continuous intrathecal baclofen infusion, using programmable pumps implanted in the lumbar subarachnoid space, have confirmed the advantages of this technique in the management of positive symptoms. For example, Penn *et al.* (1989) have reported that the acute effects of intrathecal baclofen on muscle tone, spasm, and bladder function can be maintained for over 18 months in patients previously unresponsive to oral baclofen. In addition, the ability to achieve higher, more stable concentrations in CSF enables baclofen to have a role in the treatment of cerebral spasticity, which is more common than that of spinal origin but not usually affected by oral therapy (Young, 1989). More comprehensive and comparative trials of intrathecal baclofen are required to establish whether or not this innovative therapy, which may eventually obviate the need for more invasive procedures, will be compromised by long-term side-effects such as tolerance, overdose, or infection. In this respect, initial evidence appears highly promising (Ochs *et al.*, 1989). The use of such implantable pumps is now expanding to other therapeutic areas and a variety of chronic neurological disorders may in future be treated more effectively in this way, particularly in the case of drugs with low brain permeability.

DEMENTIA

The increase in life expectancy that has occurred during the 20th century has been accompanied by a dramatic increase in the incidence of dementia. The importance of finding an effective treatment for this condition is underlined by figures from the National Institute of Ageing; it is estimated that the annual cost of caring for the chronically demented in the USA will rise to $30 billion (1978-dollars) by the year 2030 (Plum, 1979). With the exception of Japan, where multi-infarct dementia is frequently diagnosed, the majority of cases are caused by Alzheimer's disease (Plum, 1979) and, consequently, many of the potential therapies are based on advances that have been made in understanding the pathology of this disorder. The drugs that are currently prescribed for improving cognition were originally proposed as vasodilators (e.g. hydergine) or as metabolic enhancers (e.g. nootropics), but the majority of agents now under development are designed to increase cholinergic input to the cortex and hippocampus. This approach is based on consistent findings of damage to ascending cholinergic projections in the brains of patients with Alzheimer's disease (Bowen *et al.*, 1976). Although later studies have reported a depletion of several other neurotransmitters at post mortem (Rossor and Iversen, 1986), a limited number of *in vivo* biopsy studies have confirmed the importance of a cholinergic deficit in the early stages of the disease (Lowe *et al.*, 1988).

An increase in cholinergic activity may be achieved by the presynaptic enhancement of acetylcholine synthesis/release, by the inhibition of acetylcholine breakdown (anticholinesterases), and by the administration of agonists acting on the postsynaptic muscarinic receptor.

Presynaptic mechanisms

On the assumption that the uptake of choline into presynaptic terminals is the rate limiting step in the synthesis of acetylcholine, numerous trials have been carried out employing precursor loading with either lecithin or choline. However, in their review of 17 studies examining a wide range of doses, Bartus *et al.* (1982) concluded that such treatment is benign but of no value.

In vitro, an increase in acetylcholine release may be achieved by a variety of drugs including antagonists at the muscarinic autoreceptor, agonists at presynaptic nicotinic receptors, and potassium channel blockers (e.g. 4-aminopyridine). It has been argued that presynaptic stimulation of acetylcholine release may offer the advantage of mimicking the normal phasic action of cholinergic neurones, but the benefit of this approach has yet to be demonstrated in clinical studies. Indeed, trials of 4-aminopyridine in patients with probable Alzheimer's disease have been disappointing (Davidson *et al.*, 1988), and adequate studies of other potential candidates (e.g. DUP 996 and nicotine) are still required.

Anticholinesterases

Anticholinesterases, in particular physostigmine and tetrahydroaminoacridine (THA), have been the most widely used experimental agents for the treatment of Alzheimer's disease, although the majority of trials have been brief and of doubtful clinical relevance (Becker and Giacobini, 1988). Recently two groups (Stern, Sano, and Mayeux, 1988; Thal *et al.*, 1989) have reported that chronic treatment with oral physostigmine causes sustained improvements in new learning, which are too small to achieve functionally important benefits. The value of physostigmine is limited by variable bioavailability, a brief half-life, and a narrow therapeutic index (Becker and Giacobini, 1988), and there is a clear need for trials of other anticholinesterases with an improved pharmacokinetic profile. In a widely publicised report, Summers *et al.*, (1986) claimed remarkable results after chronic treatment with THA, but their study has been criticised on a number of grounds including the use of vague inclusion and exclusion criteria as well as the doubtful validity of their outcome measures (Byrne and Airie, 1989). Subsequent studies with THA have not substantiated the original claims by Summers *et al.* (1986) (Chatalier and Lacomblez, 1990). Although a large multicentre study sponsored by the National Institute of Ageing has demonstrated some clinical benefit, thus far this has not been regarded as sufficient evidence for registration in view of the drug's known hepatotoxicity.

Cholinergic agonists

The action of drugs that increase acetylcholine release or inhibit its breakdown relies on sufficient residual function in the remaining cholinergic neurones, but muscarinic agonists bypass such mechanisms and stimulate directly the preserved postsynaptic receptors in Alzheimer's disease (Cross *et al.*, 1984). Experience with a number of agonists including arecoline, pilocarpine, oxotremorine, RS86, and bethanechol has been variable, but in no study to date has there been clinically useful improvement (Gray, Enz, and Spiegel, 1989).

It might be argued that the potential of cholinergic replacement therapy has not been adequately tested because the dose range of various experimental agents has been limited by intolerable side-effects. Unfortunately, attempts at increasing the therapeutic window by intraventricular infusion of a cholinergic agonist (Penn *et al.*, 1988) or by the co-administration of peripherally acting muscarinic antagonists (Mouridian *et al.*, 1988) have not met with success. It must be hoped that the rapid advances that have recently been made in the characterization of different muscarinic receptor subtypes (Bonner, 1989) will allow the development of highly specific agonists with lower toxicity.

Other approaches

In the light of data indicating multiple neurotransmitter deficits in Alzheimer's disease, there have been a number of limited studies examining the effects of non-cholinergic intervention (Altman, Normille, and Gershon, 1987). Such treatments have included the manipulation of monoamine, GABA, and neuropeptide systems (e.g. ACTH, somatostatin and vasopressin). These procedures have improved memory in a variety of animal models but have as yet yielded only disappointing clinical results. The majority of proposed treatments for Alzheimer's disease are based on the hope that neurotransmitter replacement therapy may provide some degree of palliation. An alternative approach is to prevent the progressive neuronal degeneration that is characteristic of this disease. To this end, the finding that nerve growth factor (NGF) can prevent the death of cholinergic neurones after experimental lesions suggests that, in the future, trophic agents may be useful in the treatment of Alzheimer's disease (Hefti and Wiener, 1986). While there is clearly an urgent need for such novel therapies, all current hypotheses remain highly speculative.

EPILEPSY

Rather than a single disease state, epilepsy describes a group of related CNS disorders characterized by seizures that can adopt a variety of forms and which are variously sensitive to one or more of the current range of anticonvulsant drugs. Although approximately 80% of newly diagnosed patients can be rendered seizure-free by existing pharmacotherapy, the high incidence of epilepsy (0.5–1.0%) means there is a substantial number in whom treatment is unsatisfactory, either because of limited efficacy or intolerable side-effects.

For many years, the most productive approach to identifying novel anticonvulsants relied upon screening with rodent models of epilepsy. Besides promoting a rapid escalation in efficacious compounds, including phenytoin (Merritt and Putnam, 1938), this screen also provided the first evidence that such drugs might act by different mechanisms. Those effective against absence seizures in man were shown to raise seizure thresholds in animals, whereas clinical efficacy against partial and generalized tonic-clonic seizures was related to the prevention of seizure spread. Only in the last decade has a more rational approach to the pharmacological control of epilepsy evolved, based on an increased understanding of neurotransmission and those pathophysiological changes that underlie seizure activity. Much research has been directed towards the elucidation of the mechanisms of existing drugs, but for most currently available anticonvulsants, multiple biochemical and physiological actions have been demonstrated, and it is still unclear which of them are fundamental to antiseizure activity.

The primary cellular event responsible for seizure initiation is thought to be a paroxysmal depolarization shift (PDS) of neuronal membrane potential, with an associated 'burst discharge' (Prince and Wong, 1981). The output from a neurone showing such a burst discharge will subject the surrounding normal neurones to an excessive excitatory input leading, on ictal occasions, to recruitment. The genesis and spread of such discharges is thought to involve excitatory neurotransmitters (glutamate and aspartate), whereas seizure termination is probably controlled by the inhibitory transmitter, GABA. Normal brain function relies on a balance between these two opposing systems, which when disrupted leads to epileptic activity, and may also determine the primary clinical features and pharmacological susceptibilities of various types of epilepsy. Although a single abnormality is unlikely to be common to the whole spectrum of epilepsies, consideration of this simple theory has greatly assisted the development of new drugs.

Manipulation of inhibitory synaptic processes

An impairment of the inhibitory GABA system has long been viewed as a prime cause of seizure activity, not least because a number of established anticonvulsants (valproate, benzodiazepines, and barbiturates) are thought to work, in part, by enhancing the actions of this neurotransmitter (DeLorenzo, 1988). By increasing membrane chloride conductance, GABA hyperpolarizes the resting membrane potential, which has the effect of preventing burst discharge output. As GABA penetrates the blood–brain barrier very poorly, attempts have been made to develop GABA prodrugs (e.g. progabide) and synthetic GABA agonists (e.g. THIP); unfortunately, despite encouraging activity in animal models, neither approach has proved clinically useful (Dam, Gram, and Philbert, 1983; Petersen, Jensen, and Dam, 1983). Furthermore, inhibiting GABA uptake into nerve terminals and glial cells has provided few positive signs of efficacy. In contrast, a more successful approach seems to lie with the synthesis of specific, enzyme-activated, irreversible inhibitors of GABA-transaminase, the enzyme responsible for metabolizing GABA in neuronal tissue. One such compound, γ-vinyl-GABA (vigabatrin), has demonstrable efficacy in refractory patients and although development has preceded cautiously because of toxicological concerns (intramyelinic odema) in certain species, experience in over a thousand patients has inspired confidence in its use (Lewis and Richens, 1989). It now seems likely that this compound will be one of the newest to join the anticonvulsant armoury.

Undoubtedly the most appropriate pharmacological manipulation of the GABA system is provided by compounds that enhance the postsynaptic action of synaptically released GABA via an allosteric interaction with the GABA receptor. The various subunits that make up the $GABA_A$ receptor complex ($GABA_A$ recognition site, chloride ionophore, and benzodiazepine recognition site) have been well characterized (Hafeley and Polc, 1986) and remain central to many postulated mechanisms of anticonvulsant action. Conventional benzodiazepines produce an allosteric modulation of the GABA receptor, such that GABA binding is enhanced and the number of chloride channels opened is increased in response to a given concentration of GABA (Study and Barker, 1981). This mechanism appears optimal, because it is selective for the physiological activation of the system and therefore interference with normal function is, theoretically, minimal. Indeed, benzodiazepines are highly potent anticonvulsants with an impressive spectrum of clinical activity, although this may also reflect secondary actions on ion conductance and repetitive firing.

Unfortunately their clinical use is severely limited by sedation and, more importantly, the development of tolerance, which occurs in a significant proportion of patients (Haigh and Feely, 1988). Barbiturates act both directly to open the chloride ionophore and, in the presence of GABA, to prolong channel opening time. The relevance of these mechanisms to the anticonvulsant efficacy of barbiturates has yet to be established, but a separate action from benzodiazepines is supported by their different spectrum of clinical activity.

An additional binding site for valproate has also been postulated, albeit less convincingly, within the postsynaptic GABA receptor complex in an attempt to explain the broad range of efficacy displayed by this drug. Along with a number of other GABA-related mechanisms it has never achieved popular support and attention has now turned to the effects of valproate on brain aspartate levels (see Chapman *et al.*, 1982). This change reflects the increasing importance of excitatory processes in the development of novel antiepileptic compounds.

Manipulation of excitatory synaptic processes

Since the elucidation of excitatory amino acid receptor subtypes, suppression of excitation has become the major area of anticonvulsant research. Glutamate and aspartate act at membrane receptor sites to open ion channels (sodium, calcium, and possibly potassium), depolarising the resting membrane and initiating action potentials; seizure spread between regions depends on such activity. At present, the synthetic and metabolic pathways of important excitatory amino acids are relatively poorly understood and attempts to inhibit enzymatic synthesis have been unsuccessful. More useful as targets are the many mechanisms controlling the synaptic release of such excitants. Indeed, one particular compound, lamotrigine, which has been in successful clinical development for some years, is believed to inhibit principally glutamate release by an action at voltage sensitive sodium channels (Leach, Marden, and Miller, 1986).

The excitatory postsynaptic actions of dicarboxylic amino acids can of course be blocked by receptor antagonists and in this respect the N-methyl-D-aspartate (NMDA) receptor subtype has been the most intensively studied. This receptor operates ionic channels which have distinctive properties, leading to PDS and burst firing similar to that seen within an epileptic focus. Numerous compounds from a range of chemical series have been tested as potential antagonists at this receptor, both competitive (e.g. CGS 19755) and non competitive (voltage dependent ion channel blockers, e.g. MK-801). Efficacy is certainly apparent in animal models, but limited clinical trials with MK-801 revealed compromising psychotomimetic side-effects. However, as the sophistication of the NMDA receptor complex is further elucidated, more potential sites of action are revealed. Recently, a strychnine-insensitive glycine modulatory site has been isolated, activation of which appears to potentiate NMDA responses by increasing the frequency of channel opening (Johnson and Ascher, 1987). It remains to be seen how effective antagonists (e.g. HA 966; Foster and Kemp, 1989) may be as anticonvulsants at this site.

Membrane stabilization

Apart from modulatory neurotransmission, drugs acting directly on either membrane permeability or ionic transport and conductance mechanisms may reduce neuronal excitability. Compelling evidence exists that some well established anticonvulsants, notably phenytoin and carbamazepine, function in this way by altering resting and acting potentials. Such drugs will however, by virtue of this mechanism, demonstrate secondary actions on neurotransmission (see above). Phenytoin has numerous effects on the active transport of sodium, calcium and potassium ions (Yaari, Selzer, and Pincus, 1986), its modulation of the latter seemingly responsible for suppressing post-tetanic potentiation. In addition phenytoin can, like some other anticonvulsants, attenuate high frequency repetitive firing, most probably by a use dependent blockade of sodium conductance channels which increases channel inactivation. Predictably, the relative importance of some of these actions to the anticonvulsive efficacy of phenytoin remains to be established.

Other approaches

The development of novel drugs still offers the most rational approach to treating the majority of patients with uncontrolled seizures. Non-pharmacological therapies, such as the surgical removal of the epileptic focus, can provide dramatic improvements, but expense and the heterogeneity of both patients and lesions means that this procedure is uncommon (see Chapter 17). The utility of a variety of mechanisms (e.g. calcium antagonism) has still to be explored and, to this end, unprecedented numbers of novel compounds have been synthesized in the recent past (see Meldrum and Porter, 1986) as the limitations of established drugs have become increasingly apparent. The fact that many of these new structures possess only limited efficacy, or have unacceptable side-effects, has also focused attention on the modification of existing pharmacotherapy. For example, oxcarbazepine, the 10-keto analogue of carbamazepine, retains the clinical efficacy of its established predecessor but, by virtue of a different metabolic pathway, has less influence on oxidative processes and thus carries a lower risk of promoting pharmacokinetic drug interactions via enzyme induction (Gram and Philbert, 1986). Partial agonist benzodiazepines show lower tolerance-inducing potential and less sedation/muscle relaxation in animal models than do conventional benzodiazepines (see Haigh and Feely, 1988); if such findings can be reproduced clinically, these compounds would undoubtedly play a major role in the future treatment of epilepsy. Unfortunately, all innovation is threatened by the restrictions imposed upon clinical testing (adjunctive therapy and refractory patients) with the result that many compounds representing an advance on established treatments may be overlooked.

STROKE

Although the incidence of stroke is declining, it still remains the third most common cause of death in the western world. Because at least 80% of strokes are thromboembolic in origin (Mohr *et al.*, 1978), the majority of therapeutic approaches have been aimed at limiting the extent of cerebral infarction following vessel occlusion.

At present there is no generally accepted medical or surgical treatment for acute ischaemic stroke, although numerous forms of therapy have been tried or suggested. However, recent advances in the understanding of ischaemic neuronal damage have raised the possibility of rational therapeutic intervention. In particular there is both experimental and clinical evidence that following a stroke, areas of dense ischaemia may be surrounded by a penumbra in which local blood flow is impaired but oxygen metabolism preserved (Astrup, Siesjo, and Symon, 1981). Such findings have generated a number of therapeutic strategies aimed at raising tissue perfusion in the ischaemic penumbra above precarious levels. In addition, a number of pathophysiological studies in primates have shown that reversible occlusion of the middle cerebral artery for up to six hours is not necessarily associated with irreversible neuronal damage (Graham, 1988), which opens a possible window of therapeutic opportunity.

A large volume of preclinical data suggests that the era of therapeutic nihilism concerning the treatment of stroke may be coming to an end. Nevertheless, until the predictive value of animal models of stroke is confirmed in large clinical trials, an attitude of caution must be maintained.

Cerebral blood flow

Attempts to improve focal cerebral hypoperfusion have involved a number of techniques including the use of haemodilution (as well as other methods of lowering whole blood viscosity), thrombolytic therapy, and vasodilators.

LOWERING BLOOD VISCOSITY
A number of preclinical and clinical studies have confirmed that cerebral blood flow is inversely related to haematocrit, although the optimal levels and methods of haemodilution required to deliver maximum oxygenation to ischaemic tissue have not been defined. In spite of a considerable body of promising experimental data (Heros and Korosue, 1989), two multicentre trials of isovolaemic haemodilution in acute stroke have been negative (Scandinavian Stroke Study Group, 1987; Italian Acute Stroke Study Group, 1988). Although it might be argued that in the Swedish study therapeutic intervention was too slow and too late (only 28% of patients were entered within 12 hours of the stroke), the results from the Italian study are especially disappointing as all the patients were treated within 12 hours of the stroke and the majority within six hours. Haemodilution still retains its advocates who argue that treatment should be carried out more urgently and aggressively than was done in these multicentre trials (Heros and Korosue, 1989), but for the present, its role in the management of stroke is undefined.

Other attempts at treating ischaemic stroke by lowering whole blood viscosity have included the depletion of fibrinogen with ancrod (Hossman *et al.*, 1983), and the alteration of red cell deformability with pentoxifylline (Hse *et al.*, 1988). Overall, the benefits of these treatments were found to be small and transitory, but as with haemodilution the question remains as to whether the initiation of therapy was sufficiently early or aggressive.

THROMBOLYTIC TREATMENT

Early pilot studies with urokinase and streptokinase were disappointing in terms of efficacy and were complicated by an unacceptable incidence of cerebral haemorrhage (Fletcher, Alkjaersig, and Lewis, 1976). However, the success of thrombolytic treatment in the management of myocardial infarction and the development of relatively clot specific agents such as tissue plasminogen activator (tPA) have led to a renewed interest in this form of therapy. Studies in rabbits and baboons, as well as pilot clinical trials (Zeumer, 1985), have suggested the potential of thrombolysis but concern still persists with regard to the possibility of haemorrhagic transformation of the infarct on restoration of blood flow. Theoretically, early treatment (within 90 minutes of the stroke) should lessen the risk of cerebral haemorrhage, a possibility that is currently being addressed in a multicentre clinical trial (Brott *et al.*, 1988). Even if this study proves positive, the general applicability of such urgent therapy for stroke must remain limited.

VASODILATORS

A number of vasodilators, including papaverine, prostacyclin, and CO_2 inhalation, have been tested clinically in the hope that the outcome of ischaemic stroke might be improved by increasing tissue perfusion to the affected area (Grotta, 1987). Although the negative findings of these trials may to some extent be attributed to poor study design, there are theoretical limitations to the use of vasodilator therapy for stroke. In particular, following thromboembolic stroke local autoregulation is lost with resulting dilatation of cerebral resistance vessels in the ischaemic region. Under these circumstances the administration of a vasodilator may paradoxically reduce blood flow to the affected area by means of a 'steal' phenomenon in which perfusion is diverted to normal tissue (Cook and James, 1981). Recently there has been considerable interest in the potential role of calcium antagonists in the treatment of stroke, which apart from other mechanisms, may act as cerebral vasodilators. The possible neuroprotective actions of calcium antagonists are discussed in more detail below.

Neuroprotective agents

In recent years a body of evidence has developed indicating that an ischaemic insult may initiate a series of biochemical disturbances that ultimately lead to neuronal death. A variety of different classes of drugs, including calcium antagonists, excitatory amino acid antagonists, and free radical scavengers, have been proposed as neuroprotective agents in the hope that they may inhibit such toxic processes (see Chapter 4).

CALCIUM ANTAGONISTS

A number of investigators have reported a benefit of calcium antagonists on the extent of ischaemic damage in animal models of stroke; however, if the drugs are administered after the occlusion, improvement is usually only modest (Hossman, 1989). By contrast these agents (e.g. nimodipine) are of proven value when given before the ischaemic insult, as in the prevention of some of the late sequelae of subarachnoid haemorrhage (Pickard *et al.*, 1989). Both a vasodilator effect on cerebral vasculature and a direct action on ischaemic neurones have been suggested to account for the putative neuroprotective properties of these drugs. *In vitro*, a number of calcium antagonists dilate cerebral blood vessels preconstricted by agents including potassium, 5HT, and noradrenaline (Allen and Banghart, 1979), but *in vivo*, their effects on flow in focal cerebral ischaemia are controversial (Meyer *et al.*, 1987).

Increases in free calcium levels in the cytosol, which have been demonstrated in injured neurones after the induction of focal ischaemia (Uematsu *et al.*, 1989), have been implicated in a number of toxic processes by mechanisms that remain speculative. These include excessive activation of lipases and proteases with irreversible damage to mitochondria and other cell organelles. Although it has been argued that the administration of calcium antagonists may inhibit such toxic processes, these agents have no demonstrable effects on ischaemia-induced rises in cytosolic free calcium (Hossman, 1989).

A preliminary study by Gelmers *et al.* (1988), suggests that nimodipine may be beneficial in the treatment of acute ischaemic stroke, but a definite verdict on the value of calcium antagonists for this indication is dependent on the results of large multicentre studies, which are in progress.

EXCITATORY AMINO ACIDS

It has been known for many years that excessive stimulation by excitatory amino acids such as glutamate and aspartate, can lead to neural degeneration (Rothman and Olney, 1986). Following a number of cerebral insults, including ischaemia, there is a dramatic rise in the levels of extracellular glutamate and aspartate, presumably owing to the failure of energy requiring uptake systems (Beneviste *et al.*, 1984), and it has been postulated that this increase leads to 'excitotoxic' damage.

Amino acid receptors are classified into three or more subtypes according to their preferred agonist, N-methyl-D-aspartate (NMDA), quisqualate, or kainate (Monaghan, Mohr, and Williams, 1989). Studies employing selective antagonists indicate a major role for the NMDA receptor in the mediation of ischaemic neuronal damage. For example, NMDA antagonists have been shown to protect neurones in culture from anoxia (Rothman and Olney 1986), and have proved effective in a variety of experimental models of ischaemic stroke, including the rat and cat, when given up to two hours after vessel occlusion (Park *et al.*, 1988). The NMDA receptor is linked to an ion channel, which opens to allow the passage of sodium and calcium into the cell, when an agonist binds to its recognition site; it is the excessive entry of these ions into neurones that is thought to underlie NMDA receptor mediated neurotoxicity. Such overstimulation may be prevented by antagonists that bind to the agonist recognition site (e.g. CGS 19755 and CGP 37849), to the ion channel (e.g. ketamine and MK-801), or to a modulatory glycine recognition site associated with the NMDA complex (e.g. HA 966), although it is uncertain which is the optimal method of NMDA antagonism for clinical use (Cotman and Iversen, 1987).

The evidence that blockade of the NMDA receptor can partially limit focal ischaemic damage is impressive, but it remains to be demonstrated that such neuroprotective effects can be achieved at clinically tolerable dose levels.

FREE RADICAL SCAVENGERS

Highly reactive oxygen free radicals can be generated from a number of sources within ischaemic tissue and may attack various cell constituents (Southern and Powis, 1988). Antioxidants, such as superoxide dismutase and ascorbic acid, have been shown to limit ischaemic damage in the heart but are of doubtful benefit in stroke (Suzuki *et al.*, 1984). Recently, the development of a new series of compounds, the 21-aminosteroids (lazeroids) has led to renewed interest in the role of free radicals in ischaemic neuronal damage (Braughler *et al.*, 1989). Lazeroids, which have been shown to scavenge free radicals *in vitro*, are reported to reduce infarction and vasogenic oedema following middle cerebral artery occlusion in the cat as well as in a number of models of trauma. Reports of the clinical efficacy of lazeroids are awaited.

CONCLUSIONS

The pharmacotherapy of neurological disorders has been restricted by the complexity of the CNS, its limited capacity for repair, and its tendency to accommodate pharmacological intervention (tolerance). The concept of replacement therapy, which has been applied to the treatment of Parkinson's disease, has not so far been successful in other areas, although this may change if muscarinic agonists are shown to be of value in the management of Alzheimer's disease. The notion of tissue replacement, rather than neurotransmitter replacement, is still at an early stage. By contrast, the modulation of neurotransmitter processes has already achieved recognition in the treatment of various disease states, including epilepsy and spasticity. At present this approach is centred on the GABA$_A$ receptor complex, but there is increasing evidence that modulation of the NMDA receptor may provide substantial opportunities in the therapy of stroke and epilepsy. The realization that many insults are mediated by mechanisms involving delayed cascade and amplification, has led to the proposal that neuronal damage may be limited by antagonists of putative toxic processes (e.g. free radical scavengers). Furthermore, the ability to promote repair by the administration of trophic factors (e.g. NGF) has provided another theoretical approach to the alleviation of neurological disease. However, many of these novel concepts await further preclinical development before the evaluation of their potential in a clinical setting.

References

Allen GS and Banghart SB (1979) Cerebral arterial spasm. Part 9. In vitro effects of nifedipine on serotonin-, phenylephrine- and potassium-induced contractions of canine basilar and femoral arteries, *Neurosurgery*, **4**, 32–42

Altman HJ, Normille HJ, and Gershon S (1987) Non-cholinergic pharmacology in human cognitive disorders, In Stahl SM, Iversen SD, and Goodman EC, eds *Cognitive Neurochemistry*, Oxford, Oxford University Press, 346–71

Astrup J, Siesjo B, and Symon L (1981) Thresholds in cerebral ischemia: the ischemic penumbra, *Stroke*, **12**, 723–5

Bartus R, Dean R, Beer B, Lippa A (1982) The cholinergic hypothesis of geriatric memory dysfunction, *Science*, **217**, 408–23

Becker RE and Giacobini E (1988) Mechanism of cholinesterase inhibition in senile dementia of the Alzheimer type: clinical, pharmacological and therapeutic aspects, *Drug Dev Res*, **12**, 163–95

Beneviste H, Drejer J, Schousboe A, and Diemer NH (1984) Elevation of extracellular concentrations of glutamate and aspartate in rat hippocampus during transient cerebral ischaemia monitored by microdialysis, *J Neurochem*, **43**, 1369–74

Bjorklund A and Stenevi U (1979) Reconstruction of the nigro-striatal pathway by intracerebral nigral transplants, *Brain Res*, **177**, 555–60

Blaxter TJ and Carlen PL (1985) Pre and post synaptic effects of baclofen in the rat hippocampal slice, *Brain Res*, **345**, 195–9

Bonner TI (1989) The molecular basis of muscarinic receptor diversity. *Trends in Neurosciences*, **12**, 148–51

Bowen DM, Smith CB, White P, and Davison AN (1976) Neurotransmitter-related enzymes and indices of hypoxia in senile dementias and other abiotrophies, *Brain*, **99**, 459–96

Braughler JM, Hall ED, Jacobsen EJ, McCall JM, and Means ED (1989) The 21-aminosteroids: potent inhibitors of lipid peroxidation for the treatment of central nervous system trauma and ischemia, *Drug Dev Res*, **14**, 143–52

Brott T, Haley EC, Levy DE, Barsan WG, Reed RL, Olinger CP *et al.* (1988) Very early therapy for cerebral infarction with tissue plasminogen activator, *Stroke*, **19**, 133

Byrne J and Airie TC (1989) Tetrahydroaminoacridine (THA) in Alzheimer's disease, *Br Med J*, **298**, 845–6

Chapman AG, Keane PE, Meldrum BS, Simiand J, and Vernieres JC (1982) Mechanism of anticonvulsant action of valproate, *Prog Neurobiol*, **19**, 315–59

Chatelier G and Lacomblez L (1990) Tacrine (tetrahydroaminoacridine; THA) and lecithin in senile dementia of the Alzheimer's type: a multicentre trial, *Br Med J*, **300**, 495–8

Cook P and James I (1981) Cerebral vasodilators, *N Engl J Med*, **305**, 1508–13

Cotman C and Iversen L (1987) Excitatory amino acids in the brain. *Trends in Neurosciences*, **10**, 263–5

Cross AJ, Crow TJ, Johnson JA, Perry EK, Perry RH, Blessed G *et al.* (1984) Studies on neurotransmitter receptor systems in neocortex and hippocampus in senile dementia of the Alzheimer type, *J Neurol Sci*, **64**, 109–17

Curtis L, Lees AJ, Stern GM, and Marmot MG (1984) Effect of L-dopa on the course of Parkinson's disease, *Lancet*, **2**, 211–2

Dam M, Gram L, and Philbert A (1983) Progabide: a controlled trial in partial epilepsy, *Epilepsia*, **24**, 127–34

Davidson M, Zemishlany Z, Mohs RC, Horvath TB, Powchik P, Blass JP *et al.* (1988) 4-Aminopyridine in the treatment of Alzheimer's disease, *Biol Psych*, **23**, 485–90

DeLorenzo RJ (1988) Mechanisms of action of anticonvulsant drugs, *Epilepsia*, **29** (Suppl 2), S35–S47

Fahn S and Bressman S (1984) Should levodopa therapy for Parkinsonism be started early or late?, *Can J Neurol*, **30** (Suppl 1) 200–5

Fletcher AP, Alkjaersig N, and Lewis M (1976) A pilot study of urokinase therapy in cerebral infarction, *Stroke*, **7**, 135–42

Foster AC and Kemp JA (1989) HA-966 antagonises N-methyl-D-aspartate receptors through a selective interaction with the glycine modulatory site, *J Neurosci*, **9**, 2191–6

Gelmers H, Gorter K, De Weerdt C, and Wizer H (1988) A controlled trial of nimodipine in acute stroke, *N Engl J Med*, **318**, 203–7

Goetz CG, Olanow CW, Koller W, Penn RD, Cahill D, Morantz R *et al.* (1989) Multicenter study of autologous adrenal medullary transplantation to the corpus striatum in patients with advanced Parkinson's disease, *N Engl J Med*, **320**, 337–41

Graham DI (1988) Focal cerebral infarction, *J Cereb Blood Flow Metab*, **8**, 769–73

Gram L and Philbert A (1986) Oxcarbazepine. In Meldrum BS and Porter RJ, eds, *Current Problems in Epilepsy. 4: New Anticonvulsant Drugs*, London, John Libbey, 229–35

Gray JA, Enz A, and Spiegel R (1989) Muscarinic agonists for senile dementia: past experience and future trends, *Trends Pharmacol Sci*, In press

Grotta J (1987) Can raising cerebral blood flow improve outcome after acute cerebral infarction?, *Stroke*, **18**, 264–7

Haefely W and Polc P (1986) Physiology of GABA enhancement by benzodiazepines and barbiturates. In Olsen RW and Venter JC, eds, *Benzodiazepine/GABA Receptors and Chloride Channels: Structural and Functional Properties*, New York, Alan R Liss, 97–133

Haigh JRM and Feely M (1988) Tolerance to the anticonvulsant effect of benzodiazepines, *Trends Pharmacol Sci*, **9**, 361–6

Hardie RJ, Lees AJ, and Stern GM (1984) 'On-off' fluctuations in Parkinson's disease. A clinical and neuropharmacological study, *Brain*, **107**, 487–506

Hefti F and Weiner WJ (1986) Nerve growth factor in Alzheimer's disease, *Ann Neurol*, **20**, 275–81

Heros R and Korosue K (1989) Hemodilution for cerebral ischemia, *Stroke*, **20**, 423–7

Hossman KA (1989) Calcium antagonists for the treatment of brain ischaemia: a critical appraisal, In Krieglstein J, ed, *Pharmacology of Cerebral Ischaemia 1988*, Boca Rouge, CRC, 53–63

Hossman V, Heiss W, Bewermeyer H, and Wiedman G (1983) Controlled trial of ancrod in ischemic stroke, *Arch Neurol*, **46**, 803–8

Hsu CY, Norris J, Hogan E, Bladin P, Dinsdale HB, Yatsu FM *et al.* (1988) Pentoxifylline in acute nonhaemorrhagic stroke, *Stroke*, **19**, 716–22

Hunt KR, Shaw JM, Laurence DR, and Stern GM (1973) Sustained levodopa therapy in Parkinsonism, *Lancet*, **2**, 928–30

Italian Acute Stroke Study Group (1988) Haemodilution in acute stroke: results of the Italian haemodilution trial, *Lancet*, **1**, 318–21

Johnson JW and Ascher P (1987) Glycine potentiates the NMDA response in cultured mouse brain neurones, *Nature*, **325**, 529–31

Kurlan R (1988) International symposium on early dopamine agonist therapy of Parkinson's disease, *Arch Neurol*, **45**, 204–8

Leach MJ, Marden CM, and Miller AA (1986) Pharmacological studies on lamotrigine, a novel potential antiepileptic drug: II. Neurochemical studies on the mechanism of action, *Epilepsia*, **27**, 490–7

Lees AJ (1986) L-dopa treatment in Parkinson's disease, *Q J Med*, **59**, 535–47

Lees AJ (1989) The 'On-Off' phenomenon, *J Neurol Neurosurg Psychiatry*, **Special Suppl**, 29–37

Lewis PJ and Richens A (1989) Vigabatrin: a new antiepileptic, *Br J Clin Pharmacol*, **27** (Suppl 1)

Lindvall O (1989) Transplantation into the human brain: Present status and future possibilities, *J Neurol Neurosurg Psychiatry*, **Special Suppl**, 39–54

Lindvall O, Rehncrona S, Brundin P, Gustavii B, Astedt B, Widner H *et al.* (1989) Human foetal dopamine neurons grafted into the striatum in two patients with severe Parkinson's disease, *Arch Neurol*, **46**, 615–31

Lowe SL, Francis PT, Proctor AW, Palmer AM, Davison AN, and Bowen DM (1988) Gamma-aminobutyric acid concentrations in brain tissue at two stages of Alzheimer's disease, *Brain*, **111**, 785–99

Madrazo I, Drucker-Colin R and Torres C (1988) Long term (more than one year) evolution of patients with adrenal medullary autografts for the caudate nucleus for the treatment of Parkinson's disease, *Proceedings of the XVI CINP Congress*, Munich

Madrazo I, Leon V, Torres C, Aguilera C, Varela G, Alvarez F *et al.* (1988) Transplantation of foetal substantia nigra and adrenal medulla to the caudate nucleus in two patients with Parkinson's disease, *N Engl J Med*, **318**, 51

Markham C and Diamond S (1981) Evidence to support early levodopa therapy in Parkinson's disease, *Neurology*, **31**, 125–31

Meldrum BS and Porter RJ (1986) Current problems in Epilepsy 4. New anticonvulsant drugs, London, John Libbey

Merritt HH and Putman TJ (1938) Sodium diphenylhydantoinate in the treatment of convulsive disorders, *JAMA*, **111**, 1068–73

Meyer FB, Sundt TM, Yanajagihara T, and Anderson R (1987) Focal cerebral ischemia: pathophysiological mechanisms and rationale for future avenues of treatment, *Mayo Clin Proc*, **62**, 35–55

Mohr JP, Caplan L, Melski JW, Goldstein RJ, Duncan GW, Kistler JP *et al.* (1978) The Harvard Co-operative Stroke Registry: A prospective study, *Neurology*, **28**, 754–62

Monaghan D, Bridges R, and Cotman C (1989) The excitatory amino acid receptors: their classes, pharmacology and distinct properties in the function of the central nervous system, *Annu Rev Pharmacol Toxicol*, **29**, 365–402

Mouridian MM, Mohr E, Williams JA, and Chase TN (1988) No response to high dose muscarinic agonist therapy in Alzheimer's disease, *Neurology*, **38**, 606–8

Ochs G, Struppler A, Meyerson BA, Linderoth B, Gybels J, Gardner BP *et al.* (1989) Intrathecal baclofen for long-term treatment of spasticity: a multi-centre study, *J Neurol Neurosurg Psychiatry*, **52**, 933–9

Park CK, Nehls D, Graham D, Teasdale GN, and McCulloch J (1988) Focal cerebral ischaemia in the cat: treatment with the glutamate antagonist MK-801 after the induction of ischaemia, *J Cereb Blood Flow Metab*, **8**, 757–62

Parkinson Study Group (1989) Effect of deprenyl on the progression of disability in early Parkinson's disease, *New Engl J Med*, **321**, 1364–71

Penn RD (1988) Intrathecal baclofen for severe spasticity, *Ann NY Acad Sci*, **581**, 157–66

Penn RD, Martin EM, Wilson RS, Fox JH, and Sovoy SM (1988) Intraventricular bethanechol infusion for Alzheimer's disease – results of double-blind and escalating dose trials, *Neurology*, **38**, 219–22

Penn RD, Savoy SM, Corcos D, Latash M, Gottlieb G, Parke B, and Kroin JS (1989) Intrathecal baclofen for severe spinal spasticity, *N Engl J Med*, **320**, 1517–21

Perlow M, Freed W, Hoffer BJ, Olsen L, and Wyatt R (1979) Brain grafts reduce motor abnormalities by destruction of nigro-striatal dopamine system, *Science*, **204**, 643–7

Petersen HR, Jensen I, and Dam M (1983) THIP: a single blind controlled trial in patients with epilepsy, *Acta Neurol Scand*, **67**, 114–7

Pickard JD, Murray G, Illingworth R, Shaw MDM, Teasdale GM, Foy PM *et al.* (1989) Effect of oral nimodipine on cerebral infarction and outcome after subarachnoid haemorrhage: British aneurism nimodipine trial. *Br Med J*, **298**, 636–42

Plum F (1979) Dementia: an approaching epidemic, *Nature*, **279**, 372–3

Price GW, Wilkin GP, Turnbull MJ, and Bowery NG (1984) Are baclofen-sensitive GABA$_B$ receptors present on primary afferent terminals of the spinal cord, *Nature*, **307**, 71–3

Prince DA and Wong RKS (1981) Human epileptic neurones studied in vitro, *Brain Res*, **210**, 323–33

Quinn N, Parkes JD, and Marsden CD (1984) Control of on/off phenomenon by continuous intravenous infusion of levodopa, *Neurology*, **34**, 1131–6

Rinne UK (1987) Early combination of bromocriptine and levodopa in the treatment of Parkinson's disease: a five year follow up, *Neurology*, **37**, 826–8

Rossor M and Iversen L (1986) Non-cholinergic neurotransmitter abnormalities in Alzheimer's disease, *Br Med Bull*, **42**(1), 70–5

Rothman SM and Olney JW (1986) Glutamate and the pathophysiology of hypoxic-ischemic brain damage, *Ann Neurol*, **19**, 105–11

Scandinavian Stroke Study Group (1987) Multicenter trial of hemodilution in acute ischemic stroke. I. Results in the total patient population, *Stroke*, **18**, 691–9

Sladek JR, Redmond DE, Collier TJ, Blaint JP, Elsworth JD, Taylor JR, and Roth RH (1988) Foetal dopamine neural grafts: extended reversal of methylphenyltetrahydropyridine-induced parkinsonism in monkeys, *Prog Brain Res*, **78**, 497–506

Southern PA and Powis G (1988) Free radicals in medicine II. Involvement in human disease, *Mayo Clin Proc*, **63**, 390–408

Stern Y, Sano M, and Mayeux R (1988) Long-term administration of oral physostigmine in Alzheimer's disease, *Neurology*, **38**, 1837–41

Stibe C, Kempster P, Lees A, and Stern GM (1988) Subcutaneous apomorphine in parkinsonian 'on-off' oscillations, *Lancet*, **1**, 403–6

Stromberg I, Herrera-Marschitz M, Ungerstedt U, Ebendal T, and Olson L (1985) Chronic implants of chromaffin tissue into dopamine denervated striatum. Effects of NGF on graft survival, fiber and rotational behavior, *Exp Brain Res*, **60**, 335–49

Study RE and Barker JL (1981) Diazepam and (-) pentobarbital: fluctuation analysis reveals different mechanisms for potentiation of γ-aminobutyric acid responses in cultured neurones, *Proc Natl Acad Sci*, **78**, 7180–4

Summers WK, Majorski LV, Marsh GM, Tachiki K, and King A (1986) Oral tetrahydroaminoacridine in long-term treatment of senile dementia, Alzheimer's type, *N Engl J Med*, **315**, 1241–5

Suzuki J, Fujimoto S, Mizoi K, and Oba M (1984) The protective effect of combined administration of anti-oxidants and perfluoro chemicals on cerebral ischemia, *Stroke*, **15**, 672–9

Tetrud JW and Langston JW (1989) The effect of deprenyl (selegiline) on the natural history of Parkinson's disease, *Science*, **245**, 519–22

Thal LJ, Masur DM, Blau AD, Field PA, and Klauber MR (1989) Chronic oral physostigmine without lecithin improves memory in Alzheimer's disease, *J Am Geriatr Soc*, **37**, 42–8

Uematsu D, Greenberg J, Reivich M, and Hickey W (1989) Direct evidence for calcium-induced ischemic and reperfusion injury, *Ann Neurol*, **26**, 280–3

Van Winkle WB (1976) Calcium release from skeletal muscle sarcoplasmic reticulum: site of action of dantrolene sodium, *Science*, **193**, 1130–1

Yaari Y, Selzer ME, and Pincus JH (1986) Phenytoin: mechanisms of its anticonvulsant action, *Ann Neurol*, **20**, 171–84

Young RR (1989) Treatment of spastic paresis, *N Engl J Med*, **320**, 1553–5

Young RR and Delwaide PJ (1981) Spasticity, *N Engl J Med*, **304**, 28–33

Zeumer H (1985) Survey of progress: vascular recanalising techniques in interventional neuroradiology, *J Neurol*, **231**, 287–92

7
Compensating for impaired or lost function—biomechanical or rehabilitation engineering

Richard A. L. Macdonell and Michael Swash

Loss of function caused by disorders of the nervous system often produces permanent disability. At present, it is not possible to replace or promote the regrowth of any part of the central nervous system. Consequently, the patient with neurologic disability must rely on biomechanical devices designed to work in conjunction with remaining neuromuscular function. It is the purpose of this chapter to review recent developments in this field in relation to some common neurological disabilities.

ORTHOSES AND PROSTHESES

Orthoses are used to redistribute load, support an unstable joint, and provide a mechanical means of compensating for lost function. They may be static, such as orthoses to prevent joint contracture, or dynamic, where the orthosis applies forces to a joint weakened by paralysis of the muscles that normally control it. Dynamic orthoses have joints that allow free movement or are lockable to restrict movement (Goodwill, 1988). They may be used in conjunction with transcutaneous or intramuscular electrical stimulation of appropriate muscles or nerves to improve function.

Prostheses are artificial substitutes for missing body parts, which are used for functional or cosmetic reasons, or both. Artificial limbs are probably the most commonly used prosthesis, which are used for patients whose limbs are either congenitally absent, maldeveloped, or who have had a limb amputated.

It is not possible to provide an extensive review of orthoses and prostheses in the space available. Instead we have elected to concentrate on recent advances in such devices that improve common disabilities.

Orthoses

FOOT DROP
Weakness of dorsiflexion at the ankle producing 'foot drop' is a common neurological problem. It may be caused by lesions ranging throughout the neuraxis, from a common peroneal nerve palsy to stroke. The abnormality of gait produced, and the choice of orthosis to overcome it, depend on whether the foot drop is caused by

flaccid or spastic paralysis. In flaccid paralysis, such as following a common peroneal nerve palsy, abnormalities are produced in both the stance and swing phases of gait. There is a reduction in the length of the heelstrike phase, and a reduction in both the plantar- and dorsiflexion movements. In addition, there is an increase in inversion-eversion suggesting medial-lateral instability (Lehmann *et al.*, 1986). In overcoming this disability, the patient tends to elevate the pelvis and increase flexion at the knee and hip such that the toes may now clear the ground. This produces the characteristic 'steppage gait' of the disorder. The device most commonly used to improve this gait abnormality is an ankle-foot orthosis (AFO), usually moulded from ortholen or polypropylene. An alternative is a single inside metal upright with a piston ankle joint, which contains a coil spring pushing down behind the axis of the ankle joint. The rationale behind such devices is that they produce a dorsiflexion force at the ankle. The optimum position for the ankle joint is the minimum required for foot clearance. This reduces the potential for increased knee flexion during the heelstrike and pushoff phases of gait (Lehmann *et al.*, 1986).

Foot drop caused by spastic paralysis presents a more difficult problem. In addition to foot dragging, there is also a spastic equinovarus at the ankle to overcome. An AFO may be useful if the predominant leg weakness is at the hip (Goodwill, 1988). Several types are available, including double metal uprights with piston ankle joints, double metal uprights with double stop ankle joints, or polypropylene or ortholen orthoses.

Functional electrical stimulation (FES) used in conjunction with orthotic devices may also help to overcome the disability of either type of foot drop providing the muscle is not severely denervated (Turk and Obreza, 1985). Stimulating electrodes are placed over the peroneal nerve at the knee and a switch is located within the heel of the shoe. During the stance phase of gait, the stimulator is switched off. At heel lift off, the stimulator is triggered stimulating the common peroneal nerve and producing dorsiflexion during the swing phase of gait (Roberts and Porter, 1988). This allows the foot to clear the ground and also inhibits spasticity in plantar flexor muscles in patients with a spastic foot drop (Turk and Obreza, 1985). FES has proved quite useful in the management of foot drop, but in spastic foot drop it should be reserved for the patient who is able to walk relatively well (Liberson *et al.*, 1961).

A further approach in spastic foot drop may be to use an injection of botulinum toxin into the muscles causing spastic plantar flexion and equinovarus at the ankle. The injection weakens these muscles causing the foot drop to become flaccid, and allowing treatment with orthotic devices or FES. The reduction of spasticity produced by a single injection of botulinum toxin may last several weeks or months (Das and Park, 1989).

PARAPLEGIC WALKING

Paraplegics with lesions at or above the level of the thoracic cord are handicapped by their inability to walk. Swing through gait, using crutches with legs braced in long leg callipers, knee-ankle-foot orthoses (KAFO), or hip-knee-ankle-foot orthoses (HKAFO), has been used for many years. The major problem with this method of ambulation is that it requires high energy consumption and is only suitable for moving short distances. Swing through gait is also difficult because of the tendency for the back foot to strike the other foot or become trapped behind it. A second problem is the tendency to fall laterally, which is difficult for the patient to control. Other orthoses have been used, such as the Swivel Walker (Edbrooke, 1970; Rose and Henshaw, 1972; Stallard, Rose, and Framer, 1978) and the Parapodium (Motlock and Elliott, 1966). These devices permit low energy ambulation but are limited to flat, smooth surfaces.

Rose (1979) introduced the hip guidance orthosis, originally designed for use by paraplegic children. The device, called a Parawalker, consists of a very rigid body brace articulating through ball bearings to leg braces. This provides planar leg movement and resistance to adduction. Using the Parawalker, the tendencies to fall laterally and for foot collision are much reduced. The tendency for backwards falling is reduced by a stop limiting hip flexion; hip extension being limited naturally by the hip joint. Using this device patients are able to execute independent transfer, assumption of the upright posture and ambulation at a reasonable speed (50 feet min^{-1}) over a variety of surfaces. Most patients continue to use the Parawalker, having become used to its actions and limitations, and a number have now been using it for many years. Although originally designed for children, it has been adapted for use by adults. A problem with its use by adults, is that some adduction of the legs cannot be prevented and an extra burden is placed on the supporting arms (Nene and Major, 1987). This can be relieved by using percutaneous FES of leg and gluteal muscles to reduce energy consumption (McClelland *et al.*, 1987; Nene and Jennings, 1989). FES is also useful in reducing the energy expenditure of patients who use a swing through gait and long leg orthoses. This allows the patient to travel greater distances than with swing through ambulation alone (Marsolais and Edwards, 1988).

Prostheses

Lower limb prostheses derive their power from the users body energy in combination with gravity to produce useful movement and function. At present, attempts to improve their function by control through the patient's neuromuscular system have proved disappointing. In contrast, upper limb prostheses, which have to operate to some degree against gravity, have been developed to work under the direction of proximal neuromusculature. The body powered prosthesis is attached to the limb stump and connected to the torso by a harness. The terminal device, made in the shape of a hand or one of a variety of hooks, is opened by tension placed on a central control cable. It is closed by rubber bands or springs (Bender, 1982). Patients prefer a hook as the terminal device rather than the cable driven hand because it has proved to be more functional (Millstein, Heger, and Hunter, 1986). Recent refinements of the hand may improve its acceptability (Lamb, Dick, and Douglas, 1988). In patients with above elbow amputations, a single central cable control system can be used to flex the elbow as well as operate the terminal device (Ober 1982; Lamb, Dick, and Douglas, 1988).

Externally powered prostheses are battery driven (6 or 12 Volt) and operate either through myoelectric control, microswitches, or a combination of both. Myoelectric systems use surface recording electrodes to monitor the electrical activity of selected skeletal muscles or muscle groups while they contract. The EMG signal is fed to an amplifier and from there to a signal processor before passing to the direct current motor of a mechanical hand or elbow. With training, the patient can be taught to open and close the hand, and move the elbow through contraction of appropriate muscles (Scott and Parker, 1988). In order to be considered for such a prosthesis, the patient must be capable of eliciting and controlling myoelectric signals. In addition, the patient must be able to sustain different levels of muscle tension to make the prosthetic hand work effectively. Microswitch devices work similarly, except that rather than EMG activity triggering the electric motor, the motor is triggered by the patient compressing a microswitch using the proximal arm stump or shoulder. The pressure required to operate these switches is quite small, seven grams or less, and most patients do not find this difficult. Several different switches may be incorporated into the device, producing movement in different directions and increasing the range of functions. Microswitch and myoelectric systems can be combined, which is particularly useful in above elbow prostheses. Here the microswitch is used to flex the elbow while the hand is controlled by a myoelectric system (Sauter, 1981).

Most users prefer the externally powered upper limb prostheses to those that are body powered because they provide an increased range of function and are more cosmetically acceptable (Stein and Walley, 1983; Mendez, 1985; Millstein, Heger, and Hunter, 1986). This is particularly so for patients with amputations above the elbow, where body powered devices have not proved to be particularly successful (Sauter, 1981; Millstein, Heger, and Hunter, 1986). Main drawbacks of externally powered prostheses are their cost and speed. Myoelectrically controlled arms can take up to five times as long to perform tasks as a normal arm, and two and a half times as long as a body powered prosthetic arm (Stein and Walley, 1983).

Further improvements in the area of limb prostheses must include speeding up the function of externally driven devices and the incorporation of some type of sensory feedback system to improve their function (Cotoyannis *et al.*, 1988; Scott and Parker, 1988).

VISION

The provision of artificial vision by electrocortical stimulation has been investigated for over 20 years (Brindley and Lewin, 1968; Lewin, 1971; Dobelle, Mladejevsky, and Girvin, 1974). As yet, no useful device has been constructed and hence visual prostheses should be regarded as being purely experimental. The aims of research in this area are to produce a prosthesis capable of providing the blind with independent mobility. Interested readers are referred to an excellent review by Girvin (1988).

AUDITORY LOSS AND HEARING AIDS

Various kinds of devices have been used through the years to improve the hearing of the totally or partially deaf. Considerable progress has been made and it is now possible to offer the totally deaf some prospect of speech perception (Clark *et al.*, 1987). Hearing aids are used by patients with a sensorineural component to their deafness. Pure conductive deafness is best treated medically and there is an 80–95% chance that hearing will be restored to normal or near normal levels (Paparella and Davis, 1978).

Hearing aids range from externally worn aids, whose prime function is to amplify the auditory input to the affected ear, to cochlear implants, which directly stimulate the acoustic nerve.

Externally worn hearing aids

Externally worn hearing aids are appropriate primarily for patients with mild to moderate sensorineural hearing loss. A number of factors determine whether a patient needs an aid. The most important of these is the individuals own perception of hearing impairment. Even relatively mild hearing loss, as judged by an audiogram, can be quite disabling for some patients and they can benefit from amplification

(Cunningham and Ganzel, 1986). In assessing the likely benefit to be gained from a hearing aid, the audiogram may be quite helpful. In general, the more marked the degree of loss of higher frequency sounds relative to low frequency sounds, the more benefit the patient will derive from an aid. Hearing loss is commonly bilateral, such as in the common, age related deafness (presbyacusis) and this is best treated with binaural hearing aids (Wilson and Wilson, 1988).

Over recent years hearing aid technology has improved considerably. The most dramatic strides have been taken in size reduction. The integrated circuit, microchip, and smaller power units have enabled the construction of a hearing aid that can fit discretely into the ear canal. Other types of aid fit in the ear or over the ear with attached ear moulds. These latter aids are preferred to the in-canal type for patients whose auditory canal is small or when a greater amount of amplification is required than is possible with currently existing in-canal aids (Wilson and Wilson, 1988).

Patients who have difficulty manipulating the small control knobs on ear mounted aids, or who need considerable amplification, may prefer the older style, body worn aid. This type of aid produces a greater amplification of sound than aural aids and has controls that are easier for the less dextrous to manipulate. The aid is connected to an earpiece mounted on an earmould by a cord. Those patients who cannot use an ear mould fitting in the external ear canal because of chronic otorrhoea can be fitted with a bone conductor (Corrado, 1988).

A major problem confronting users of all types of hearing aids is understanding speech in noisy environments. This is because aids amplify all noise regardless of its source, whereas the normal ear can discriminate and preferentially amplify speech. Directional microphones, which only detect sound in the direction they are pointing, are used to overcome this. If placed so that they are directed forwards, the speech of persons speaking to the aid user may be amplified while sound coming from other directions is amplified to a lesser extent.

At present, such microphones are limited by the short distance over which they are effective and by their inability to respond to changes in the level of background noise. One approach has been to use more than one directional microphone in the aid, aimed in different directions. This has been found to improve speech recognition in noisy environments (Peterson *et al.*, 1987). Future development of microphones will be directed towards finding an optimum number and direction of microphones compatible with preserving a cosmetically acceptable on-ear aid.

Amplification in patients with sensorineural hearing loss can also be complicated by a phenomenon known as recruitment (Cunningham and Ganzel, 1986). This causes an enormously increased sensation of loudness for only a modest increase in the intensity of the sound (Fowler 1936; Ballantyne, 1977). This hypersensitivity to loud sounds may make an amplified sound uncomfortable or unintelligible, which makes the fitting of hearing aids more difficult. In patients where recruitment is a problem, an automatic compression circuit can be fitted to the aid. This reduces the amplification produced by an aid immediately a loud sound occurs in the listening environment (Steinberg and Gardner, 1937; Riko, Pichora-Fuller, and Albert, 1986; Cunningham and Ganzel, 1986). It is now feasible to construct a low distortion, frequency dependent multichannel compression system, which may further improve speech intelligibility in most environments. At present, such devices are too bulky to win patient acceptance but further improvements should lead to reduction in size in the near future (Riko, Pichora-Fuller, and Albert, 1986).

Despite these major improvements in hearing aids over the last decade, patient acceptance is still low. In a survey of 200 patients, only 34% declared that they were very satisfied with their aid after six months of use; 66% declared that they were dissatisfied or only moderately satisfied with their device (Littlejohns and John, 1987). Therefore, there is still room for considerable improvement in hearing aid perform-ance. Patients need to be given a clear indication of what they can expect from their aid.

In the next decade the major improvements in hearing aid technology will probably come from the application of digital technology. Digital hearing aids promise many advantages including control of acoustic feedback and the use of advanced signal processing techniques for noise reduction (Levitt, 1987). A further research approach has been to investigate the feasibility of an implantable middle ear hearing device. One approach has been to use an electromagnetic transducer cemented to the head of the stapes (Maniglia *et al.*, 1988). This device acts by responding to incoming noise, producing a frequency and amplitude coded vibration, which stimulates the ossicular chain in the middle ear and hence the cochlear. At present this device has only been used experimentally in animals but it does show potential for further development.

Despite these improvements in hearing aid technology, patients with severe or total sensorineural deafness will not benefit by improvement in the amplification character-istics of hearing aids alone. In such patients, the development of a multi-electrode cochlear prosthetic implant to stimulate the auditory nerve has opened up the possibility of restoring some degree of hearing (Clark *et al.*, 1987).

Cochlear implants

The first reports of electrical stimulation of the acoustic nerve in man date from the late 1930s but it was not until 1968 that animal studies demonstrated that intracoch-lear electrodes could be maintained safely and remain functional for long periods of time (Michelson, 1971). The most successful of the multichannel cochlear implants so far was developed by an Australian group (Clark *et al.*, 1987). Their approach was to design a multichannel electrode in which only one channel is activated at a time (Pickett and McFarland, 1985). The electrode is inserted along the scala tympani after entering it through the round window. It is connected to a receiver–stimulator that is sited in a subcutaneous pocket located in a groove drilled over the mastoid and sutured into place. Using this device, many postlingually deaf adults can obtain significant help in understanding speech, when combined with lipreading, compared with lipreading alone. About 50% of patients are able to understand some speech using the device without the benefit of lipreading. The average patient should be able to understand considerable amounts of running speech using the cochlear implant in combination with lip reading (Pyman *et al.*, 1983; Clark *et al.*, 1984; Clark *et al.*, 1987).

For the most part, these devices have only been used in adults who have developed profound or total hearing loss after four years of age (postlingual deafness). In a recent preliminary study, it was found that prelingually deaf subjects may also receive some benefit from this device. They were able to understand words and running speech better when using the cochlear implant with lipreading compared to lipreading alone (Clark *et al.*, 1987).

Tactile aids

Another approach to aid the hearing of patients with profound or total deafness has been the development of tactile aids (Sherrick 1984; Pickett and McFarland, 1985). A number of different devices have been described. They may be used to stimulate the digital nerves of the hand or skin of the abdomen (Lynch *et al.*, 1989). One such device works in conjunction with the speech processor developed for use with the cochlear prosthetic implant. Eight electrodes are used, one on each side of each digit on one hand excluding the thumb. With training, patients are able to obtain useful information regarding the spoken word using tactile stimulation alone. The device supplements lipreading and can be used in conjunction with other types of hearing aids (Blamey *et al.*, 1988). Similar results have been reported for other types of tactile hearing aids (Lynch *et al.*, 1989). A related approach has been to locate a vibrating element within an earmould (Weisenberger, Heidbreder, and Miller, 1987).

IMPOTENCE AND PENILE PROSTHESES

Impotence is quite common and its prevalence increases with age. Between adolescence and 35 years of age, it is found in 0–2% of the male population. After this age, it becomes increasingly common and by 80 years of age, 75% of men describe themselves as impotent (Kinsey, Pomeroy, and Martin, 1947). Only a small proportion of these will request or require a penile prosthetic implant as their definitive management.

Impotence may be organic or psychogenic in origin. Distinguishing between them as causes of impotence needs careful history taking, examination, and appropriate laboratory investigations. The erectile mechanism in patients with psychogenic impotence is intact, but they are unable to sustain erections as a result of factors such as stress, anxiety, and depression (Krane, 1988; Smith, 1988). Treatment of this disorder should be directed towards the underlying cause, and clearly penile prostheses are inappropriate. Organic impotence may be due to a structural cause, such as Peyronie's disease or chordee, defects in the hormonal, vascular, or neurological mechanisms leading to erection, a side-effect of prescribed drug use, or a result of acute or chronic excessive alcohol intake (Krane, 1986; Wein and Van Arsdalen, 1988). The commonest cause of organic impotence is diabetes mellitus. The basis for this is probably an autonomic neuropathy but in some patients, large and small vessel disease may also contribute (Saenz de Tajeda and Goldstein, 1988). If the underlying cause of neurogenic impotence is not reversible and the patient desires erections, he should be treated initially using intracavernosis pharmacotherapy (Sidi, 1988). The patient self-injects the corpora cavernosa with agents (e.g. prostaglandins or papaverine) to produce erections. The injections need to be administered cautiously. Denervation hypersensitivity may result in an abrupt and sustained increase in corporal body pressure with the risk of inducing priapism if an excessive dose is administered. Penile prostheses should be reserved for patients with neurologic impotence when intracavernosis pharmacotherapy has either failed or proved unsatisfactory.

Penile prostheses

There are a large number of different types of penile prostheses on the market (Montague, 1989). Unfortunately they are expensive, particularly the inflatable types, and carry risks, such as infection, associated with their implantation. Before proceeding to implant a prosthesis, it is important to have detailed discussion with both the patient and his sexual partner. Patient expectation of the likely performance of the prosthesis is often unrealistically high, and he should be counselled in detail of what to expect from each type of available device. His sexual partner also needs to know what to expect, and be given the opportunity to express preferences and feelings towards the various types of prosthetic implants.

If it is decided to proceed, a choice of implant must then be made. This is essentially between a semirigid and an inflatable device. There are many different varieties of each on the market and the final choice probably depends as much to what the urologist is familiar with and has had success with, as on the individual merits of each device (Krane, 1989). In general, patients prefer the simpler, semirigid device and tend to avoid the apparently more complicated inflatable devices.

SEMIRIGID PROSTHESES

The major advantage of semirigid devices is the relative ease of surgery to implant them and the simplicity of use for the patient. The major drawback is that they do not provide extra length or width to the penis when in the activated state.

A semirigid device is the device of choice in patients with some remaining functional erectile tissue. Erectile tissue can aid the use of these devices by augmenting erection and providing extra length and width to the penis. Such patients can also use intracavernous pharmacotherapy to further augment erection. Inflatable devices are contra-indicated in such patients because most, if not all, erectile tissue must be removed during implantation (Krane, 1989).

The acceptance level of semirigid devices is quite high. In one survey of the Subrini implant, 70% of patients and their spouses were satisfied or very satisfied with intercourse (Subrini, 1982).

INFLATABLE DEVICES

The major advantage of an inflatable device, particularly those with a separate pump and reservoir, is the appearance of the penis, which closely resembles that of the natural organ in both the erect and flaccid state. Inflatable devices function like an inner tube within the corpora cavernosa. The device consists of two cylinders implanted within the corpora, which are connected by silicon tubing to a reservoir located in the paravesical space. The reservoir is in turn connected by tubing to a pump located in an intrascrotal pocket. The pump inflates the cylinders, which causes distention of the corpora with resultant rigidity; deflation produces a return to normal flaccidity. The major disadvantage of such multicomponent inflatable devices has been their tendency for component failure, which requires further surgery to correct the fault.

The situations where an inflatable prosthesis should be considered are: neurogenic impotence with no residual functioning erectile tissue; if the patient desires full flaccidity in the resting state; and if the patient requires repeat endoscopic procedures for other urological problems. Inflatable prostheses should not be used in patients with a history of priapism. In such patients, semirigid devices should be used.

Although patients are less likely to choose an inflatable device than a semirigid device when given the choice, patients with inflatable devices are generally happy with the results as are their partners (Apte, Gregory, and Purcell, 1984; Hollander and Diokno, 1984).

In an attempt to combine the simplicity of semirigid devices with the advantages of inflatable devices, self-contained inflatable devices have been introduced. These contain an inner compartment made of non-distensible material, an outer compartment of pliable silicon, and a proximal reservoir. Compression of a pump located in the tip of the cylinders, transfers fluid from the reservoir to the inner chamber thereby stiffening the cylinders. Deflation is accomplished by either squeezing a valve or by a downward flexion motion (Krane, 1988).

References

Apte SM, Gregory JG, Purcell MH (1984) The inflatable penile prosthesis, reoperation and patient satisfaction: A comparison of statistics obtained from patient record review with statistics obtained from intensive follow up search, *J Urol*, **131**, 894–5

Ballantyne J (1977) *Deafness*, 3rd Edn, Edinburgh, Churchill Livingstone, 61–80

Bender LF (1982) Upper extremity prostheses. In Kottke FJ, Stillwell GK, and Lehmann JF, eds, *Krusen's Handbook of Physical Medicine and Rehabilitation*, 3rd Edn, Philadelphia, WB Saunders, 906–20

Blamey PJ, Cowan RSC, Alcantara JI and Clark GM (1988) Phonemic information transmitted by a multichannel electrotactile speech processor, *J Speech Hear Res*, **31**, 620–9

Brindley GS and Lewin WS (1968) The sensations produced by electrical stimulation of the visual cortex, *J Physiol*, **196**, 479–93

Clark GM, Blamey PJ, Brown AM, Busby PA, Dowell RC, Franz BK-H et al. (1987) The University of Melbourne – Nucleus Multi-electrode cochlear implant, *Adv Oto-Rhino-Laryngology*, **38**

Clark GM, Dowell RC, Pyman BC, Brown AM, Webb RL, Tong YC et al. (1984) Clinical trial of multichannel cochlear prosthesis. Results on 10 postlingually deaf patients, *Aust NZ J Surg*, **54**, 519–26

Corrado OJ (1988) Hearing aids, *Br Med J*, **296**, 33–5

Cotoyannis B, Blackney H, Angliss V, and Fahrer M (1988) A modified electric hand, *J Rehabil Res Dev*, **25**(Suppl), 37

Cunningham DR and Ganzel TM (1986) Hearing aids for adults: A primer for the physician. *J Ky Med Assoc*, **84**, 549–53

Das TK and Park DM (1989) Effect of treatment with botulinum toxin on spasticity. *Postgrad Med J*, **65**, 208–10

Dobelle WH, Mladejevsky MG, and Girvin JP (1974) Artificial vision for the blind: electrical stimulation of visual cortex offers hope for a functional prosthesis, *Science*, **183**, 440–4

Edbrooke H (1970) The Royal Salop Infirmary clicking splint, *Physiotherapy*, **56**, 148–52

Fowler EP (1936) Methods for early detection of otosclerosis; study of sounds well above threshold, *Arch Otolaryngol*, **24**, 731–41

Girvin JP (1988) Current status of artificial vision by electrocortical stimulation, *Can J Neurol Sci*, **15**, 58–62

Goodwill JC (1988) Orthotics (Callipers & Appliances). In Goodwill JC and Chamberlain MA, eds, *Rehabilitation of the physically disabled adult*, London, Croom Helm, 741–74

Hollander JB and Diokno AC (1984) Success with penile prothesis from patient's viewpoint, *Urology*, **23**, 141–3

Kinsey AC, Pomeroy WB, and Martin CE (1948) In *Sexual behaviour in the human male*, Philadelphia, WB Saunders, 235–8

Krane RJ (1986) Sexual function and dysfunction. In Walsh PC, Gittes RF, Perlmutter AD, and Stamey TA, eds, *Urology* Vol 3, 5th Edn, Philadelphia, WB Saunders, 700–10

Krane RJ (1988) Penile prostheses, *Urol Clin North Am*, **15**, 103–9

Krane RJ (1989) Malleable and mechanical penile prostheses. In Carlton CE, ed, *Controversies in Urology*, Chicago, Year Book Medical, 120–5

Lamb DW, Dick TD, and Douglas WB (1988) A new prosthesis for the upper limb, *J Bone Joint Surg*, **70-B**, 140–4

Lehmann JF, Condon SM, deLateur BJ, and Price R (1986) Gait abnormalities in peroneal nerve paralysis and their corrections by orthoses, *Arch Phys Med Rehabil*, **67**, 380–6

Levitt H (1987) Digital hearing aids: A tutorial review, *J Rehabil Res Dev*, **24**, 7–20

Lewin W (1971) Towards a visual prosthesis, *Clin Neurosurg*, **18**, 155–65

Liberson WT, Holmquest HJ, Scot D, and Dow M (1961) Functional electrotherapy: Stimulation of the peroneal nerve synchronized with the swing phase of the gait of hemiplegic patients, *Arch Phys Med Rehabil*, **42**, 101–5

Littlejohns P and John AC (1987) Auditory rehabilitation; should we listen to the patient?, *Lancet*, **294**, 1063–4

Lynch MP, Eilers RE, Oller DK, and Cobo-Lewis A (1989) Multisensory speech perception by profoundly hearing impaired children, *J Speech Hear Disord*, **54**, 57–67

Maniglia AJ, Ko WH, Zhang RX, Dolgin SR, Rosenbaum ML, and Montague FW (1988) Electromagnetic implantable middle ear hearing device of the ossicular-stimulating type; principles, designs and experiments, *Ann Otol Rhinol Laryngol*, **97** (Suppl 136), 1–16

Marsolais EB and Edwards BG (1988) Energy costs of walking and standing with functional neuromuscular stimulation and long leg braces, *Arch Phys Med Rehabil*, **69**, 243–9

McClelland M, Andrews BJ, Patrick JH, Freeman PA, and El Masri WS (1987) Augmentation of the Oswestry Parawalker orthosis by means of surface electrical stimulation. Gait analysis of three patients, *Paraplegia*, **25**, 32–8

Mendez MA (1985) Evaluation of a myoelectric hand prosthesis for children with a below elbow absence, *Prosthet Orthot Int*, **9**, 137–40

Michelson RP (1971) Electrical stimulation of the human cochlea, *Arch Otolaryngol*, **93**, 317–23

Millstein SG, Heger H, and Hunter GA (1986) Prosthetic use in adult upper limb amputees. A comparison of the body powered and electrically powered prostheses, *Prosthet Orthot Int*, **10**, 27–34

Montague DK (1989), ed, Genitourinary prostheses, *Urol Clin North Am*, **16**

Motlock WJ and Elliott J (1966) Fitting and training children with swivel walkers, *Artif Limbs*, **10**, 27–38

Nene AV and Jennings SJ (1989) Hybrid paraplegic locomotion with the Parawalker using intramuscular stimulation. A single subject study, *Paraplegia*, **27**, 125–32

Nene AV and Major RE (1987) Dynamics of reciprocal gait of adult paraplegics using the Parawalker (Hip guidance orthosis), *Prosthet Orthot Int*, **11**, 124–7

Ober JK (1982) Upper limb prosthetics for high level arm amputation, *Prosthet Orthot Int*, **6**, 17–20

Paparella MM and Davis H (1978) Medical and Surgical treatment of hearing loss, In Davis H and Silverman SR, eds, *Hearing and Deafness*, 4th Edn, New York, Holt, Rinehart and Winston, 162–76

Peterson PM, Durlach NI, Rabinowitz WM, and Zurek PM (1987) Multimicrophone adaptive beamforming for interference reduction in hearing aids, *J Rehabil Res Dev*, **24**, 103–10

Pickett JM and McFarland W (1985) Auditory implants and tactile aids for the profoundly deaf, *J Speech Hear Res*, **28**, 134–50

Pyman BC, Clark GM, Webb RL, Brown AM, Bailey QE, and Luscombe SM (1983) The clinical trial of multichannel cochlear prosthesis, *J Otolaryngol Soc Aust*, **5**, 43–6

Roberts C and Porter D (1988) Bioengineering in Rehabilitation, In Goodwill JC and Chamberlain MA, eds, *Rehabilitation of the physically disabled adult*, London, Croom Helm, 741–74

Riko K, Pichora-Fuller MK, and Albert PW (1986) Clinical evaluation of a two-channel amplitude compression hearing aid, *Laryngoscope*, **96**, 1226–30

Rose GK (1979) The principles and practice of hip guidance articulations, *Prosthet Orthot Int*, **3**, 37–43

Rose GK and Henshaw JT (1972) A swivel walker for paraplegics; medical and technical considerations, *Biomed Eng*, **7**, 420–5

Saenz de Tejada I and Goldstein I (1988) Diabetic penile neuropathy, *Urol Clin North Am*, **15**, 17–22

Sauter WF (1981) Myoelectric and microswitch controlled upper extremity prostheses. In Kostuik JP, ed, *Amputation Surgery and Rehabilitation: The Toronto Experience*, New York, Churchill Livingstone, 367–83

Scott RN and Parker PA (1988) Myoelectric prostheses: State of the art, *J Med Eng Technol*, **12**, 143–51

Sidi AA (1988) Vasoactive intracavernous pharmacotherapy, *Urol Clin North Am*, **15**, 95–101

Sherrick CE (1984) Basic and applied research on tactile aids for deaf people. Progress and prospects, *J Acoust Soc Am*, **75**, 1325–42

Smith AD (1988) Psychologic factors in the multidisciplinary evaluation and treatment of erectile dysfunction, *Urol Clin North Am*, **15**, 41–52

Stallard J, Rose GK, and Farmer IR (1978) The ORLAU swivel walker, *Prosthet Orthot Int*, **2**, 35–42

Stein RB and Walley M (1983) Functional comparison of upper extremity amputees using myoelectric and conventional prostheses, *Arch Phys Med Rehabil*, **64**, 243–8

Steinberg JC and Gardner MB (1937) The dependence of hearing impairment on sound intensity, *J Acoust Soc Am*, **56**, 1601–11

Subrini L (1982) Subrini penile implants. Surgical, sexual and psychological results, *Eur Urol*, **8**, 222–6

Turk R and Obreza P (1985) Functional electrical stimulation as an orthotic means for the rehabilitation of paraplegic patients, *Paraplegia*, **23**, 344–8

Wein AJ, Van Arsdalen KN (1988) Drug induced male sexual dysfunction, *Urol Clin North Am*, **15**, 23–32

Weisenberger JM, Heidbreder AF, and Miller JD (1987) Development and evaluation of an earmould sound-to-tactile aid for the hearing impaired, *J Rehabil Res Dev*, **24**, 51–66

Wilson LA and Wilson KS (1988) Hearing aids, *Postgrad Med*, **83**, 249–56

8
Bio-feedback and principles of motor learning in the rehabilitation of movement disorders

Aftab E. Patla and Ronald G. Marteniuk

The term bio-feedback is generic and is used to characterize any form of 'augmented' feedback of some parameter(s) of a biological system. The demonstration of control and regulation of variables, that were hitherto considered under autonomic control and hence inaccessible, provided the impetus for research in bio-feedback as a tool for treatment of various disorders. One of the most common and probably easiest demonstrations of bio-feedback is the reduction in muscle activity around the temporal region to relieve tension headache. Applying similar principles to the rehabilitation of movement disorders is a natural extension. The focus of this chapter is to examine the various uses of bio-feedback in the treatment of movement disorders, and use the successes and failures to highlight important issues in this area.

To provide a framework for classifying the large variety of movement disorders that are encountered, it is important to review current knowledge of control of movement. Humans have developed a vast repertoire of movements, a legacy of evolution that did not commit the upper limb to specific functions. To perform these movements, humans have a complex control and effector system. Researchers have tried to understand how the various structures within the nervous system control movement, and how this harnesses the large degrees of freedom found within the effector system. Although neurophysiological studies have been successful in characterizing functions of various subsystems in isolation, understanding of even the simplest functional movement, such as control of upper arm flexion extension at the elbow joint, is far from complete (cf. Gottlieb, Corcos, and Agarwal, 1988).

There are a few known general aspects related to movement control that can be stated. First, the feedback from visual, vestibular, and proprioceptive systems is essential for control of movement. This is not only in corrective action, but also in the execution of normal movement. For example, during locomotion, even on a treadmill which represents a rather sterile and stereotyped environment, research has shown that absence of peripheral feedback has an effect on activation profiles of certain muscles (Belanger, Drew, and Rossignol, 1988). Second, the execution of movement not only involves setting the appropriate motor commands to the muscles, but also pre-setting the sensory system. For example, during locomotion the gain of the stretch reflex is set such that functionally appropriate, rather than stimulus dependent, response is elicited during gait (Stein and Capaday, 1987). Third, stereotypical rhythmic movements, such as locomotion, can be restructured to meet the demands of the environment, goal of the animal, or both (Drew, 1988; Patla *et al.*, 1989, 1990). These changes are not a simple modification of the basic pattern, but represent substantial changes to the movement pattern to achieve the desired goal. This flexibility in the basic movement patterns bodes well for treatment of movement disorders. The emphasis on examples from the locomotion literature is partially because this movement, unlike other episodic movement, has been studied most extensively, and also because independent locomotor ability has occupied a large portion of the rehabilitative efforts.

Therefore, movement disorders can be classified broadly into three categories: those resulting from damage to one or more of the sensory modalities; those caused by damage of structures within the nervous system that are responsible for planning sensory-motor commands; and those resulting from damage to the effector system. Examples of movement disorders from each of these categories highlight important issues in the use of bio-feedback in rehabilitation of movement disorders.

REHABILITATION OF MOVEMENT DISORDERS CAUSED BY DAMAGE TO SENSORY MODALITIES

Damage to the visual system, whether partial or complete, is one of the more common and debilitating deteriorations of a sensory modality, which has a dire consequence on learning and execution of voluntary movements. Particularly affected are orientation and mobility skills. The National Accreditation Council for Agencies Serving the Blind and Visually Handicapped defines orientation and mobility skills as the ability to 'move from one place to another with confidence, safety, and purpose'. The majority of research on mobility skills has been conducted on individuals who are totally blind (Strelow, 1985; Brown and Brabyn, 1987) and hence see no forms, colour, or motion. The emphasis is, as expected, on substituting for the loss of visual information on sensory modalities, and developing training programs for teaching the use of substitute information for guiding locomotion. Legal blindness is simply predicated on 6/60 (20/200) as an arbitrary level of best acuity performance, or 20 degrees as the maximum dimension of the visual field. Researchers estimate that as many as 90% of the legally blind population retain some level of usable vision (Riley, 1969; Kahn and Moorehead, 1973; Bailey, 1978; Genesky, 1978). Low vision describes a condition of diminished visual capability, which cannot be improved by routine medical, surgical, or refractive intervention to a sufficient level that would enable an individual to adequately perform common tasks requiring vision. More people have visual impairment than those who are legally blind (Riley, 1969; Bailey, 1978; Genesky, 1978). Mobility programs developed for the blind are by default applied to individuals who have retained some visual function. This is due to paucity of research on minimum visual capacity required for mobility (Beggs, 1986; Brown and Brabyn, 1987), which has an important bearing on the nature of substitution of visual information required for those who are totally blind.

It is clear that no external device can match the richness of information provided by the visual system. The travelling aids developed produce impoverished, albeit useful, information for purposeful travel. The types of travelling aids developed, their successes, and failure highlight issues related to bio-feedback as a tool for sensory substitution.

The travelling aid that comes closest to the visual system is the one originally proposed by a Polish researcher in 1897 (Jansson, 1990) involving transformation of visual into cutaneous stimuli. The principle of operation is relatively simple. Capture an image, process it for salient features, convert this into a matrix of on-off patterns, and stimulate the skin electrically via an array of electrodes or mechanically via an array of vibrators attached to the skin, with the matrix array ranging from 400 to 1024 (cf. Bach-y-Rita *et al.*, 1969; Bach-y-Rita, 1972; Kurcz, 1974; Palacz, 1975; Collins, 1985). The use of such aids for travel has not progressed beyond the laboratory environment with the majority of studies dealing with the ability of subjects to recognize the scene when provided the cutaneous stimuli. Of particular relevance is the kind of information fed back to the subject. The on-off patterns are most conducive to providing edge and core features that allow the subject to recognize presence of obstacles or openings such as doors. If that is not the goal then simpler devices will suffice.

The most successful travelling aid for the blind is the simple long cane. Haptic exploration extended and facilitated by the long cane allows the blind to scan their immediate environment and identify low, small obstacles, unevenness in the surface, and curbs (Welsh and Blasch, 1980). The use of echoes created by the cane (and footsteps) to detect obstacles and some features of the surface characteristics is an important skill developed by the blind (cf. Rice and Feinstein, 1965; Schenkman, 1985, 1986; Schenkman and Jansson, 1986); although Strelow and Brabyn (1982) found this to be limited to larger size obstacles. The one area where the cane is deficient is in detection of obstacles above waist level. Also the preview of the environment is limited by the length of the cane. To overcome these problems, researchers have developed electronic travel aids that the subject either carries in the hand or can be attached to the head. A widely used hand held device is a Mowat's sensor (Pressey, 1977), which uses the haptic system to convey information. The Sonic guide, which can be mounted on the head or chest, uses the auditory channel (cf. Kay, 1974).

All of these devices discussed above work as a clear path finder for safe travel rather than providing a detailed image of the environment. Blind people augment this immediate information with cognitive spatial maps developed to chart their travel course. The regularity and predictability of city and town environment greatly facilitates their travel. It is interesting to note the problems that visually impaired people have identified. They are uncomfortable in unfamiliar neighbourhoods suggesting a problem with orientation (and spatial maps); they have difficulty with small and horizontal objects, and uneven surfaces in the path of travel; they have no problems with large objects; and they have difficulty with night travel and going from broad daylight to dimly lit areas (Genesky *et al.*, 1979; Passini, Dupre, and Langlois, 1986).

The learning or training time for purposeful travel for the blind is important from the rehabilitation perspective. The National Institutes for the Blind have developed training courses for instructors who train the blind. These are three months long followed by a two-month practical course where essentially they would have to travel in a familiar city or town environment blindfolded. The earliest training for the blind begins at approximately five years of age and would involve a minimum 100 hours of instruction. Developing cane skills requires additional time which is usually a minimum of 50 hours. The two important aspects that emerge from this are commitment for long training and early intervention. When rehabilitation protocols are not successful, lack of attention to these two factors are often responsible. We should not be surprised by the long training period. Most of our movement skills are developed over long duration of trial and error, and is clear when one observes motor skill development in children. Early intervention is important to offset any self-selection of undesirable patterns of movement and posture. In fact, in spinal cord injured patients, lack of demonstration of rhythmic movement elicitation by pharmacologic means (to release the inherent motor patterns) is attributed to the delay in treatment (cf. Rossignol, 1988).

Rehabilitation of patients who have problems with sensory modalities other than vision is also a challenging problem. For example, people with inner ear problems have tremendous problems maintaining balance when they turn abruptly during travel. Most people learn to live with this and adapt movement patterns to avoid these situations. Loss of proprioceptive information, such as in patients with diabetic neuropathy, has a profound influence on movements. Diabetic patients get ulcers on their feet from repeated stress on the injured area (cf. Cavanagh *et al.*, 1986); they are also more prone to falls because of a delayed or absent corrective response when gait is obstructed. Bio-feedback of pressure patterns under the feet to change their foot fall patterns to avoid ulcers would be an interesting area of research.

REHABILITATION OF MOVEMENT DISORDERS CAUSED BY DAMAGE TO THE CENTRAL NERVOUS SYSTEM

In trauma of the central nervous system, both motor outflow and sensory system priming are affected. The effect on the motor system is secondary and usually follows from disuse. The challenge for rehabilitation is enormous. We will use the rehabilitation of stroke patients to illustrate salient issues.

Strokes have a debilitating impact on ambulatory skills, and therefore major effort is directed towards improving locomotor capability. Blind people in the earlier examples could locomote well when they are escorted by another person. Changes in gait patterns that result are caused by loss of visual information. In contrast, the stroke patient has to basically recalibrate and learn to perform most movements, including locomotion, in a different way. The traditional rehabilitation method relies on neuromuscular facilitation through passive movements (cf. Bobath, 1970; Brunnstrom, 1970), strengthening of specific muscle groups, and asking the patients to perform various movements repeatedly. In most cases, isolated movements are practiced rather than locomotion, which is of interest. Evaluation of efficacy of this treatment is confounded by normal recovery process. The feedback that the subject receives is non-specific and most often related to some overall measure of movement outcome. In the case of locomotion, it is the distance travelled and time taken to traverse the distance giving an estimate of average velocity.

The use of more specific feedback may result in better improvement in performance, faster rehabilitation, or both. There is some basis for this hypothesis. Controlled trials on stroke patients have shown that movement related specific feedback led to a clinically significant improvement and was better than traditional exercise programs (cf. Burnside, Tobias, and Bursill, 1982; Shahani, Connors, and Mohr, 1977; Hogue and McCandless, 1983). There are several issues that have to be considered in this mode of treatment.

First, and perhaps most important, is the selection of appropriate parameters for feedback, in which biomechanical analyses of movement can help. For example, Olney and co-workers have examined hemiplegic gait from an energy perspective (Olney and Grondin, 1988; Olney *et al.*, 1988), specifically identifying deficits in propulsive power that can slow down the gait. These studies have identified reduced push-off action in the late stance phase to account for most of the speed reduction.

Since push-off action in the late stance phase is primarily achieved by the plantar-flexor group, feedback of the relevant muscle activity for possible regulation would be appropriate, and is currently pursued by this research group. In an earlier study they used joint angle feedback to increase knee flexion during push-off and early pull-off, and showed objective improvement in gait (Olney, Colborne, and Martin, 1989).

Second, the training of individual muscles or a muscle group assumes that the nervous system controls their activation. Researchers in motor control agree that the locus of control in any movement does lie at the individual muscle level simply because the control of large degrees of freedom would be tremendous. How the nervous system reduces the potentially large degrees of freedom is a major question in motor control. There are numerous connections between various muscle groups, which can be used to coordinate activity of groups of muscles. For example, Ia facilitatory connections between the triceps surae group could coordinate the push-off action at the ankle in the stance phase with the pull-off action in the early swing phase (cf. Pierrot-Deseilligny, Bergego, and Mazieres, 1983). Similarly, extension braking action at the knee by the hamstrings during late swing can be coordinated with the quadriceps action in the early swing through connections between antagonist muscles. This suggests that feedback and control of a single muscle group during locomotion may have effects on activation levels of other muscles, which has to be recognized in the evaluation of treatment.

Third, bio-feedback training should be performed during the execution of an actual movement of interest (locomotion) rather than training the patients to control the activation of the muscle during isolated movement of the joint. From an instrumentation perspective, it is easier to do feedback training while the subject is seated than during locomotion. Studies have shown that improvements following training are task-specific and show poor transfer to other functions. This is not surprising because the use of multiple muscles in various movements is highly task-specific. For example, during walking the major source of power is from the plantarflexor muscles, whereas during stair climbing, the quadriceps group becomes dominant. One problem of using task- and phase-specific feedback is that it can only be given in the subsequent cycle following processing of the data. If that feedback is not received in the beginning of the next cycle, then the response will be delayed by two cycles because of reaction and planning time limitations. An important issue is the ability of subjects to control not only level of activation or inhibition, but also the shape of the profile, which has an effect on the net output. The latter may be much more difficult, especially for patients, and may require extensive training. Most of the studies on bio-feedback have been restricted to training subjects to regulate the level of activation.

So far we have talked mainly about affecting motor output. Sensory priming on the other hand is less amenable to bio-feedback. It is known that spinal cord injured patients do not show the same modulation of stretch reflex as normal subjects: the gain is higher, which can impede their movements. Here researchers are attempting to use another reflex, the flexion reflex, to provide functional improvement. But this aspect of regulation is probably not amenable to voluntary control.

REHABILITATION OF MOVEMENT DISORDERS CAUSED BY DAMAGE TO THE MOTOR SYSTEM

In this category of movement disorders, we are primarily dealing with patients whose limb segments are amputated. The most common form of rehabilitation is the prescription of a prosthesis. Lower limb prostheses are mainly passive devices, which have to be controlled by the residual musculature. For upper limbs, powered prostheses are much more common. This may in part be due to the larger repertoire of possible movements with the upper limbs compared to lower limbs. The use of passive prostheses during locomotion is greatly facilitated by the dynamics, mainly the pendular action during swing phase. The harnessing of the dynamics, and compensation by the other muscles to provide propulsive power and stability, allows subjects to travel relatively easily. Clearly, the learning curve and training aspects would be different for the two types of prostheses.

One of the major concerns of patients using a prosthesis is the lack of feedback. This is particularly acute for lower limb prostheses where use of vision is not possible. Above-knee amputees have always expressed their fear of tripping because of lack of knowledge of the artificial limb segment position. This forces them to overcompensate to ensure adequate ground clearance, which entails higher energy cost. It is here that assistive feedback can help, although the problem is not trivial. During normal locomotion, most subjects clear the ground by less than one centimetre (Winter, 1987). The position of the toe at that point can be affected by actions of both the stance and swing limb. The degrees of freedom are large. Normally this is done with ease, which results from the complex control system for locomotion, although normal subjects are also prone to tripping by small unevenness in the terrain if anticipatory action is not taken; they can easily recover from a trip by taking a stumbling, corrective action. The problem for the above-knee, or even below-knee amputees, is far more serious. The potential for knee collapse causing falls is greater. This has to be considered when training patients to use a prosthesis. It may be that more varied terrains should be incorporated in their training regime, and in a controlled environment, they can be taught how to recover from a trip, which is similar to downhill skiing lessons. This reflects the variability issue in learning, which is evident when observing an infant learning to walk; the child is exposed to different terrains and learns, over a relatively long period, to adapt the locomotor patterns for different environments.

The control of upper limb powered prostheses normally involves using residual muscles to trigger specific functions (Parker and Scott, 1986; Scott, 1990a, 1990b). There are two alternatives in the use of powered prostheses. Firstly, several muscles can be used, with activation of each tied to a specific function of the prosthesis. The problems with this mode of control are: multiple muscles may not be easily available; learning to activate different muscles requires more training; and the normal use of these muscles around the residual body segments is affected if they are to be used to activate a specific function when they are supposed to be inhibited. Secondly, the use of a single muscle site, which alleviates some of the problems mentioned above. Usually, level of activation is used to trigger specific functions. But there are problems. Because of the inherent variability in raw EMG, it is impossible to have a large number of levels of activation. Reducing the variability by processing the signal, such as filtering, affects the response time. The probability of errors increases with the number of levels required. So far, a three state control has proved to be most robust in terms of minimum errors in performance, but this limits the number of functions that can be controlled. The proportional control of specific functions is still in the early stages. Therefore, a prosthesis that can match even some of the versatility of the human hand needs more research. Particularly, building better processing of control signals to maximize the use of existing functions in current prostheses is needed. The problem of lack of feedback is similar to the lower limb. In this case, the parameter that needs to be fedback is the level of force applied by the manipulated object to ensure no unfortunate accidents occur. To provide unobtrusive control, transduction of the force signal into audio-feedback is not desirable. Researchers have used cutaneous receptors to transmit the appropriate information, and relieve the load on the visual system.

The above discussion highlights some of the fundamental control and learning issues that have to be considered when using bio-feedback in the rehabilitation of movement disorders. How to evaluate the success of these procedures, and trying to sort out other confounding factors, such as motivation, placebo effect, and normal recovery process, is an important but separate issue (cf. Wolf, 1983). Since learning plays such an integral part in all aspects of rehabilitation, we need to understand basic principles of human learning, which has potential implications for improvement of patient performance. This is discussed under motor learning principles, below.

MOTOR LEARNING PRINCIPLES

Principles for the use of bio-feedback in enhancing rehabilitation must be consistent with principles of motor learning. Two issues in motor learning research that have direct relevance to facilitating learning in a rehabilitation setting are the sensorimotor basis for motor learning and the specificity of learning.

The sensorimotor basis for motor learning

Any attempt at understanding the principles involved in the acquisition of coordinated movement must address how the central nervous system deals with the large number of degrees of freedom represented by the joints, and the permissible motions of the complex biokinematic chains that are represented in the musculoskeletal system. There are two concerns here. First, the observation that despite the apparent complexity involved in controlling the large number of degrees of freedom, the mature, normal person has no problem in mastering complex skills. Second, highly skilled individuals exhibit flexibility in that they can realize the same result in a large number of ways (e.g. one can throw an object in a large number of different ways but still hit the target).

Traditionally, mastering of the degrees of freedom in motor control while allowing for flexibility in skill attainment, has been explained by the acquisition of motor programs (Schmidt, 1975). From this view, classes of movement have generalized motor programs and before execution these programs are parameterized with movement parameters specific to the needs of the task. Motor programming theory has been criticized on the grounds that one central controller (the motor program) cannot possibly compute the necessary detail to plan and execute movements with large degrees of freedom. To overcome this limitation, distributed processing views are advocated (Allport, 1980) where the control of movement is distributed over autonomous subsystems. These subsystems have the ability to control certain aspects of the total movement and the responsibility of the central controller is to coordinate appropriate subsystems so that the complete task can be carried out. The central controller in a distributed processing system does not directly enter into the control process (executive ignorance) and hence its computational load is relatively light.

While distributed processing views have come from disciplines like artificial intelligence, psychologists have approached the degrees of freedom problem in a similar way. Bruner (1971), for example, described skilled activity as a program specifying an objective to be obtained and requiring the serial ordering of a set of modular subroutines. The subroutines initially come from an innate repertoire of reflex-based patterns. These patterns are evoked by appropriate interaction with the environment, and are derived from the differentiation of initially gross acts into component elements that achieve independence from their original context. A similar approach has been advocated by Fitts (1964) where he maintains that past six years of age, all human beings have the necessary subroutines (automatic sequences of activity) to learn any novel movement.

Therefore, one way of viewing coordinated performance would be to postulate that, for example, the upper limbs are two relatively independent subsystems and, perhaps, each has subsystems within it. Evidence for this comes from the work of Jeannerod (1981) who has shown two components to a single arm reaching task; one component concerned with moving the hand to the object and another with orienting the hand to the object. Also, as Greene (1982) points out, arm movements can be likened to a spring model of control that allows the relatively easy specifications of such movement parameters as end location and speed. Therefore, by invoking the concept of relatively autonomous subsystems underlying movement control, one aspect of the degrees of freedom problem (the large number) for coordinated performance can be solved. That is, relatively large numbers of degrees of freedom are controlled collectively through an autonomous subsystem. However, to explain the flexibility a skilled person demonstrates in achieving a given goal requires further elaboration.

This latter problem deals with the question of how the various subsystems are brought together to produce flexible but coordinated movement. The contention here is that this problem, central to understanding motor coordination, can be understood by considering that at the base of all coordinated movement is an integrated store of sensory and motor information, which defines relations among body parts for the achievement of goals (see MacKenzie and Marteniuk, 1985a, 1985b). The actual expression of coordinated movement, however, is modified by an interplay of motor and sensory information that fine tunes movement to the specific content of the situation. Therefore, motor coordination can be described as a type of multimovement coordination, where the process of sensorimotor integration underlies coordination of movement components. The term multimovement coordination, from Abbs, Gracco, and Cole (1984), is used to describe this kind of coordination.

An example of multimovement coordination can be found in insect flight. Altman (1982) has discussed the relationship between the concepts of the central pattern generator and sensory inputs in terms of their contributions to insect flight. Evidence shows that phasic sensory inputs play a crucial role in regulating the output of the central pattern generator. These sensory inputs come not only from wing receptors, but also from the head, tail, and, perhaps, the entire body surface. More importantly, the inputs from the central pattern generator and sensory receptors during flight summate to produce a stable yet flexible motor output. In fact, Altman raises the possibility that there may be no such thing as a central pattern generator but rather a flying insect might be more properly thought of as a combination of components, mechanical, sensory, and central neurons, all oscillating in resonance at flight frequency.

Analogous examples to the above can be found in human motor behavior. The work of Abbs and his colleagues, summarized in Abbs and Gracco (1983), shows that coordination of multiple speech movements is not entirely preprogrammed but is subject to refinement through sensorimotor feedforward adjustments. Evidence for this comes from data showing that during speech, when the lower lip is perturbed, compensations occur in synergistic movements of the upper lip. This is significant since the lower and upper lip are controlled independently, thus ruling out a closed-loop process. It is believed that the basis for this open-loop adjustment is a sensorimotor translation, established through prior experience, between the lower-lip afferent signals and upper-lip motor actions. Abbs and Gracco call this sensorimotor translation a predictive or feedforward process.

Feedforward processes have also been implicated in the interaction of postural muscles with muscles involved in rapid arm movements. Work has shown that leg stabilizers produce EMG responses about 50 milliseconds prior to EMG appearance in an arm that must be rapidly moved (Nashner and Cordo, 1981). Data like these implicate a feedforward anticipation of the kinematic consequences of the muscular contractions in the prime mover.

The nature of feedforward processes is such that a movement is generated to cancel a previously generated error, before that error can cause a functional disturbance in the motor output (Ito, 1975). Houk and Rymer (1981) postulate that in multimovement coordination, the feedforward controller consists of a neural model of the motor system that translates a predicted error in one component of the movement to an adjustment in a synergistic movement, which cancels the effect of the error on the functional output of the multicomponent movement.

Abbs, Gracco, and Cole (1984) and MacKenzie and Marteniuk (1985a, 1985b) have commented on how such a system might be acquired. Prediction in such a system is derived from past experience where the relationship between afferent signals from muscles comprising the system are related to efferent signals to the same muscles. In other words, sensory events are coded in efferent terms. The establishment of this representation (the neural model) is specific for each learned task. Abbs, Gracco, and Cole (1984) point out that to implement the interdependent actions that make up a compound motor gesture, a motor program is constructed, which results in the establishment of pertinent sensorimotor contingencies that ensure coordination of the multiple movement to one common goal. When executed, the movement is dependent on the exact demands of the environment, in that the program only sets up the correct patterns of interaction among the components of the movement. Hence, it is the result of the initial planning and the resulting interaction among the components of the multimovement that determine the exact nature of the motor output. In this way, it makes sense to not build conceptually too much into the motor program because feedback and feedforward processes can efficiently and rapidly guide movement to accomplish the goal.

The above account of motor learning has direct relevance to rehabilitation settings. The fact that a sensorimotor store of pertinent information is developed over learning, implies that this store would need to be recalibrated if normal sensory or motor information were eliminated, such as in the use of prosthetic limbs, or in stroke patients where some aspects of the motor command is lost. The emphasis for the therapist, therefore, would be to identify or create new sources of augmented feedback that the patient can use for motor control purposes and for learning to interrelate with appropriate efferent information. It is not until a modified sensorimotor store is created, allowing feedforward as well as feedback processes to operate, that relatively efficient movement will be realized.

Decisions regarding what sources of feedback should be used in rehabilitating movement must be guided by the next most important principle of motor learning, the specificity of learning.

The specificity of motor learning

When an individual is deprived of a normal source of feedback as a result of injury or amputation, feedback for movement relearning must come from a different source of intrinsic feedback (e.g. using vision exclusively to guide a prosthetic limb, with kinesthesis being non-existent) or augmented feedback must be used (e.g. as previously mentioned, use of joint angle feedback to increase knee flexion during push-off and early pull-off in the late stance phase of gait). We have indicated that a biomechanical analysis of movement may aid in the selection of appropriate parameters for feedback, but there is also the problem of determining whether the selected feedback will actually support performance as it occurs in everyday life. In other words, whereas some sources of feedback may work in the rehabilitation setting, in that improvement of movement coordination is observed, it may be that once the patient leaves the clinic, and attempts to incorporate the newly acquired movement into every day activities, the movement cannot be performed as efficiently. This type of situation demonstrates the specificity of motor learning, which has been amply supported by research.

Proteau and co-workers have written on the theory of the specificity of motor learning and produced some intriguing evidence in support of it (Proteau *et al.*, 1987). In their study, they had one group of people practise an arm pointing task without being able to see their arm or where their hands hit the target (people were given oral feedback by the experimenter on how close they had come to the target). Another group practised with full vision of their arms and the target acquisition. After four days of practise, the full vision group were transferred to the condition of the other group and their performance, which had been vastly superior with vision, immediately degraded to a level worse than that of the group that had been practising without vision all along. This study not only demonstrated that vision is necessary even for skills that are highly practised, but because performance without vision was so poor, it showed that learning was quite specific to the feedback conditions present during skill acquisition. Although kinesthesis was obviously present for this group as they practised the skill with full vision of their movements, this latter sensory information was not used in the same way as in the condition where subjects practised without vision. In terms of the sensorimotor view of learning described above, it appears that the sensorimotor store, which is established through learning, is very sensitive to the context of the learning situation. When the context changes, as for example when different types of feedback are used, the sensorimotor store must undergo recalibration, which takes an additional period of practise.

To reinforce the above results and interpretation, Proteau, Marteniuk, and Levesque (1990) conducted a similar study but this time they had two groups of subjects practise for two days in the no-vision condition described above. After considerable practise and improvement, one group was transferred to the full-vision condition. Whilst vision is usually thought to be very powerful in its contribution to motor control, the results showed just the opposite. The performance of the transferred group not only immediately became much slower but it also became very inaccurate. In fact, their performance became worse than what it was when they were tested prior to the experiment with full vision. These results are quite conclusive in showing that learning results in an integration of efferent and sensory information about the movement being learned; if the learning conditions are changed, performance suffers dramatically.

Another example of the above principal can be derived from an experiment in speech training for the deaf (Nickerson, Kalikow, and Stevens, 1976). Visual targets were displayed on an oscilloscope screen and then selected attributes of the person's utterance were extracted and also displayed for comparison to the targets. An example of this is where the pitch of the voice is used to control the upward and downward motion of a 'ball' on the screen. At the beginning of a trial the ball would be displayed on the left hand part of the screen and then begin moving to the right. The ball would then encounter a vertical wall with a small hole in it. The task of the learner would be to vary voice pitch so that the ball would go up or down to the level of the hole and allow its passage. By having more than one wall on the screen, pitch patterns could be learned when the holes in the walls were at different heights. Whilst the various training methods proved successful for the practised utterances when transferred to a setting without the scope display, this improvement did not transfer to utterances not practised with the system. Again, specificity of practise appears to have been operational.

The above results collectively support specificity of motor learning, and when combined with a sensorimotor view of learning, suggest that learning results in the use of afferent and efferent information for the formation of an integrated representation of movement. After this representation has been formed, feedback normally available during the execution of the movement can be compared to the representation to ensure rapid and accurate control of movement. Furthermore, this representation is so specific to the conditions present during learning that changing the feedback (or efferent) information available to the performer causes an immediate decrease in performance. Performance will continue to suffer until a recalibration of available feedback with efferent sources of information can take place.

References

Abbs JH and Gracco VL (1983) Sensorimotor actions in the control of multimovement speech gestures, *Trends Neurosci*, **6**, 391–5

Abbs JH, Gracco VL, and Cole KJ (1984) Control of multimovement coordination: sensorimotor mechanisms in speech motor programming, *J Motor Behav*, **16**, 195–231

Allport AA (1980) Patterns and actions: Cognitive mechanisms are content-specific, In Claxton G, ed, *Cognitive Psychology*, London, Routledge & Kegan Paul

Altman J (1982) The role of sensory inputs in insect flight motor pattern generation, *Trends Neurosci*, **5**, 257–60

Bach-y-Rita P (1972) Brain mechanisms in sensory substitution, New York, Academic

Bach-y-Rita P, Collins CC, Saunders F, White B, and Scadden L (1969) Vision substitution by tactile image projection, *Nature*, **221**, 963–4

Bailey IL (1978) A profile of the low vision population, *Optometric Monthly*, **69**(5), 198–206

Beggs WDA (1986) Mobility of training today I: Dealing with the real world, *British Journal of Visual Impairment*, **(IV:3)**, 87–9

Bobath B (1970) *Adult Hemiplegia: Evaluation and Treatment*, London, Heinemann Medical

Brown B and Brabyn JA (1987) Mobility and low vision: A review, *Clin Exp Optometry*, **70**(3), 96–101

Brown B, Brabyn L, Welch L, Haegerstrom-Portnoy G, and Colenbrander A (1986) Contribution of vision variables to mobility in age-related maculopathy patients, *Am J Optom Physiol Opt*, **63**, 733–9

Bruner JS (1971) The growth and structure of skill, In Connolly KJ, ed, *Motor Skills in Infancy*, New York, Academic Press

Brunnstrom S (1970) *Movement Therapy in Hemiplegia*, New York, Harper and Row

Burnside IG, Tobias HS and Bursill D (1982) Electromyographic feedback in the remobilization of stroke patients: A controlled trial, *Arch Phys Med Rehabil*, **63**, 217–22

Cavanagh PR, Hennig EM, Rodgers MM and Sanderson DJ (1985) The measurement of pressure distribution on the plantar surface of diabetic feet, In Whittle M and Harris D, eds, *Biomechanical Measurement in Orthopaedic Practice*, Oxford, Clarendon, 159–68

Collins CC (1985) On mobility aids for the blind. In Warren DH and Strelow ER, eds, *Electronic spatial sensing for the blind*, Dordrecht, Nijhoff, 35–64

Drew T (1988) Motor cortical cell discharge during voluntary gait modification, *Brain Res*, **457**, 181–7

Genesky SM (1978) Data concerning the partially sighted and functionally blind, *Journal of Visual Impairment and Blindness*, May, 177–80

Genesky SM, Berry SH, Bikson TH and Bikson TK (1979) Visual environmental adaptation problems of the partially sighted: Final report (CPS-100-HEW), Center for Partially Sighted, Santa Monica Medical Center

Gottlieb GL, Corcos DM and Agarwal GC (1989) Strategies for the control of voluntary movements with one mechanical degree of freedom, *Behav Brain Sci*, **12**, 189–250

Government of Canada, Blind Persons Act: Chapter 371: Regulations Respecting Blind Persons

Green PH (1982) Why is it easy to control your arms? *J Motor Behav*, **14**, 260–86

Houk JC and Rymer WZ (1981) Neural control of muscle length and tension, In Brooks VB, ed, *Handbook of Physiology*, Vol. 2, Motor Control, Bethesda, American Physiological Society, 257–323

Jeannerod M (1981) Intersegmental coordination during reaching at natural visual objects, In Long J and Badderley A, eds, *Attention and Performance IX*, Hillsdale, Erlbaum

Kahn HA and Moorehead HB (1973) Statistics on Blindness in the Model Reporting Area 1969–1970, Washington, HEW Publication, U.S. Government Printing Office

Kay L (1974) A sonar aid to enhance spatial perception of the blind: Engineering design and evaluation, *Radio and Electronic Engineering*, **44**, 40–62

Kurcz E (1974) Elektroftalm-a mobility aid with a tactile display, In *Report on European Conference on Technical Aids for the Visually Handicapped*. March 1974 (Report No. 81), Stockholm, Handikappinstitutet

MacKenzie CL and Marteniuk RG (1985a) Motor skill: feedback, knowledge, and structural issues. *Can J Psychol*, **39**, 313–7

MacKenzie CL and Marteniuk RG (1985b) Bimanual coordination, In Roy EA, ed, *Neuropsychological Studies of Apraxia and Related Disorders*, Amsterdam, North-Holland

National Accreditation Council for Agencies Serving the Blind and Visually Handicapped: Orientation and mobility service standards, adopted June 1979

National Accreditation for Agencies Serving the Blind and Visually Handicapped: Low vision service standards adopted, June 1981

Nashner LM and Cordo PJ (1981) Relation of automatic postural responses and reaction-time voluntary movements of human leg muscles. *Exp Brain Res*, **43**, 395–405

Nickerson RS, Kalikow DN and Stevens KN (1976) Computer-aided speech training for the deaf, *J Speech Hear Disord*, **41**, 120–32

Olney SJ, Colborne GR and Martin CS (1989) Joint angle feedback and biomechanical gait analysis in stroke, *Phys Ther*, **69**, 863–70

Passini R, Dupre A, and Langlois C (1986) Spatial mobility of the visually handicapped active person: A descriptive study, *Journal of Visual Impairment and Blindness*, **80**(8), 904–7

Palacz O and Kurcz E (1978) Przydatnosc zmodyfikowanego elektroftalmu EL-300 wg Starkiewicza dla niewidomych (The usefulness of modified Electrophthalm designed by Starkiewicz for the blind), *Klin Oczna*, **48**, 61–3

Parker P and Scott RN (1986) Myoelectric control of prosthesis. *Crit Rev Biomed Eng*, **13**(4), 283–310

Patla AE (1989) In search of laws for the visual control of locomotion: Some observations, *J Exp Psychol [Hum Percep]*, **15**, 624–8

Pierrot-Deseilligny E, Bergego C, and Mazieres L (1983) Reflex control of bipedal gait in man. In Desmedt JE, ed, *Motor Control Mechanisms in Health and Disease*, New York, Raven, 699–776

Pressey N (1977) Mowat Sensor, *Focus*, **3**, 35–9

Proteau L, Marteniuk RG, Girouard Y, and Dugas C (1987) On the type of information used to control and learn an aiming movement after moderate and extensive training, *Can J Psychol*, **6**, 181–99

Proteau L, Marteniuk RG, and Levesque L (1990) A sensorimotor basis for motor learning: Evidence indicating specificity of practice, Submitted for publication

Rice EC and Feinstein SH (1965) Echo detection ability of the blind: Size and distance factors, *J Exp Psychol*, **70**, 246–51

Riley LH (1969) Low vision statistics, *J Am Optom Assoc*, **49**(8), 23–30

Schenkman BN (1985) Human echolocation: The detection of objects by the blind, *Acta Universitatis Uppsaliensis*, Abstracts of Uppsala Dissertations from the Faculty of Social Sciences, No. 36

Schenkman BN (1986) Identification of ground materials with the aid of tapping sounds and vibrations of long canes for the blind, *Ergonomics*, **29**, 985–98

Schenkman BN and Jansson G (1986) The detection and localization of objects by the blind with the aid of long cane tapping sounds, *Hum Factors*, **28**, 607–618

Scott RN (1990a) Myoelectric control systems research at Bioengineering Institute, New Brunswick, *Med Prog Technol*, **16**, 5–10

Scott RN (1990b) Feedback in myoelectric prosthesis, *Clinical Orthop*,

Schmidt RA (1975) A schema theory of discrete motor skill learning, *Psychol Rev*, **82**, 225–60

Shahani BT, Connors L, and Mohr JP (1977) Electromyographic audiovisual feedback training effect on the motor performance in patients with lesions of the central nervous system, *Arch Phys Med Rehabil*, **58**, 519

Stein RB and Capaday C (1988) The modulation of human reflexes during functional motor tasks, *Trends Neurosci*, **11**, 328–32

Strelow ER (1985) What is needed for a theory of mobility: Direct perception and cognitive maps – lessons from the blind, *Psychol Rev*, **92**(2), 226–48

Strelow ER and Brabyn JA (1982) Locomotion of the blind controlled by natural sound cues, *Perception*, **11**, 635–40

Welsh R and Blasch BB (1980) eds, *Foundations of Orientation and Mobility*, New York, American Foundation for the Blind

Winter DA (1987) *The Biomechanics and Motor Control of Human Gait*, Waterloo, University of Waterloo

Wolf SL (1983) Electromyographic feedback applications to stroke patients: A critical review, *Phys Ther*, **63**, 1448–59

9
Applications of principles of training to neuromuscular disorders

Joe M. Watt and Michael H. Brooke

The principles of rehabilitation in neuromuscular disorders affecting children include: fostering optimal physical and mental and emotional development; maintaining or improving function whenever possible; and preventing secondary complications, such as contractures, skin breakdown, and malalignment of the spine (Eng and Binder, 1988). Training of abnormal muscle to maintain or improve strength and endurance might assist in achieving the desired goals of rehabilitation.

Duchenne (1861) suggested that electrical stimulation of diseased muscle might be beneficial to patients with muscular dystrophy. More recently intermittent, chronic, low frequency electrical stimulation of muscles in six young ambulant children with Duchenne muscular dystrophy resulted in a significant increase in mean maximal voluntary contraction compared with the mean forces exerted by the unstimulated control muscles of the contralateral leg (Scott *et al.*, 1986). The authors proposed that the beneficial effect could be due to a slower deterioration of the existing diseased muscle fibres, a better and more rapid growth of regenerating fibres, or hypertrophy of existing healthy fibres.

Early studies (Abramson and Rogoff, 1952) of resistance exercise of older patients with Duchenne muscular dystrophy reported small improvements in strength. Vignos and Watkins (1966) studied 24 patients with muscular dystrophy. Maximum resistance exercise program was instituted for one year. Improvement in muscle strength occurred in all patients throughout the first four months of exercise regardless of the type of dystrophy. Subsequently, a plateau occurred and was maintained throughout the period of observation. Improvement of functional abilities was less than the increase in muscle strength. Patients with 'limb girdle' and facioscapulohumeral dystrophy derived the greatest benefit. These earlier studies were not randomized or controlled, and statistical methods were not used in the analysis of data. de Lateur and Gianconi (1979) studied four children with Duchenne muscular dystrophy in whom they submaximally exercised one quadriceps using a Cybex isokinetic exerciser and recorder, with the contralateral quadriceps as control. This was performed four or five days per week for six months. There was no statistically significant increase in strength during the six month exercise period. There was no evidence of over-work weakness. Scott *et al.* (1981) published a six-month feasibility study comparing a group of boys with Duchenne muscular dystrophy who performed manually resisted exercise with another group who performed exercises in response to oral commands for 15 minutes per day. No statistical difference was found between the two regimes. Hagberg, Carroll, and Brooke (1986) reported that endurance exercise training in patients with central core disease resulted in a significant increase in work capacity and maximal oxygen consumption. Fowler suggested that exercise training programs in patients with neuromuscular disease should be started early in the course of the disease, when muscle fibre degeneration and weakness are minimal, and emphasize submaximal exercise levels (Fowler and Taylor, 1982).

Endurance training consists of repetitive periods of aerobic exercise carried out on a regular basis. In normal volunteers, such a program increases the maximum work output and maximal oxygen consumption (VO_2 max). Strenuous exercise is associated with the production of lactate, hypoxanthine, and ammonia by muscle, as well as release of creatine kinase and myoglobin into the circulation. Endurance training or conditioning increases the aerobic capacity of muscle because the muscle is functioning more efficiently. Exercise in the trained state is associated with much less production of lactate, hypoxanthine, and ammonia; release of creatine kinase and myoglobin into the circulation is similarly reduced. In an attempt to determine whether patients with neuromuscular disease could benefit from the effects of training, Florence *et al.* (1984) investigated endurance training in eight patients with a variety of neuromuscular diseases, all of which were relatively non-progressive. Training consisted of 30 minutes of bicycle exercise performed three times weekly close to their maximum work capacity. This was continued for three months. At the start and end of the training period, each subject performed a prolonged exercise test consisting of 90 minutes of exercise on a bicycle with the loads set at 50% of their maximum. Of the eight patients, five showed a significant increase in their work capabilities and in the level of their VO_2 max, a normal response to training. Of these five, only one had a normal biochemical response to training. One of the five showed increased levels of lactate, hypoxanthine, and creatine kinase release, suggesting that the effect of training had been to increase the amount of stress on the muscle that the patient could tolerate. Two others showed an increase in the amount of hypoxanthine produced, again suggesting that the muscle was under greater stress in the trained state. This obviously indicates that patients differ in their responses to training. If the effect of training is simply an increased tolerance to the discomfort of maximal exercise rather than an adaptive response of the muscle, it might not be a useful therapeutic regimen. It is therefore suggested that each patient be considered on an individual basis rather than any generalization being made as to the advisability of training all patients with neuromuscular disease.

Since respiratory failure accounts for death in over 75% of Duchenne muscular dystrophy cases (Newson-Davis, 1980), specific respiratory muscle training exercises are often used to improve ventilatory endurance. Uncontrolled studies (Adams and Chandler, 1974; Siegel, 1975) showed improvement in vital capacity after a breathing exercise program. DiMarco *et al.* (1985) reported a remarkable improvement in ventilatory endurance for a heterogeneous group of neuromuscular disease patients following six weeks of inspiratory resistance training. Martin (1986) noted a significant improvement in endurance but not in strength as a result of specific respiratory muscle training. The authors suggested that this was the result of training Type I fibres, preventing deterioration caused by disuse atrophy, the disease, or both. Smith, Coakley, and Edwards (1988) were unable to reproduce these results and concluded that the benefits of inspiratory resistance training in Duchenne muscular dystrophy are small, and that distinguishing learning effects from training effects may be difficult. They further cautioned against the use of resistive training in advanced

Duchenne muscular dystrophy, as the weak respiratory muscles are working against the reduced compliance of the lungs and chest wall, and may already be close to their fatiguing threshold (Smith *et al.*, 1987). Stern *et al.* (1989) used adapted computer games in training inspiratory resistance in boys with muscular dystrophy but found no significant change after 18 months.

There have been questions raised about the possibility that exercise training may lead to over-work weakness in diseased skeletal muscle. Adult dystrophic mice did not adapt to treadmill training, resulting in high mortality (Taylor, Fowler, and Doerr, 1976). Asymmetric weakness observed in several members of a family with facioscapulohumeral dystrophy suggested that even usual daily occupations might accelerate the progression of muscle weakness, but asymmetric weakness is almost the rule in that illness (Johnson and Braddon, 1971). Previously cited studies of peripheral muscle (Vignos and Watkins, 1966; de Lateur and Gianconi, 1979; Scott *et al.*, 1981; Hagberg, Carroll, and Brooke, 1986) and respiratory muscle strengthening (Siegel, 1975; DiMarco *et al.*, 1985) of Duchenne muscular dystrophy patients did not show over-work weakness. Some authors have suggested that vigorous physiotherapy in motorneuron disease may be harmful (British Medical Journal, 1976; Sinaki and Mulder, 1978) whereas others reported conflicting results (Lenman, 1959; Bohannon, 1983).

There has been no long-term study demonstrating any effect of muscle training in altering the relentless course of progressive neuromuscular disorders. There has not been any convincing evidence of improvement in locomotor or functional ability after a training exercise program. In order to achieve the goals of rehabilitation, our neuromuscular clinic relies heavily on modalities to circumvent the handicap rather than on overcoming the weakness. Until some therapeutic intervention is shown to strengthen weakened muscles, the approaches described below will be the mainstay of treatment programs.

DUCHENNE MUSCULAR DYSTROPHY

The orthodox management of Duchenne muscular dystrophy includes the use of surgery and bracing to allow the patients to remain ambulatory for as long as possible. Studies on the natural history of Duchenne muscular dystrophy (Brooke *et al.*, 1989) indicate that boys begin to fall quite frequently and have increasing difficulty in climbing stairs between 6 to 8 years of age. From 9 to 11 years of age, they cease climbing stairs completely and are no longer able to stand up from the floor. Part of this difficulty is caused by the muscular weakness and part by contractures, which develop in the hips, knees, and ankles, and make it impossible for the child to stand with the degree of hyperextension necessary to retain balance. Contractures of the iliotibial bands and hip flexors are noted by 4 to 5 years of age and heel cord tightness follows shortly. Early therapy is therefore aimed at preventing them. Passive stretching exercises should be performed daily by the family. If this is done conscientiously, it is possible to retard but not prevent the development of these contractures. Stretching exercises done on a weekly basis are completely ineffective. In a study of therapy and management of contractures, the most effective treatment in the prevention of contractures was splinting. There was a high correlation between the use of night splints (plastic ankle-foot orthoses), which maintain the foot in dorsiflexion during the night, and preservation of movement at the ankle (Brooke *et al.*, 1989).

The time at which leg braces are used for ambulation and the type of brace used are critical to the success of braced ambulation. Only the very rare patient will ever benefit from the use of a short leg brace for walking, because the major functional weakness in the Duchenne muscular dystrophy patient is of the quadriceps. It is the collapse of this muscle that causes the patient to fall. Early in the course of the illness, Duchenne muscular dystrophy patients often fall because they are hurrying and careless about their balance. Bracing such patients will not be successful, because the brace will slow down the patient who will find it unacceptable. When falls occur during quiet standing, or when the patient is walking slowly, the child finds it much easier to tolerate bracing. We therefore use the following criteria for bracing: the child has several falls per week; can no longer climb stairs or only with great difficulty; cannot arise from the floor or does this so slowly that it is not useful; and can no longer extend the knee against gravity.

In this situation, bracing can be quite helpful. The type of brace is also important. The use of a long leg brace with knee support is essential in Duchenne muscular dystrophy. If the limb is too contracted to allow this to be used, then consideration should be given to percutaneous tenotomy with release of the iliotibial bands, hip flexors, hamstrings, and heel cords (Siegel, 1981). The type of long leg brace used is a matter of personal preference. The disadvantage of the plastic knee-ankle-foot-orthosis (KAFO) is the tendency of the patient to throw the foot into equinovarus, which sometimes results in calluses and abrasions on the outside of the foot. The metal double-upright attached to a surgical boot is cosmetically less appealing, but can be more comfortable and probably holds the ankle in a more rigid position. In clinics with an aggressive approach to surgery and bracing, it is not unusual to find patients walking at 12 to 15 years of age. One study showed that the mean age of loss of ambulation in these patients was at 12.4 years of age (Brooke *et al.*, 1989).

SPINAL MUSCULAR ATROPHY

In acute infantile Type I Wernig-Hoffman spinal muscular dystrophy (SMA), nutritional and respiratory concerns are of primary importance in the first year. The use of nasogastric or gastrostomy feeding may be necessary. Chronic assisted ventilation for this severe type is probably not warranted because of the poor prognosis. In children with less severe types of SMA, attention should be directed towards improvement of function and prevention of complications.

In order to mimic normal motor development, a custom seating device is provided at 6–8 months of age (Watt and Greenhill, 1984). A special headrest or neck orthosis can be used to support the neck so that the child can look at the world in an upright posture. At one year of age, a standing frame or A-frame is provided to promote axial loading and to stretch out contractures. Night splints for the feet are routinely used. Most of the children will be unable to propel the standing frame, and a miniature wheelchair will be provided. A spinal orthosis is used to control early scoliosis. As these children are usually very bright, powered mobility can be provided as early as two years of age. Children with Type II or Type III SMA can often walk with polypropylene light-weight ankle-foot orthoses, or knee-ankle-foot orthoses (Granata *et al.*, 1987), using a Kaye or Rollator walker. Recently, we have used Louisiana State University reciprocating orthoses with good success. These children are usually integrated into normal schools.

Besides soft tissue releases to allow brace wearing, we are not aggressive in treatment of peripheral joint contractures. Most of the older non-ambulatory children develop hip dislocation, which is usually painless. The most difficult complication to treat is scoliosis of the collapsing paralytic type (Mertini *et al.*, 1989). Luque and Moseley spinal fusion has revolutionized the treatment of paralytic scoliosis (Stevens and Beard, 1989). Patients usually wear spinal orthoses until such time as the scoliosis is shown to be progressive beyond 40°. Elective surgery with careful pre-operative pulmonary assessment and post-operative endotracheal ventilation for about 24 hours is usually successful. Post-operative bracing is usually not necessary. Patients with juvenile SMA may need a triple arthrodesis to correct planovalgus deformity.

Most of the patients will become wheelchair bound in their early teens. Respiratory care includes using an inspirometer to encourage deep breathing, chest physiotherapy, and postural drainage. Chronic ventilation through a tracheostomy can be instituted to treat respiratory failure. As they become weaker, devices such as computers, environmental control devices, and adaptive equipment will lessen the amount of care necessary to look after these severely handicapped patients.

HEREDITARY SENSORY MOTOR NEUROPATHIES

This group of heterogeneous disorders is characterized by symmetrical, slowly progressive paralysis, which develops in a proximal direction. As a result of muscle imbalance, severe foot deformities develop early in life. Upper limb muscles are similarly atrophic, especially the distal intrinsics and radially innervated muscles of the forearm. Endurance training probably improves general cardiovascular fitness and prevents disuse atrophy of unaffected muscles; stretching and bracing may retard contractures. Strategies to diminish the risk of falling, joint protection techniques, work simplification, and energy conservation methods are taught to patients early in life. Polypropylene drop-foot orthoses are used to control dynamic foot instability and to correct steppage gait when necessary. Special footwear is often necessary to accommodate foot deformities and to ensure comfort.

Most patients develop cavovarus feet unresponsive to conservative treatment (Shapiro and Bresnan, 1982). The main surgical technique had been triple arthrodesis (Jacobs and Carr, 1950; Levitt *et al.*, 1973), with various tendon transfer procedures, calcaneal tenotomies, and plantar fasciotomy in skeletally matured patients. More recent long-term follow-up studies (Wukich and Bowen, 1989) suggested that only 14% of 178 patients required this approach, which the authors regard as a salvage procedure. Another long-term study (Wetmore and Drennan, 1989) reported unsatisfactory results in most of the patients requiring this salvage procedure. Roper and Tibrewal (1989) suggested that early soft tissue surgery consisting of lengthening the calcaneal tendon, Steindler plantar fasciotomy, and tendon transfers before skeletal maturity gives better results, and can postpone or obviate the need for triple arthrodesis. Triple arthrodesis in an immature skeleton has the disadvantage of leaving a smaller foot. Young patients with very severe varus of the heel can have Dwyer calcaneal osteotomies (Dwyer, 1959).

Scoliosis develops in 10% of patients with Charcot-Marie-Tooth Disease. Spinal orthosis is often unsuccessful, and Luque or Moseley instrumentation is required. Subluxation of the hip is treated by proximal femoral varus osteotomy. Knee instability can be controlled by knee-ankle-foot orthosis. Patients with Dejerine-

Scottas disease can become wheelchair-bound in the second decade of their life and management is similar to the approach described for patients with spinal muscular atrophy.

References

Abramson AS and Rogoff J (1952) Physical Treatment in Muscular Dystrophy, Abstract of Study, *Proc Second Med Conf Musc Dystrophy Ass Am*, 123–4

Adams MA and Chandler LS (1974) Effects of Physical Therapy Program on Vital Capacity of Patients with Muscular Dystrophy, *Phys Ther*, **54**, 494–6

Bohannon RW (1983) Results of Resistance Exercise on a Patient with Amyotrophic Lateral Sclerosis, *Phys Ther*, **63**, 965–8

British Medical Journal (1976) Management of Motor Neuron Disease, *Br Med J*, **2**, 1422–3

Brooke MH, Fenichel GM, Griggs RC, Mendell JR, Moxley R, *et al.* (1989) Duchenne muscular dystrophy; patterns of clinical progression and effects of supportive therapy, *Neurology*, **39**, 475–81

de Lateur BJ and Gianconi BA (1979) Effect of Maximal Strength of Submaximal Exercise in Duchenne Muscular Dystrophy, *Am J Phys Med*, **58**(1), 26–36

DiMarco AF, DiMarco MS, Jacobs I, Shields R, and Altose MD (1985) The Effects of Inspiratory Resistive Training on Respiratory Muscle Function in Patients with Muscular Dystrophy, *Muscle Nerve*, 284–90

Duchenne GB (1861) De L'electricisation Localisee et son Application a la Pathlogre et a la Therapeutique, 2nd edn, Paris, Bailliere et Fils

Dwyer FC (1959) Osteotomy of calcaneum for pes cavus, *J Bone Joint Surg [Br]*, **41B**, 80–6

Eng GD and Binder H (1988) Rehabilitation of Infants and Children with Neuromuscular Disorders, *Pediatr Ann*, **17**(12), 745–55

Florence JM, Brooke MH, Hagberg MJ, Carroll JE (1984) Endurance Exercise in Neuromuscular Disease. Transactions of the Fifth International Congress on Neuromuscular Disease, Serratrice G *et al.*, eds, *Neuromuscular Disease*, New York, Raven

Fowler W, Gardner GW, Kazerunion HH, and Lauvstad WA (1968) Effect of Exercise on Serum Enzymes, *Arch Phys Med Rehabil*, **49**, 554–65

Fowler WM and Taylor M (1982) Rehabilitation management of muscular dystrophy and related disorders: I The role of exercise, *Arch Phys Med Rehab*, **63**, 319–21

Granata C, Cornelio F, Bonfilioi S, Mattutini P, and Merline L (1987) Promotion of ambulation of patients with spinal muscular atrophy by early fitting of knee-ankle-foot orthoses, *Dev Med Child Neurol*, **29**, 221–4

Hagberg JM, Carroll JE, and Brooke MH (1986) Endurance Exercise Training in Patients with Central Core Disease, *Neurology*, **30**, 1242–4

Jacobs JE and Carr CR (1950) Progressive muscular atrophy of the peroneal type (Charcot-Marie-Tooth disease), *J Bone Joint Surg [Am]*, **32**, 27–8

Johnson EW and Braddon R (1971) Over-work Weakness in Facioscapulohumeral Muscular Dystrophy, *Arch Phys Med Rehabil*, **52**, 333–5

Lenman JAR (1959) A Clinical and Experimental Study of the Effects of Exercise on Motor Weakness in Neurological Disease, *J Neurol Neurosurg Psychiatry*, **22**, 182–94

Levitt RL, Canale ST, Cooke AJ, and Gartland JJ (1973) The role of foot surgery in progressive neuromuscular disorders in children, *J Bone Joint Surg [Am]*, **55**, 1396–1410

Martin AG (1986) Respiratory Muscle Training in Duchenne Muscular Dystrophy, *Dev Med Child Neurol*, **28**, 314–8

Mertini L, Granata C, Bonfiglioli S, Marini ML, Cerevellati S, and Savini R (1989) Scoliosis in spinal muscular atrophy; natural history and management, *Dev Med Child Neurol*, **31**, 501–8

Newson-Davis J (1980) The Respiratory System in Muscular Dystrophy, *Br Med Bull*, **36**, 135–48

Piasecki JO, Mahinpour S, and Levine DB (1986) Long-term follow-up of spinal fusion in spinal muscular atrophy, *Clin Orthop*, **207**, 44–54

Roper BA and Tibrewal SB (1989) Soft tissue surgery in Charcot-Marie-Tooth disease, *J Bone Joint Surg [Am]*, **71B**(1), 17–20

Scott OM, Hyde SA, Goddard C, Jones R, and Dubowitz V (1981) Effect of Exercise in Duchenne Muscular Dystrophy, *Physiotherapy*, **67**(6),174–6

Scott OM, Vrbova G, Hyde SA, and Dubowitz V (1986) Response of Muscles of Patients with Duchenne Muscular Dystrophy to Chronic Electrical Stimulation, *J Neurol Neurosurg Psychiatry*, **49**, 1427–34

Shapiro F and Bresnan MNJ (1982) Orthopedic management of childhood neuromuscular disease; current concepts review; Part II: Peripheral Neuropathies, Friedreich Ataxia, and Arthrogryposis Multiplex Congenita, *J Bone Joint Surg* [*Am*], **64A**(6), 949–53

Siegel IM (1975) Pulmonary Problems in Duchenne Muscular Dystrophy. Diagnosis, Prophylaxis and Treatment, *Phys Ther*, **55**, 160–2

Siegel IM (1981) Diagnosis, management and orthopedic treatment of Muscular Dystrophy, *Am Acad Orthopedic Surg*, **30**, 3–35

Sinaki, M and Mulder DW (1978) Rehabilitation Techniques for Patients with Amyotrophic Lateral Sclerosis, *Mayo Clin Proc*

Smith PEM, Calverley PMA, Edwards RHT, Evans GA and Campbell EJM (1987) Practical Considerations of Respiratory Care of Patients with Muscular Dystrophy, *N Engl J Med*, **316**, 1197–205

Smith PEM, Coakley JH, and Edwards RHT (1988) Respiratory Muscle Training in Duchenne Muscular Dystrophy, *Muscle Nerve*, 784–5

Stern LM, Martin AJ, Jones N, Garrett R, and Yeates J (1989) Training Inspiratory Resistance in Duchenne Dystrophy using Adapted Computer Games, *Dev Med Child Neurol*, **31**, 341–500

Stevens BB and Beard C (1989) Segmental spinal instrumentation for neuromuscular spinal deformity, *Clin Orthop*, **242**, 164–8

Taylor RG, Fowler W, and Doerr L (1976) Exercise Effect on Contractile Properties of Skeletal Muscle in Mouse Muscular Dystrophy, *Arch Phys Med Rehabil*, **57**, 174–80

Vignos PJ and Watkins MP (1966) The Effect of Exercise in Muscular Dystrophy, *JAMA*, **197**(11), 121–6

Watt J and Greenhill B (1984) Rehabilitation and orthopedic management of spinal muscular atrophy. Progressive Spinal Muscular Atrophies, International Review of Child Neurology Series, New York, Raven Press, 173–88

Wetmore RS and Drennan JC (1989) Long-term results of triple arthrodesis in Charcot-Marie-Tooth disease, *J Bone Joint Surg* [*Am*], **71A**(3), 417–22

Wukich DK and Bowen JR (1989) A long-term study of triple arthrodesis for correction of pes cavovarus in Charcot-Marie-Tooth disease, *J Pediatr Orthop*, **9**(4), 433–7

10
Stroke rehabilitation: the scientific basis for a 'model' service

R. Langton Hewer

Stroke is a major cause of death and long-term physical disability. The cost of stroke-induced illness is very considerable, both for the state and for individual families. The long-term manifestations of stroke include impaired mobility, paralysis of one arm, impaired ability to communicate, depression, and, for many people, a greatly reduced quality of life. For all these reasons, the topic of stroke and its management is a matter of profound importance. Unfortunately, there has been much dissatisfaction (Consensus Conference, 1988) with stroke rehabilitation services and there is now a widespread desire to establish high quality services.

The subject of assessment and management is discussed first, because of its fundamental importance as a basis for describing outcome and the effects of therapeutic intervention. This leads to a brief discussion of the 'practical' epidemiology of stroke, and of the costs involved. Current evidence regarding the natural history of stroke is briefly reviewed. The principles of physical therapy are outlined as is the evidence that recovery within the nervous system can be influenced. The importance of spasticity and its management is emphasized. Finally, there is discussion of the organizational principles upon which a district stroke service should be based.

MEASUREMENT AND ASSESSMENT

The importance of reliable methods of assessment cannot be over-emphasized. The topic is a large one and is discussed in detail elsewhere (Wade *et al.*, 1985).

A large number of assessment tools have been developed during the last few years. Some of these are of limited value because they can only be applied by specialists; for example, the Porch test of communicability (Porch, 1971) can only, in reality, be used by a trained speech therapist. An assessment tool must have a number of characteristics, which can be summarized:

1. Relevance. The test must measure some function that is clinically relevant.
2. Validity. The test must measure whatever it is supposed to be assessing. For example, if a speech assessment shows a severe impairment, it would be anticipated that the subject could not use a telephone adequately. If the subject could, the test is probably invalid as a measure of language function.

3. Reliability. There must be consistency of results by one observer (intra-observer variation) and between observers (inter-observer variation). Similarly, the effect of time of day, fatigue, and background noise must be taken into consideration.
4. Sensitivity. The test needs to be sufficiently sensitive to detect significant change in the patient's condition. Unfortunately, sensitivity is inversely proportional to reliability. The more sensitive a test, the less, in general, the reliability, and vice versa. A balance between the two ideals must be achieved. For example, death is a highly reliable outcome measure, but clearly lacks sensitivity. On the other hand, the ability of a stroke patient to 'finger-tap' may be a sensitive indicator of hand function but is, in reality, not reliable or consistent.
5. Simplicity. The demands of validity, reliability, and sensitivity have sometimes been met by designing highly complex tests that are useless in routine clinical practice. Simplicity is vital. A test that is not understood by the operator and patient is not likely to give reliable results.
6. Communicability. The results of the assessment must be capable of being easily communicated to other members of the rehabilitation team. A numerical score is ideal. For instance, a Barthel score of 14/20 usually indicates that the patient is ready to go home, whereas a score of 6 or less indicates that the patient needs continuous nursing care.

It is not possible to discuss assessment procedures in detail here. Table 10.1 shows a selection of the tests used in the Bristol Stroke Unit (see also Wade *et al.*, 1985).

EPIDEMIOLOGY OF STROKE

Knowledge of the epidemiology of stroke (Wade and Langton Hewer, 1987a) is important because it gives an idea of the size and scope of the problem. Information relating to the incidence of stroke is reasonably well researched, but there have been remarkably few studies relating to the prevalence of stroke induced disability. The figures given in Table 10.2 relate to a notional population of 250 000 people, which is the average size of a health district, one of the units of the National Health Service in the UK. In England and Wales, there are 200 health districts, each having a median population of about a quarter of a million. Each health district has at least one district hospital with about 600 beds, four physicians practising internal medicine, and 120 'general practitioners', each of whom will have about 2000 people on their 'list'.

COST OF STROKE

Stroke illness is extremely expensive. Carstairs (1976) found that stroke consumed 4.6% of NHS resources in Scotland. An Office of Health Economics study (1988) showed that cerebrovascular disease cost the National Health Service 550 million pounds in 1985, which was 3.9% of the total NHS budget. This figure is an underestimate, because it does not include community support services, such as home nursing. A study in Bristol has shown that stroke accounts for 11% of district hospital 'bed-days'. An average health district of a quarter of a million people, spends at least £3 million per year on acute stroke care.

It is important for all those doctors who are keen to establish good quality stroke services to understand the high cost of providing such a service. The paradoxical situation, as discussed below, is that in many areas of the world, stroke care services

Table 10.1 Assessment procedures used in the Bristol Stroke Unit

Topic	Test	Reference
Cognition	Mini-Mental State	Folstein, Folstein, and McHugh, 1975
Perceptual Assessment	Rivermead Perceptual Assessment	Bhavani and Cockburn, 1983
Communication and Speech	Functional Communication Profile	Jarno, 1969
	Frenchay Aphasia Screening Test. This test is suitable for use by doctors	Enderby *et al.*, 1987
Arm Function	Frenchay Arm Test	Heller *et al.*, 1987
	Action Arm Test	Lyle (1981)
	9-hole peg test	Heller *et al.*, 1987
Mobility	Much information is contained in the Barthel Scale see below	Mahoney and Barthel, 1965
Walking	Record: 1. Safety – does he fall? 2. Speed of walking 3. Distance walked in 6 mins	Wade *et al.*, 1987
Activities of Daily Living	The Barthel Scale is used routinely	Mahoney and Barthel, 1965; Wade, Skilbeck, and Langton Hewer, 1983
	FIM test – Functional Independence Measurements	Granger and Gresham, personal communication
Depression	General Health Questionnaire	Goldberg and Hillier, 1979
	Wakefield Self Assessment Inventory	Snaith *et al.*, 1971
Social Functioning	Frenchay Activities Index – this test has been in routine use for several years. It records 3 separate factors – domestic, leisure and social. A single score is produced	Holbrook and Skilbeck, 1983

Table 10.2 Epidemiology of stroke induced disability in a notional population of 250 000 people

Clinical group	Incidence*	Prevalence†	References
New strokes each year	500		
Number who survive annually with a significant impairment	170		
Number with dysphasia	80	350	
Number with paralysed arm	130	500	
Prevalence of stroke survivors		3000	
Prevalence of disabled stroke survivors		900	

*Incidence = Number of new cases per year
†Prevalence = Number of cases existing at any one time

are generally considered to be unsatisfactory. The cost of stroke can be a powerful 'weapon' and it should certainly be argued that it is unjustified to spend large sums of money on unsatisfactory services. It is for this reason that standards of care are being widely discussed.

ORGANIZATION OF SERVICES

A consensus conference (1988) on stroke management was held in London, whose recommendations have been endorsed by a working party of the Royal College of Physicians (1989). The recommendations which are probably applicable to most developed countries, can be summarized:

1. There should be a written and widely circulated district stroke policy. This should set standards, identify services, and allocate resources.
2. A named individual should be made accountable for the implementation, monitoring of the policy, coordination with local and other authorities.
3. There should be a district stroke service, which would integrate hospital and community resources. There should be a care team working both in the hospital and in the community, and should consist of nurses, therapists, social workers, and doctors fully trained in the management of stroke disability.
4. It has subsequently been suggested that every health district should produce an annual report on its stroke service, which should include an analysis of costs.

The King's Fund conference identified six particular points, which should be considered when managing stroke patients. These can be summarized:

1. All patients should be fully assessed using standard assessment tools (see Table 10.1).
2. Great care should be taken to involve both the patient and the carer in decision making.
3. The nursing, and other, staff on the ward must be fully trained and familiar with the neurological and other deficits in stroke patients.
4. There should be a well-organized programme of management for each patient, who should know precisely what treatment is planned for the following week. Activities for the evenings and weekends for hospitalized patients should be planned. The panel noted particularly that 'doing nothing' is highly demoralizing.
5. A key worker should be identified for each patient to coordinate a care plan, and provide education and support for the patient and family.
6. Discharge from hospital to the community should be carefully planned and executed.

Long-term follow-up

It is recognized that many patients face lifelong disability. The overall objective of rehabilitation is to help the patient make the most of his residual capacities and achieve the highest possible quality of life. Studies have shown that even three to four years after the stroke (Holbrook, 1982), many patients have not been able to come to terms with their problems. It is suggested, for this reason, that the district stroke team would keep in contact with stroke patients following discharge from hospital, and every effort made to ensure that the patient does achieve maximum potential. Research is needed to assess the usefulness, or otherwise, of long-term professional follow-up. The Northwick Park study (Smith *et al.*, 1981) has shown that post-discharge rehabilitation provided for a period of six months, can be effective. In the UK, the Chest, Heart, and Stroke Association has organized a national network of Stroke Clubs, which provide long-term support. For instance, in Bristol there are 150 volunteers currently 'looking after' 450 stroke patients.

Table 10.3 comprises a checklist that can be used by doctors, and others, when assessing the needs of stroke patients.

Other disabling disorders

The notional health district discussed above will contain many patients who are disabled as a result of other neurological disorders (Wade and Langton Hewer, 1987a). For instance, there will be about 300 people with multiple sclerosis, of whom 200 are disabled; 15 with motorneuron disease; and about 400 with Parkinson's disease, of whom about 250 will be disabled. It is clear, therefore, that the stroke service must eventually be part, albeit an important one, of the district neurological disability service.

Stroke wards

It has been suggested that one way of improving stroke care would be to segregate patients into a special ward. This suggestion is receiving widespread support (Consensus Conference, 1988; Royal College of Physicians, 1989), and is discussed in detail elsewhere (Langton Hewer, 1989).

NATURAL HISTORY OF STROKE INDUCED IMPAIRMENT AND DISABILITIES

The term 'natural history', used to describe recovery following stroke, is technically incorrect because most patients receive some form of therapy. Nonetheless, it is, in practice, impossible to collect data from patients who have received no therapy at all. The data referred to in this chapter is obtained largely from patients admitted to hospital and from unselected community studies.

The process of recovery in the hemiplegic limbs was described in a classical paper by Twitchell (1951). The process of recovery in the paralysed hand and foot was described as a constantly evolving series of reactions, which follows a general pattern with some variations. With the onset of hemiplegia, the affected limbs were completely paralysed with diminution of the tendon reflexes and little resistance to passive movement. Within 48 hours, the tendon reflexes became hyperactive and resistance to passive movement increased in the wrist and finger flexors, and the plantar flexors of the ankle. Resistance became more intense over a period of time and involved other muscle groups, particularly the flexors and adductors in the upper limb, and the extensor and adductors in the lower limb. The tendon reflexes became more brisk and sometimes clonic. The return of voluntary movement appeared first as flexion at the shoulder and hip. Later, flexion of the elbow, wrist and fingers, and knee and ankle were added to these movements. At this time, any attempt at voluntary movement resulted in a flexion movement of the shoulder, elbow, wrist, and fingers, or hip, knee, and ankle together. Thus, the 'flexor synergies' of the arm and leg became manifest as total reactions. In later, but overlapping sequence, the extensor synergies of the arm and leg developed. This paper has become the basis on which current physiotherapy techniques are based. It is 'required reading' for anyone seriously interested in the subject.

Table 10.3 Checklist for use when assessing stroke survivors

1. Current medication

2. Measures to prevent a further stroke
   a) Is BP satisfactory?
      If not, what action is required?
   b) Is the patient/should he be/taking aspirin?

3. Mobility of patient
   a) Walking speed over 20 metres:
   b) Do any contractures involve the ankle and/or foot?
   c) Is he a candidate for surgery on the ankle or foot?
   d) Can he walk safely indoors?
   e) Does he fall?
   f) Does he have a wheelchair?
      If so, is it satisfactory?
   g) Is any type of walking aid used or required?
   h) Is he driving a car?
      If not driving, is there any chance of re-starting driving?

4. Housing
   Are housing alterations required?
   If so, specify

5. Toilet
   Is he continent?
   Is there adequate access to a toilet?
   Is he using a commode?

6. Communication
   Does the patient have dysphasia?
   If yes, is there scope for further treatment?
   Should he be referred for attendance at a Stroke Club or Speech Group?
   Can he write?
   Is a typewriter or other communication aid used and/or needed?

7. Vision
   Can the patient read?
   Can sight be improved by spectacles?
   Is lighting adequate?
   Can he see television?
   Is there a hemianopia?
   If so, have the implications of this impairment been explained to the patient?

8. Psychological and psychiatric problems
   Does the patient appear to have adjusted to the stroke?
   Is he depressed?
   If so, does this need treatment?

   The 'rules of recovery' are reasonably well established on the basis of a number of studies (Wade *et al.*, 1983; Skilbeck, Wade, and Langton Hewer, 1983; Wade, Wood, and Langton Hewer, 1985), which can be summarized:

Table 10.3 — continued

9. Employment and hobbies
   Is the patient back at work?
   If not, is there any chance of getting back?
   Has he got any hobbies or leisure activities?
   If not, is there any scope for any?
   Is there anything he really enjoys doing?
   (? refer to—Stroke Support Group or Gardening for the Disabled)

10. Miscellaneous problems
    Does the patient have any pain?
    Is there pain in the affected shoulder?
    Does he sleep well?
    Have any possible sexual problems been discussed?

11. Home situation
    With whom is the patient living?
    What is the health of the spouse (or carer)?

ACTION SHEET
CHANGE IN MEDICATION: REFER FOR:
HOME ALTERATIONS: STROKE SUPPORT GROUP
AIDS AND APPLIANCES: DISTRICT NURSE
MOBILITY AIDS: SPEECH GROUP
                           SOCIAL SECURITY ALLOWANCES
                           DRIVING ASSESSMENT
                           FURTHER APPOINTMENT

---

1. The ultimate level of recovery is largely dependent on the severity of the initial deficit. For instance, a study of a large number of dysphasic stroke patients whose functional communication profile (FCP) (Sarno, 1969) was measured at three weeks and at six months, showed a straight line relationship between the initial and final score. The majority of recovery occurs within the first three months.
2. Up to 10% further recovery occurs between three months and one year.
3. In most patients, there is no evidence of further measurable recovery beyond one year. There is, however, some evidence that patients continue to adapt to their disability during the second and third year.
4. There are occasional cases who 'break the rules'. Few such cases have been described in the literature and this is an area for further research.

Prognostic factors

We have already mentioned that the most important factor is the severity of the initial insult. Other important factors include the presence of initial unconsciousness or prolonged drowsiness, and persistent incontinence (Wade and Langton Hewer, 1985). Other important factors are sitting balance and age (Wade and Langton Hewer, 1987b).

There are still major problems with making an accurate prognosis at an early stage following an acute stroke. One of the Bristol studies showed that the maximum reliability was 55% (Wade, Skilbeck, and Langton Hewer, 1983).

MECHANISMS OF RECOVERY

It is necessary to distinguish between two basic types of recovery, adaptive and intrinsic. The two types of recovery cannot be absolutely separated and there is considerable overlap between them.

Adaptive recovery has been termed 'behavioural substitution' (Goldberger, 1980). There is a large scope for adaptive recovery, which can make assessment of the underlying neurological processes very difficult. For instance, almost all ADL functions can be recovered purely through adaptation. A patient may walk on a spastic leg, and dress, wash, and feed one handed. Social recovery is, likewise, clearly adaptive, and a failure of social and psychological recovery will greatly hinder the ultimate level of functioning. Occasionally, writing can be transferred to the left hand.

Intrinsic recovery

Intrinsic recovery refers to improvement in lost neurological functions. Various models exist, for instance, the hemiplegic arm and hemianopic defects following stroke can both be used to study intrinsic recovery. Gait, on the other hand, is more difficult, as some patients learn to walk at a near normal speed despite having an abnormal gait pattern.

The mechanisms of recovery within the central nervous system are, in reality, largely unknown. It is agreed that during the first few days and weeks there is resolution of oedema, but this hardly explains continued recovery up to three to six months following stroke. It is known that regeneration of interrupted axons does not play an important part in the recovery process, although experimental studies have shown that damaged axons can sprout for up to two weeks after injury. It is theoretically possible that brain function is sufficiently plastic, or adaptable, for there to be a global reorganization of roles when certain areas of the brain are damaged. Such a mechanism undoubtedly exists in small children, but the evidence in adults is not convincing (Bach-y-Rita, 1981).

It is clear from animal studies and clinical experience that some relearning does occur after acute neural damage. Prevo, Visser, and Vogelaar (1982) showed that bio-feedback can lead to changed motor function, but is limited to the specific activity being trained. Generalization does not seem to occur.

THE BASIS OF THERAPY

Although there is clearly a certain amount of 'natural' recovery, therapies to speed-up or improve this process are usually attempted. Many branches of medicine and the remedial professions have developed treatments without having a clear understanding of whether they work and if so, how and why. Although the mechanisms of recovery of lost function are currently unknown, it is worth considering how therapy might affect recovery and rehabilitation. Some possible beneficial effects of therapy include the following:

1. Prevention of complications. Contractions are a good example of a complication that used to be frequent but is now rare. The probable reason is the recognition of the importance to maintain a full range of passive movement in the paralysed limbs from an early stage. Other complications include pressure sores, fractures (sometimes occurring as a result of premature mobilization), severe depression, and a painful, stiff shoulder (sometimes caused by faulty lifting of the patient).
2. Encouraging adaptive behaviour. For example, to teach a patient with a paralysed limb to dress and wash using one arm. The patient is thus encouraged to make the best use of residual abilities.
3. Retraining of the damaged nervous system (intrinsic recovery). Many people see retraining of the affected nervous system as the main aim of therapy. However, there is little or no evidence that therapy can in fact influence intrinsic recovery. For instance, the Bobath technique is based upon a theory of neurological recovery which, it is claimed, does influence intrinsic recovery. No evidence that this is so has ever been produced.
4. A further aim of therapists is to ensure that the patient has the correct physical aids (e.g. walking aid and wheelchair) and that these are used correctly.
5. Prevention of learned non-use. It has been suggested previously (Taub, 1980) that some of the disabilities seen after stroke reflect not so much the original loss of ability but a secondary effect, in which the patient learns not to use the affected limb. This hypothesis is derived from experimental work on monkeys, but at the moment there is very little human work to support or refute the idea. However, there are an increasing number of studies that involve immobilization of the 'normal' arm in an attempt to encourage the patient to use the affected arm. The technique is certainly worthy of further study, and is probably the most promising line of research in this difficult area.

Overall, it is extremely important that all medical staff are quite clear as to the scientific evidence upon which a stroke rehabilitation programme should be based. The lack of clear evidence that intrinsic recovery can be influenced by therapy is clearly a matter of both disappointment and concern. Much further research is needed into this area.

On what basis should physical therapy be planned? The following is suggested:

1. Therapy must be properly coordinated. For instance, there can be no rigid separation between physiotherapy, occupational therapy, and speech therapy. Indeed, there is much to be said for fusing the roles of physiotherapy and occupational therapy. The practice of allocating mobility to the physiotherapist, and arm function and self-care activities to the occupational therapist has no validity and should be discouraged.
2. The objectives of rehabilitation must be clearly understood, which include achievement of the maximum possible degree of independence, and ultimately the greatest possible quality of life; to maintain the maximum improvement achieved and avoid deterioration; and avoid complications (e.g. frozen shoulder).
3. It is important that every patient is thoroughly assessed using agreed assessment tools (see above).
4. It must be remembered that many stroke patients have subtle disturbances of cognitive function that are not always easily recognized. These include disturbances of comprehension, spatial disorder, apraxia, and disturbance of intellect and memory.

5. Many stroke patients are profoundly upset psychologically by what has happened to them. One reason for this is the implied threat to life. Another is the fact that most stroke patients look abnormal, resulting from a paralysed arm and, frequently, walking with a limp. This situation is in marked contrast to the patient who has suffered a myocardial infarction, but appears outwardly normal when dressed in a smart suit and tie. A third problem is that stroke patients soon realize that they are destined for a life of continued and permanent disability.
6. Depression following stroke is very common and about a third of patients, whether studied at six months or one year following stroke, show significant depression (Wade, Legh-Smith, and Langton Hewer, 1987).
7. Spasticity is an important characteristic of the hemiplegic limb. If untreated, it can result in contractures (see above). Various techniques to improve spasticity are practiced by therapists. There is no clear evidence that oral drug therapy (e.g. baclofen) has a beneficial effect.
8. Various techniques have been used in order to correct the foot deformity that frequently occurs after a stroke. Several types of surgical procedure are used; in some centres, below-knee splints are used either alone or in combination with surgery. There has been no adequate evaluation of these techniques. In general, surgery should be considered if there has been a reasonable return of motor control to the lower limb, but the patient is unable to achieve weight bearing on the sole of the foot and the heel. Occasionally, severe ankle clonus can be a problem. This can sometimes be alleviated either by motor point injection, or by the injection of alcohol or phenol around the posterior tibial nerve in the popliteal fossa.

OUTSTANDING RESEARCH QUESTIONS

The whole area of recovery following stroke is open for research. Some examples are given above and the following topics should be considered:

1. An evaluation of the benefits of long-term follow-up (over two to three years) of disabled stroke patients.
2. An evaluation of the effects of various therapies to counteract depression.
3. The principle of learned non-use and its relevance, particularly, to the paralysed hemiplegic arm.
4. A careful evaluation of the effects of surgical intervention, splinting for patients with foot deformity, or both.
5. A critical evaluation of the King's Fund consensus proposals for a 'model' stroke service.

CONCLUSIONS

This has been a brief review of the scientific basis underlying various aspects of stroke rehabilitation. It is not comprehensive and various topics have been omitted. For instance, there has been little discussion of speech and language deficits following stroke, or of the various sexual problems that can occur. Stroke-induced disability is not only expensive, but also a cause of untold misery to many hundreds of thousands of people around the world. For both scientific and humanitarian reasons, it is a subject of importance.

References

Bach-y-Rita P (1981) Central nervous system lesions: sprouting and unmasking in rehabilitation, *Arch Phys Med Rehabil*, **62**, 413–7

Bhavani G and Cockburn J (1983) The viability of the Rivermead Perceptual Assessment and implications for some commonly used assessments of perception, *Br J Occ Ther*, **46**, 17–9

Carstairs V (1976) Stroke: resource consumption and the cost to the community. In Gillingham FJ, Mawdsley C, and Williams AE, eds, *Stroke*, Edinburgh, Churchill Livingstone, 516–28

Consensus Conference (1988) King's Fund Forum, Treatment of Stroke, *Br Med J*, **297**, 126–8

Enderby PM, Wood VA, Wade DT, and Langton Hewer R (1987) The Frenchay Aphasia Screening Test: a short, simple test, for aphasia appropriate for non-specialists, *Int Rehabil Med*, **8**, 166–70

Folstein MF, Folstein SF, and McHugh PR (1975) Mini-mental state: a practical method for grading the cognitive state of patients for the clinician, *J Psychiatr Res*, **12**, 189–98

Goldberg DP and Hillier VF (1979) A scaled version of the General Health Questionnaire, *Psychol Med*, **9**, 139–45

Goldberger ME (1980) Motor recovery after lesions, *TINS*, Nov, 288–91

Granger CV and Gresham GE, Functional Independence Measure, Personal Communication

Heller A, Wade DT, Wood VA, Sunderland A, Langton Hewer R, and Ward E (1987) Arm function after stroke: measurement and recovery over the first three months, *J Neurol Neurosurg Psychiatry*, **50**, 714–9

Holbrook M (1982) Stroke: social and emotional outcome, *J R Coll Physicians Lond*, **16**, 100–4

Holbrook M and Skilbeck CE (1983) An activities index for use with stroke patients, *Age Ageing*, **12**, 166–70

Langton Hewer R (1989) *World Congress of Neurology, Rehabilitation in Stroke Units – Effects and Outcome*, New Delhi

Lyle RC (1981) A performance test for assessment of upper limb function in physical rehabilitation and research, *Int J Rehabil Res*, **4**, 483–92

Mahoney FI and Barthel DW (1965) Functional evaluation: the Barthel Index, *Md Med J*, **14**, 61–5

Office of Health Economics (1988) *Stroke*, London

Porch BE (1971) *The Porch Index of Communicative Ability: Administration, Scoring and Interpretation*, Consulting Psychologists, Palo Alto, California

Prevo AJH, Visser SL, and Vogelaar TW (1982) Effect of EMG feedback on paretic muscles and abnormal co-contraction in the hemiplegic arm, compared with conventional physical therapy, *Scand J Rehabil Med*, **14**, 121–31

Royal College of Physicians (1989) *Stroke: Report of Working Party*, London

Sarno MT (1969) *The Functional Communication Profile: Manual of Directions. Rehabilitation Monograph 42*, Institute of Rehabilitation Medicine, New York

Skilbeck CE, Wade DT, and Langton Hewer R (1983) Recovery after stroke, *J Neurol Neurosurg Psychiatry*, **46**, 5–8

Smith DS, Goldenberg E, Ashburn A, Kinsella G, Sheikh K, Brennan Meade TW *et al.* (1981) Remedial Therapy after Stroke: a randomised controlled trial, *Br Med J*, **282**, 517–8

Snaith RP, Ahmed SN, Mehta S, and Hamilton M (1971) Assessment of the severity of primary depressive illness: Wakefield self-assessment depression inventory, *Psychol Med*, **1**, 143–9

Taub E (1980) Somatosensory deafferention research with monkeys: implications for rehabilitation medicine. In Ince LP, ed, *Behavioural Psychology in Rehabilitation Medicine: Clinical Applications*, Baltimore, Williams & Wilkins, 371–401

Twitchell TE (1951) The restoration of motor function following hemiplegia in man, *Brain*, **74**, 443–80

Wade DT and Langton Hewer R (1985) Outlook after an Acute Stroke: urinary incontinence and loss of consciousness compared in 532 patients, *Q J Med*, **221**, 601–8

Wade DT and Langton Hewer R (1987a) Epidemiology of some neurological diseases with special reference to work load on the NHS, *Int Rehabil Med*, **8**, 129–37

Wade DT and Langton Hewer R (1987b) Functional abilities after stroke: measurement, natural history and prognosis, *J Neurol Neurosurg Psychiatry*, **50**, 177–82

Wade DT, Langton Hewer R, Skilbeck CE, and David RM (1985) *Stroke. A Critical Approach to Diagnosis, Treatment and Management*, London, Chapman & Hall Medical

Wade DT, Langton Hewer R, Wood VA, Skilbeck CE, and Ismail HM (1983) The hemiplegic arm after stroke: measurement and recovery, *J Neurol Neurosurg Psychiatry*, **46**, 521–4

Wade DT, Legh-Smith J, and Langton Hewer R (1987) Depressed mood after stroke. A community study of its frequency, *Br J Psychiatry*, **151**, 200–5

Wade DT, Skilbeck CE, and Langton Hewer R (1983) Predicting Barthel ADL Score at 6 months after an acute stroke, *Arch Phys Med Rehabil*, **64**, 24–8

Wade DT, Wood VA, Heller A, Maggs J, and Langton Hewer R (1987) Walking after stroke. Measurement and recovery of the first three months, *Scand J Rehabil Med*, **19**, 25–30

Wade DT, Wood VA, and Langton Hewer R (1985) Recovery after stroke – the first three months, *J Neurol Neurosurg Psychiatry*, **48**, 7–13

11
Acute and long-term care of patients with spinal cord injury or impairment

Robert R. Young and Mehdi Sarkarati

Before World War II and the discovery of antibiotics, very few quadriplegic or paraplegic patients survived to reach the first anniversary of their injuries. Repeated infections, particularly of the urinary tract and kidneys, and renal failure resulted in the fatal outcome. Presently, with comprehensive multi-disciplinary care provided by specialized centers, life-expectancy following injury, even for complete quadriplegics, is measured in decades. Acute spinal cord injury units have been shown to provide more effective, less costly care than even the best general hospitals (Duncan et al., 1987; Tator, 1990). Although precise data are not available, approximately 8000 new spinal cord injured patients are seen each year in the USA with a prevalence of about 200 000. At least 85% of spinal cord injuries arise in men, most of them young. Medical costs of acute and long-term care for such patients are at least $1.5 billion per year, which does not include loss of productivity/income, and costs for carers, and environmental modifications. The medical, psychological, and economic burdens borne by these patients, their families, and society at large is enormous.

This chapter will review some of the highlights of the field known as spinal cord injury (SCI), which has been enriched by input over the years from neurosurgeons, orthopedists, urologists, psychiatrists, and neurologists. The care and management of these patients represents a particularly well-developed area within restorative neurology (Ozer, 1988). Much can be learned at SCI centers that is applicable to the care of other neurologic patients; care for an SCI patient is virtually identical to that for a patient whose multiple sclerosis or infarct affects primarily the cord. Even though care for SCI patients has improved, practically everything we really need to know about minimizing neural damage and rational treatment of this catastrophic disorder remains to be learned.

ACUTE MANAGEMENT

Most SCI patients are injured as a result of reckless behavior, often in a motor vehicle accident, when diving, or in a fall, sometimes by a gun shot, and occasionally during sport such as horseback riding, rugby, or football. Prevention of such injuries, many of which are associated with intoxication, is most important. Campaigns against drinking and driving, and the increased use of seatbelts and airbags, have probably reduced the incidence of SCI but careful epidemiologic studies remain to be performed.

Campaigns have also been effective in training police officers, Emergency Medical Technicians (EMTs), and lay people in careful immobilization of the spine while patients are being removed from the scene of the accident and taken to the nearest general hospital or acute trauma center (Green, Eismont, and O'Heir, 1987). The spinal cord is seldom completely transected by the initial injury (Kakulas, 1984) and some recovery is usually possible; therefore, all conceivable efforts should be made to avoid secondary trauma to the cord at that time. Similarly, compression or swelling of the cord, vascular damage with ischemia, ongoing injury secondary to release of excitotoxins, free radicals, peroxides, and other tissue changes, such as increased cellular potassium efflux and calcium influx must be avoided or reduced whenever possible (De La Torre, 1980; Janssen and Hansebout, 1989). Recent clinical studies (Bracken *et al.*, 1990) document the efficacy of megadose intravenous steroids administered within the first eight hours after acute spinal cord injury. Methylprednisolone 30 mg kg^{-1} as an IV bolus, followed by 5.4 mg kg^{-1} hr^{-1} for 23 hours was shown to improve neurologic recovery. Although this therapy improves long-term function only to a modest extent, it is the first in what should be a progressively more efficacious group of acute therapies designed to minimize eventual disability, which is determined by the number of axons and neurons damaged by the initial mechanical event. These new and more effective therapies will only be developed as research provides increased understanding of the cascade of molecular events triggered by tissue damage.

By the time the acutely injured patient reaches the hospital, immobilization and steroid therapy should have been instituted together with attention to the airway, breathing, and cardiovascular function (Green, Eismont, and O'Heir 1987; Meyer, 1989). By the time the neurologist or neurosurgeon sees the patient, other general medical and surgical responses will be underway to treat traumatic damage outside the nervous system. Very careful neurologic examinations must be instituted as early as possible to determine the level of lesion, and degree of completeness of deficit below the level, as well as to monitor subtle changes in those parameters. Of particular importance is determination of completeness of deficit. For a tabular review of key sensory areas and muscles for classification of levels, see *Standards for Neurologic Classification of Spinal Injury Patients* published by the American Spinal Injury Association (ASIA, 1990). Prognosis, and particularly the need for immediate surgical decompression of the cord and stabilization of the spine, depend upon whether the lesion is clinically complete or not. Generally accepted wisdom suggests that nothing can be done to restore function below a complete spinal injury, whereas intra- and post-operative risks are justified if even a little motor or sensory function remains caudal to the lesion (Tator *et al.*, 1987). Imaging studies (CT, MRI, and occasionally contrast myelography) will demonstrate extra-axial compression caused by bone fragments, disc material, or epidural hematoma, which should be removed if the lesion is not complete. In patients with complete lesions, a separate decision can be made later concerning orthopedic surgery to produce a stable spine so that the patient can be mobilized as soon as possible for rehabilitation, without producing further deficit, progressive deformity, or pain (Braakman, 1986; Ducker *et al.*, 1984; Wagner and Chehrazi, 1980; White and Panjabi, 1984).

Care must be taken as soon as possible to preserve and facilitate vital functions. The urinary bladder should be emptied by intermittent catheterization (usually every six hours) before it becomes overdistended (Wyndaele and De Taeye, 1990); alimentation can be started if the bowels are working, otherwise intravenous fluid replacement will be needed. Gastro-intestinal bleeding may result from stress ulcers (Kiwerski, 1986). Vagally induced cardiac arrhythmias (Lehmann *et al.*, 1987) may occur in quadriplegic patients whose sympathetic outflow to the heart and elsewhere is paralysed. The patient must be turned from side to side every two hours or placed on a rotating bed to prevent pressure sores. Episodic mini-dose heparin plus electrical stimulation of calf muscles should be started to reduce the likelihood of deep vein thrombosis and pulmonary emboli (Merli *et al.*, 1988). Because a spinal cord injury is catastrophic for the patient and his family, and sometimes for his carers, experienced and intensive acute psychologic counselling is needed on a daily basis. Psychosocial support is essential if rehabilitation is to be fully successful.

The incidence of deep vein thrombosis is much reduced six weeks after the injury. Mobilization of mineral from bone with resultant hypercalcemia (Claus-Walker *et al.*, 1982) and phosphatemia caused by disuse often develops several weeks after the injury and may produce nausea and anorexia requiring treatment with increased IV fluids. The increased fluid intake may necessitate Foley catheterization on a temporary basis. Because of spinal shock (a complex, poorly understood syndrome), the bladder will almost always be flaccid, a situation that may last for many weeks or months. On the other hand, the bulbocavernosus reflex returns almost immediately, although other skeletal muscle reflexes do not return for days or weeks. Research is needed to understand spinal shock and how to manipulate it, discover ways to reduce demineralization in this setting (it being almost impossible to reverse later), and aid in preventing deep vein thrombosis and pulmonary emboli.

Full passive range of motion and positioning of paralysed limbs with joints at functional angles should be undertaken at least daily. The acute management phase overlaps with the active rehabilitation phase, which continues throughout the months before the patient is discharged. It often takes four or more months for paraplegics, and eight or more for quadriplegics, to achieve maximal benefit from hospitalization. The realistic goals of rehabilitation of an SCI patient depend on various individual factors such as motivation, general health, and age, but are particularly dependent on the level of lesion. For example, someone with a level at C7 can be independent in transfers, activities of daily living, driving a car, and dressing, whereas someone with a level at C5 is completely dependent on others for all these activities. Ozer (1988) describes a tabular summary of 'functional goals by level of impairment'.

Just as very few injured cords are completely transected, few have damage restricted to a short length (several millimeters) in the rostro-caudal dimension. Usually at least one, and often several, segments are involved in the injury zone. Whereas the cord is intact somewhere below the injury zone (but disconnected from higher centers), it is damaged at and just below the level by the original injury. As a consequence, motorneurons in this injury zone are often destroyed and their muscles denervated. Reflex connections through these cord segments may be permanently inoperative whereas those below eventually become hyperactive. Recovery of strength is possible in muscles at the level of injury because axons from any surviving motorneurons sprout to reinnervate muscle fibres that have been denervated in the same muscle (Little *et al.*, 1989). If those motorneurons, at the rostral edge of the lesion, are still under voluntary control, as they often are, strength and function increase just as they do with reinnervation following damage caused by acute poliomyelitis.

The autonomic nervous system in the isolated cord also recovers over several weeks from an initial hyporeflexic state. With lesions above T6, the sympathetic system is effectively disconnected from intracranial control. Orthostatic hypotension, which is prominent early, decreases as patients are 'trained' to sit upright, perhaps as a result of increased alpha-adrenergic activity and intravascular volume. In patients with levels at or above T6, a type of spasticity of circulatory control, termed autonomic dysreflexia (Comarr, 1984; Lindan, Joiner, and Freehafer, 1980; Colachis, 1992), develops after a few more weeks. Various noxious circumstances below the level of lesion, such as a full bladder, distention of bowel, pressure sores, ingrown toenails, and so on, produce a massive sympathetic outflow. This causes sweating, profound hypertension, and headache; it can lead to death from intracranial hemorrhage (Hanowell and Wilmot, 1988). This emergency must be treated acutely with nifedipine (10 mg to be chewed and swallowed) plus attention to relieve the causative factors.

Unless the sacral cord (conus) or cauda equina has been severely damaged in the injury, bladder function recovers so that detrussor contractions eventually occur when urine distends the bladder. This would produce automatic urination except detrussor–sphincter dyssynergia has usually also developed (Madersbacher, 1990). The external urethral sphincter, a striated muscle that behaves like a flexor muscle in the limb, also contracts, rather than relaxing as it normally does, when detrussor contraction occurs or when the body caudal to the spinal level is stimulated in a variety of ways. This spasticity of the sphincter results in urinary retention and increased intravesicle pressure, which produces reflux of urine up the ureters, infection, kidney stones, hydronephrosis, and renal failure unless treated. Long-term intermittent catheterization, perhaps together with anticholinergic paralysis of the detrussor is a reasonable option, particularly for women for whom an effective external collecting device does not exist (Wyndaele, 1990; Brendler, Radebaugh, and Mohler, 1989). It is also useful for those with damage to the sacral cord or its roots in whom a 'balanced bladder' (periodic reflex emptying without either a post-voiding residual of more than 100 ml or high intravesicular pressures) is impossible. As an alternative to long-term intermittent catheterization or to transurethral transection of the sphincter, the two main approaches to alleviating urinary retention caused by dyssynergia, botulinum toxin can be injected into the external sphincter (Dykstra *et al.*, 1988). When the sphincter is weakened, either pharmacologically or surgically, automatic contraction of the detrussor when the bladder fills to a certain volume will then expel urine through a condom catheter into a leg bag. The male patient will thus be continent, or at least dry, without a permanent indwelling catheter. A permanent indwelling catheter is to be avoided if possible because it increases the risks of urinary tract infection and of squamous cell cancer of the bladder (Benjany, Lockhart, and Rhamy, 1987), but for women it may be the only viable option if they are to remain dry.

ACTIVE REHABILITATION

During the month after injury, the patient and his care givers gradually spend more time restoring function by rehabilitation and less on acute care. Ideally, neurorehabilitation should begin soon after the injury and continue smoothly, without discontinuities in care, until the patient can be discharged home or to a home-like community facility. Very few SCI patients cannot go home and need to remain in a chronic hospital or nursing home. As research provides the means, neurorehabilitation will become increasingly involved with regeneration of the cord and redirection of axons, which will result in a full or nearly full recovery. Until that time, we are concerned with minimizing secondary damage to the cord (see Chapter 4) and maximizing functional abilities as determined by the spinal level of injury. Maximizing functional abilities depends upon technology for assistance with powered wheelchairs, hydraulic lifts in vans, and environmental control units, which enable a quadriplegic patient to control such things as room lights, telephone, or television by movements of head/ chin or by sip-and-puff (a simplified Morse code of negative or positive pressures in the mouth conveyed through a tube to the control device). Newer techniques use infra-red or laser devices to permit quadriplegics to control a computer with their eyes. Transfers of information and devices from engineering centers to spinal cord centers have been very important in permitting the utilization of new technologies to improve patient functions and independence. This is an area of active research and development.

Ischemic necrosis of skin, subcutaneous tissue, and muscle caused by ischeal pressure when seated, sacral pressure when lying supine or reclining, trochanteric pressure when lying on the side, or pressure elsewhere (pressure sores) can be prevented by arrangements for spreading the force caused by gravity over wider areas so that nowhere will the tissue pressure exceed capillary filling pressure. These devices include special cushions, air or water-filled mattresses, and beds containing air fluidized silicon beads; a technological problem for which a number of useful solutions have been developed to complement the equally effective method of pressure relief by turning at least every two hours in bed and lifting oneself (in the case of paraplegic patients) off the sitting surface for 15–30 seconds every 15 minutes (Pressure Relief Behavior). Pressure sores should be prevented but if they occur, they will usually heal once pressure upon them is eliminated. Antiseptic dressings and plastic surgery may also be required (Reichart, 1986; Woolsey and McGarry, 1991; Lee, 1991).

Muscles below the injury zone are largely innervated and can be excited to contract by stimulation of their alpha motor axons in peripheral nerves or at their motor points as they enter the muscle. Denervation potentials can be recorded electromyographically from many of these muscles but such denervation is minor unless peripheral nerves have been damaged by intermittent or chronic pressure upon them, subsequent accidents and so on. Whether denervation is also secondary to degeneration of motorneurons following damage to descending tracts, or similar CNS atrophic influences, remains to be proven. At any rate, muscles below the injury zone that are paralysed to voluntary activation can be made to contract by reflex inputs or electrical stimulation of their axons. When muscles have become atrophic with disuse, electrical stimulation may initially produce little or no visible contraction but when stimulation is continued daily, contractile activity improves and functional contractions usually result.

Phrenic nerve pacemakers, an electrode surrounding each phrenic nerve that is stimulated transcutaneously, produce fully functional diaphragm contractions in patients with cords damaged above C4, allowing them to live independent of mechanical ventilators (Glenn and Phelps, 1985). A circular radio transmitter, taped to the skin over each side of the chest, activates a receiver implanted beneath the skin under each transmitter. This receiver/demodulator is connected to the phrenic electrode; the transmitter is connected to a battery powered stimulator that fits under the wheelchair or on the bedside table. Each inspiratory contraction is produced by a

1.2 second train of 20 Hz stimuli that ramp up during the first 0.3 seconds of each train to produce smoothly graded respiratory movements. Without the stimulus ramping, a myoclonic or hiccough-like inspiration would be produced. This type of functional electrical stimulation (FES) is useful for patients whose phrenic motoneurons are disconnected from the brainstem but were not damaged in the injury zone. Useful respiratory excursions have been produced in a large number of patients for many years. Patients prefer this more natural type of respiration because they can smell things, taste their food, and have their tracheostomy tubes capped.

When FES techniques are applied to improve function of the upper limb, things become much more complex. Patients with lesions at C5/6 are able to flex the elbow voluntarily and perhaps dorsiflex the wrist but have no functional control of grasp or other useful finger movement. Muscles in the forearm can be electrically stimulated to extend the fingers, abduct the thumb, and then to flex all five fingers to grip a glass, eating utensil, or pencil. The entire upper limb can then be manipulated by proximal muscles, which are under voluntary control. Technical problems include difficulty with electrodes, which are placed into individual muscles. When these muscles contract, electrodes move or eventually break. Multiple muscles must be activated sequentially if the movement (e.g. palmar or key pinch) is to be truly functional, which requires multiple programmable stimulators; they need to be programmed on-line according to the movement being produced. Activators or control units for these stimulators must be developed so patients can use their unaffected muscles to operate the FES system. Ideally there would be some sort of continuous feedback modifying the strength of muscle according to the task being performed. The Rehabilitation Engineering Center of Case Western Reserve University (Keith *et al.*, 1989) has developed a system of upper extremity FES that restores clinically useful function to the forearms and hands of quadriplegic patients. This complex technology is now being transferred to certain special centers around the USA.

Attempts have also been made to use FES to enable paraplegics to walk (Marsolais and Kobetic, 1983; Cybulski, Penn, and Jaeger, 1984). Although functional use of lower limbs may seem simpler than upper limbs, several problems have prevented FES from being as clinically useful in the legs as it is in the arms of SCI patients. To stand and walk requires considerable contraction of anti-gravity muscles. Normally small Type I motor units are recruited, according to Henneman's size principle, to produce the force necessary to stand and walk. These units are notably fatigue-resistant and aerobic in metabolism. On the other hand, electrical stimulation preferentially recruits the largest Type II motor units, which are powerful but they fatigue very quickly and are metabolically anaerobic. Even well-conditioned young paraplegic patients find FES-mediated gait for short distances extremely exhausting. It is difficult electrically to stimulate selectively smaller diameter alpha motor axons, which supply small Type I motor units. A second problem has to do with maintaining balance and adapting the gait to irregularities of the surface upon which the person tries to walk. FES is still open-loop; that is, the motor output is not controlled as it should be by feedback of joint angles, limb position, muscle length and force, and cutaneous pressure. FES is being used to produce standing and walking with support for balance over short distances in the laboratory but has not yet become clinically useful in the way upper extremity FES has.

A serious practical drawback to high-tech solutions for neurorehabilitation problems concerns patient acceptability. For example, powered metal exoskeletons for lower limbs to produce walking of a sort with the SCI patient inside the mobile frame and similar devices for the paralysed or amputated arm have been developed but are not in general use because patients prefer wheelchairs or the assistance of attendants; they are not willing to use complex high-tech devices routinely, largely because of cosmetic factors and the excessive effort required to put such an apparatus on and take it off. Simple solutions to problems of this sort are favored. Wheelchairs (ordinary, electric and marathon types), which can be adapted for events such as basketball, tennis, or road racing, are very popular and, with new environmental access regulations, can be used in many public areas for work, recreation, and entertainment. Electrically powered wheelchairs can be driven by high quadriplegic patients whose voluntary motor performance is limited to the cranial nerves and neck muscles.

An even simpler device has been employed to enable complete paraplegic patients to stand and walk using crutches or canes for balance (Lee *et al.*, 1991). This stabilizing orthosis is a custom fit, firm leather boot reaching up to just below the fibular head. Like a ski-boot, it fixes the ankle but in 15–20° of plantar flexion. When paraplegics stand in these boots, their center of gravity falls behind the hip joint and in front of the knee thereby locking both joints without need for muscle contractions. The paraplegic then walks by shifting body weight over one leg and rotating the trunk to swing the unweighted leg forward. Using these orthoses, completely paralysed patients (with levels in the thoracic or lumbar region) walk long distances using canes for balance, and can go up and down stairs. Simplicity, ease of use, and cosmetic suitability make these orthoses very useful once patients have spent several weeks training to use them. This sort of exercise and loading of bones in the trunk and lower extremities, if begun early after injury, should reduce bone demineralization and aid in general fitness. In addition, these orthoses provide patients with access to areas in which wheelchair use is impractical and enhance morale. They complement but do not replace wheelchairs.

Sexual function, particularly in males, is seriously disrupted by SCI. Many male patients who desire children and whose injuries are above the sacral cord or thoracolumbar spine can make use of reflex ejaculation with vibratory (Szasz and Carpenter, 1989) or electrical (Bennett *et al.*, 1988) stimulation to produce sperm for use in artificial insemination. Various aids exist to produce erections, including penile prostheses (which often extrude or become infected in insensate SCI patients) and intracorporeal injections of prostaglandins (Lee, Stevenson, and Szasz, 1989). See also Chapter 7.

CONTINUING CARE

Some of the late effects of SCI begin to develop during the phase of active rehabilitation, others emerge after the patient has been discharged home. Although few of these medical problems are unique to SCI, the patient population in which they cluster is best cared for by an SCI/neurorehabilitation physician. Continuing care for the SCI patient is very important; the rarity of terminal renal failure in SCI patients is due in large part to yearly check-ups, using ultrasound to look for hydronephrosis and renal stones.

Urinary tract infections are common in SCI patients. Practically all have urine continually colonized with bacteria but fever, elevated WBC, and other symptoms only occur sporadically. Antibiotic treatment is usually effective (Stover *et al.*, 1989). Gallstones are 10 times more common in SCI patients than in the general population

(Apstein and Dalecki-Chipperfield, 1987); some bouts of fever treated as though they were caused by urinary tract infections may actually result from cholecystitis.

Pressure sores usually require patients to be hospitalized for pressure relief (using special mattresses), debridement, and often plastic surgery. Paraplegics develop more pressure sores than do quadriplegics, perhaps because the former are less careful about pressure relief. Certain patients develop repeated pressure sores, most never have any. Some pressure sores are produced by the patient for reasons of secondary gain such as hospitalization.

Bones in paralysed limbs become demineralized (Biering-Sorensen, Bohr, and Schaadt, 1988; Elias and Gwinup, 1992), very brittle, and fracture with little trauma. Such fractures usually heal with simple immobilization, and alignment is less crucial than in patients who will use the limb. Plaster or similar casts must never be applied to insensate limbs because serious pressure sores may be produced, which require extensive hospitalization.

Careful neurologic examinations should be repeated at 6–12 month intervals or more often if alterations are suspected. The most common cause of neurologic deterioration many months or years after the initial injury is post-traumatic syringomyelia (Rossier *et al.*, 1985; Williams, 1990). Intramedullary cysts develop in the injury zone, expand, coalesce, and reduce function of the uninjured cord above and below the lesion; it may also develop far rostral to the original level of zone. Typically, such a cyst produces pain at the level of injury and loss of function in one or more segments rostral to the lesion, which initially are unilateral. This situation is disastrous especially for patients with cervical lesions; for example, a syrinx may convert someone to a C5 completely dependent patient who has been a C7 independent one for years after rehabilitation. Draining these cysts with a percutaneous needle may help temporarily but indwelling shunts rarely help in the long run (Tator, Meguro, and Rowed, 1982). Studies of glial response to CNS injury and the development of these cysts should make their prevention and treatment more efficacious.

Other rarer causes of neurologic deterioration years after injury (Braakman and Vinken, 1967; Bosch, Stauffer, and Nickel, 1971) include re-injury with a second traumatic fracture, myelopathy caused by a spondylotic bar, spinal deformity, or ruptured disc and compression injury to peripheral nerves. Chronic pain and depression also reduce the function of SCI patients both during rehabilitation and months or years later. Depression is sometimes difficult to diagnose but it responds to usual pharmacologic therapies or, if not, to electroconvulsive therapy. Chronic pain (Davis and Martin, 1947; Burke, 1973; Waisbrod, Hansen, and Gerbershagen, 1984; Woolsey, 1986) often develops in the first few weeks after injury and is very common throughout the patients life. It usually occurs at or just rostral to the level of injury, responds poorly to analgesics, and is usually something the patient must learn to live with.

Pain may also accompany flexor spasms, a manifestation of spasticity seen particularly with spinal cord lesions, demyelinative or traumatic. Spasticity, in the form of flexor (and sometimes is extensor) spasms, dystonia, or contractures, is often more troublesome when lesions are incomplete.

Patients learn to use flexor spasms to help them put on their trousers. Spasms may also increase venous return from the legs cutting down on the incidence of deep vein thrombosis and pulmonary emboli. In short, spasticity may not always require therapy. Although spasticity has been defined as exaggerated stretch reflexes (Lance, 1980), there is much more to it than that (Young and Wiegner, 1987). Cutaneous and autonomic reflexes are also exaggerated, particularly in patients with lesions of the cord. Most of the disability experienced by such patients is not due to hyperactive reflexes; it is due to paresis, lack of dexterity, fatiguability, and other manifestations, consequent to disconnection of cerebral motor centers from the spinal segmental motor apparatus. Whereas therapies exist to reduce hyperactive reflexes, very little can be done to encourage regeneration and thereby restore function. Investigators must evaluate available therapies, using quantitative techniques such as those described by Delwaide (1985) and in Chapter 3 to identify those that are effective.

Baclofen, diazepam and tizanidine reduce flexor spasms or contractures in SCI patients but do little for bladder or other automatic hyperreflexia, and do nothing to improve function. Intrathecal baclofen, via continuous infusion from subcutaneous pumps, may be needed in patients who are not satisfactorily treated with oral therapy (Penn *et al.*, 1989). Phenol, alcohol or botulinum toxin injections of nerve terminals in muscles, percutaneous selective dorsal rhizotomies (Kadson and Llathi, 1984), or lesions of the dorsal root entry zone (Sindou and Jeanmonod, 1989) (see also Chapter 13) made intradurally, all relieve hyperreflexia by damaging neural elements (particularly afferents) in the reflex arcs. They are invasive, often irreversible, and not frequently employed. As years go by, spastic SCI patients gradually become less so. How this happens isn't clear. Do nerves in limbs become progressively compressed and damaged by sitting on toilet or other seats?

SUMMARY

The care of SCI patients is complex and rewarding. These patients live high quality lives for long periods of time and so the challenge of their care is demanding, but outcomes are usually satisfactory to patient and physician. SCI care is a particularly well developed area within restorative neurology. We appear to be at the threshold of exciting new developments in technology transfer, functional neurosurgery, and pharmacotherapy. Neurobiological research will provide the miracles of tomorrow.

References

Apstein MD and Dalecki-Chipperfield K (1987) Spinal cord injury is a risk factor for gallstone disease, *Gastroenterology*, **92**, 966–8

ASIA (American Spinal Injury Association) (1990) Standards for neurological classification of spinal injury patients. ASIA, Georgia

Benjany DE, Lockhart JL, and Rhamy RK (1987) Malignant vesical tumors following spinal cord injury, *J Urol* **138**, 1390–1392

Bennett CJ, Seager SW, Vasher EA *et al.* (1988) Sexual dysfunction and electroejaculation in men with spinal cord injury: Review, *J Urol*, **139**, 453

Biering-Sorensen F, Bohr H, and Schaadt O (1988) Bone mineral content of the lumbar spine and lower extremities years after spinal cord lesion, *Paraplegia*, **26**, 293–301

Bosch A, Stauffer ES, and Nickel VL (1971) Incomplete traumatic quadriplegia, A ten-year review, *JAMA*, **216**, 473–8

Braakman R (1986) The values of more aggressive management in traumatic paraplegia, *Neurosurg Rev*, **9**, 141–7

Braakman R and Vinken PJ (1967) Unilateral facet interlocking in the lower cervical spine, *J Bone Joint Surg*, **49**, 249–57

Bracken MB, Shepard MJ, Collins WF, Holford TR, Young W, Baskin DS, Eisenberg HM, Flamm E *et al.* (1990) A randomized, controlled trial of methylprednisolone or naloxone in the treatment of acute spinal cord injury – Results of the Second National Acute Spinal Cord Injury Study, *N Engl J Med*, **322**, 1405–11

Brendler CB, Radebaugh LC, and Mohler JL (1989) Topical oxybutynin chloride for relaxation of dysfunctional bladders, *J Urol*, **141**, 1350–2

Burke DC (1973) Pain in paraplegia, *Paraplegia*, **10**, 297–313

Claus-Walker J, Halstead L, Rodriguez GR, and Henry YK (1982) Spinal cord injury hypercalcemia: Therapeutic profile, *Arch Phys Med Rehabil*, **63**, 106–15

Colachis SC III (1992) Autonomic hyperreflexia with spinal cord injury, *J Am Paraplegia Soc*, **15**, 171–86

Comarr AE (1984) Autonomic dysreflexia (hyperreflexia), *J Am Paraplegia Soc*, **3**, 53–7

Cybulski GR, Penn RD, and Jaeger RJ (1984) Lower extremity functional neuromuscular stimulation in cases of spinal cord injury, *Neurosurgery*, **15**, 132–40

Davis L and Martin J (1947) Studies upon spinal cord injuries. II – The nature and treatment of pain, *J Neurosurg*, **4**, 483–91

De La Torre JC (1980) Chemotherapy of spinal cord trauma. In Windle W, ed, *The Spinal Cord And Its Reaction to Traumatic Injury*, New York, Marcel Dekker, 291–310

Delwaide PJ (1985) Electrophysiological analysis of the mode of action of muscle relaxants in spasticity, *Ann Neurol*, **17**, 90–5

Ducker TB, Bellarigue R, Salcman M, and Walleck C (1984) Timing of operative care in cervical spinal cord injury, *Spine*, **9**, 525–31

Duncan EG, Tator CH, Edmonds VE, Lapczak LI, and Andrews DE (1987) Treatment in specialized unit improves three measures of outcomes after acute spinal cord injury: statistical analysis of 552 cases, *Surgical Forum*, **38**, 501–3

Dykstra DD, Sidi AA, Scott AB, Pagel JM, and Goldish GD (1988) Effects of Botulinum A toxin on detrusor–sphincter dyssynergism in spinal cord injury patients, *J Urol*, **139**, 919–22

Elias AN and Gwinup G (1992) Immobilization osteoporosis in paraplegia, *J Am Paraplegia Soc*, **15**, 163–70

Glenn WWL and Phelps ML (1985) Diaphragm pacing by electrical stimulation of the phrenic nerve, *Neurosurgery*, **17**, 974–89

Green BA, Eismont FJ, and O'Heir JT (1987) Spinal cord injury – A systems approach: prevention, emergency medical services, and emergency room management, *Crit Care Clin*, **3**, 471–93

Hanowell LH and Wilmot C (1988) Spinal cord injury leading to intracranial hemorrhage, *Crit Care Med*, **16**, 911–2

Janssen L and Hansebout RR (1989) Pathogenesis of spinal cord injury and newer treatments: A review, *Spine*, **14**, 23–32

Kasdon DL and Lathi ES (1984) A prospective study of radio frequency rhizotomy in the treatment of post-traumatic spasticity, *Neurosurgery*, **15**, 526–9

Kakulas BA (1984) Pathology of spinal injuries, *Central Nervous System Trauma*, **1**, 117–29

Keith MW, Peckham PH, Thrope GB, Stroh KC, Smith B, Buckett JR *et al.* (1989) Implantable functional neuromuscular stimulation in the tetraplegic hand, *J Hand Surg [Am]*, **14A**, 524–30

Kiwerski J (1986) Bleeding from the alimentary canal during the management of spinal cord injury patients, *Paraplegia*, **24**, 92–6

Lance JW (1980) Symposium Synopsis. In Feldman RG, Young RR, and Koella WP, eds, *Spasticity Disordered Motor Control*, Chicago, Yearbook Medical, 485–94

Lee BY (1991) Plastic surgery for pressure sores. In Lee BY, Ostrander LE, Cochran GV, and Shaw WM, eds, *The Spinal Cord Injured Patient*, Philadelphia, Saunders, 223–30

Lee IY, Craffey E, Davidson D, Durso V, Tun CG, Walsh N, and Young RR (1991) Complete paraplegics can walk using a below-the-knee orthosis, *Neurology*, **41**, 221

Lee LM, Stevenson RWB, and Szasz G (1989) Prostaglandin E-1 versus phenolamine/papaverine for the treatment of erectile impotence: A double-blind comparison, *J Urol*, **141**, 549–50

Lehmann KG, Lane JG, Piepmeier JM, and Batsford WP (1987) Cardiovascular abnormalities accompanying acute spinal cord injury in humans: Incidence, time course and severity, *J Am Coll Cardiol*, **10**, 46–52

Lindan R, Joiner E, and Freehafer AA (1980) Incidence and clinical features of autonomic dysreflexia in patients with spinal cord injury, *Paraplegia*, **18**, 285–92

Little JW, Moore D, Brook M, and Powers R (1989) Electromyographic evidence for motor axon sprouting in recovering upper extremities of acute quadriplegia, (American Paraplegia Society – Abstract), *J Am Paraplegia Soc*, **13**, 16

Madersbacher H (1990) The various types of neurogenic bladder dysfunction: An update of current therapeutic concepts, *Paraplegia*, **28**, 217–9

Marsolais EB and Kobetic R (1983) Functional walking in paralyzed patients by means of electrical stimulation, *Clin Orthop*, **175**, 30–6

Merli GJ, Herbison GJ, Ditunno JF, Weitz HH, Henzes JH, Park CH *et al.* (1988) Deep vein thrombosis: Prophylaxis in acute spinal cord injured patients, *Arch Phys Med Rehabil*, **69**, 661–4

Meyer PR (1989) Emergency room assessment: Management of spinal cord and associated injuries, In Meyer PR, ed, *Surgery of Spine Trauma*, New York, Churchill Livingstone, 23–59

Ozer MN (1988) *The management of persons with spinal cord injury*, New York, Demos

Penn RD, Savory MNS, Corcos D, Latash M, Gottlieb G, Parke B *et al.* (1989) Intrathecal baclofen for severe spinal spasticity, *N Engl J Med*, **320**, 1517–21

Reichart H (1986) Surgical treatment of pressure sores in paraplegics and possible prevention of their recurrence, *Scand J Plast Reconstr Surg Hand Surg*, **20**, 125–7

Rossier AB, Foo D, Shillito J, and Dyro FM (1985) Posttraumatic syringomyelia – Incidence, clinical presentation, electrophysiological studies, syrinx protein and results of conservative and operative treatment, *Brain*, **108**, 439–61

Sindou M and Jeanmonod D (1989) Microsurgical DREZ-otomy for treatment of spasticity and pain in the lower limbs, *Neurosurgery*, **24**, 655–70

Stickler DJ and Chawla JC (1988) An appraisal of antibiotic policies for urinary tract infections in patients with spinal cord injuries undergoing long-term intermittent catheterization, *Paraplegia*, **26**, 215–25

Stover SL, Lloyd LK, Waites KB, and Jackson AB (1989) Urinary tract infection in spinal cord injury, *Arch Phys Med Rehabil*, **70**, 47–54

Szasz G and Carpenter C (1989) Clinical observations in vibratory stimulation of the penis of men with spinal cord injury, *Arch Sex Behav*, **18**, 461–75

Tator CH (1990) Acute management of spinal cord injury, *Br J Surg*, **77**, 485–6

Tator CH, Duncan EG, Edmonds VE, Lapczak LI, and Andrews DF (1987) Comparison of surgical and conservative management in 208 patients with acute spinal cord injury, *Can J Neurol Sci*, **14**, 60–9

Tator CH, Meguro K, and Rowed DW (1982) Favorable results with syringo-subarachnoid shunts for treatment of syringomyelia, *J Neurosurg*, **56**, 517–23

Wagner FC and Chehrazi B (1980) Spinal cord injury: Indications for operative intervention, *Surg Clin North Am*, **60**, 1980

Waisbrod H, Hansen D, and Gerbershagen HU (1984) Chronic pain in paraplegics, *Neurosurgery*, **15**, 933–4

White AA and Panjabi MM (1984) The role of stabilization in the treatment of cervical spine injuries, *Spine*, **9**, 512–22

Williams B (1990) Post traumatic syringomyelia. An update, *Paraplegia*, **28**, 296–313

Woolsey RM (1986) Chronic pain following spinal cord injury, *J Am Paraplegia Soc*, **9**, 39–41

Woolsey RM and McGarry JD (1991) The cause, prevention and treatment of pressure sores. In Woodsey RM and Young RR, eds, *Neurologic Clinics – Disorders of the Spinal Cord*, Philadelphia, Saunders, 797–808

Wyndaele JJ (1990) Pharmacotherapy for urinary bladder dysfunction in spinal cord injury patients, *Paraplegia*, **28**, 146–50

Wyndaele JJ and De Taeye N (1990) Early intermittent self catheterization after spinal cord injury, *Paraplegia*, **28**, 76–80

Young RR and Wiegner AW (1987) Spasticity, *Clin Orthop*, **219**, 50–62

12
Multiple sclerosis—treatment and rehabilitation

Rene Elkin and Labe Scheinberg

Multiple sclerosis (MS) is the most common demyelinating disease of the central nervous system (CNS) in the USA and in most temperate zones of the world. MS is amongst the commonest diseases causing severe disability in the young adult population. The cause of MS is unknown and the course of the disease is unpredictable. No therapy has been unequivocally shown to alter this course. Ideal restoration of function after chronic impairment is dependent on restoration of central myelin, which is not currently feasible.

IMMUNOPATHOLOGY OF MULTIPLE SCLEROSIS

MS, clearly defined clinically more than a century ago, remains an enigma in terms of pathogenesis, etiology, and meaningful therapy (Charcot, 1868). In essence, MS is an inflammatory disease in which lymphocytes and mononuclear cells penetrate the parenchyma of the CNS with myelin destruction and relative axonal sparing. Oligodendrocytes are damaged, astrocytes proliferate, and the residual demyelinated area constitutes a plaque that fails to remyelinate. There is a predilection for plaques to occur in the periventricular regions, brainstem, spinal cord, and optic nerves, but they are randomly distributed in time and space throughout the CNS (Powell and Lampert, 1983; Prineas, 1985).

Available evidence suggests that MS may be triggered by an infectious agent (e.g. virus), and may result from the action of immune mechanisms on the nervous system in susceptible individuals. Although many viruses have been implicated, attempts to identify a single infectious agent as the cause of MS has been unsuccessful (Johnson, 1982).

The immunology of MS has been extensively reviewed (Bloom, 1980; Oger, Roos, and Antel, 1983; Rodriguez, 1989). Rodriguez summarizes the immune hypotheses for the cause of MS, namely, immune-mediated demyelination triggered by viral infection (Rodriguez, 1989).

CLINICAL FEATURES

MS may produce a variety of symptoms, usually lasting for days or weeks before improving, which tends to occur over 4 to 12 weeks. About two thirds of patients have a remitting–relapsing course. In approximately 15% of patients, the course of the disease is relentlessly progressive without remissions (Prineas, 1985).

The diagnosis is based on symptoms and objective evidence of white matter lesions in the CNS, disseminated in time and space. Disturbances of sensation and gait, and monocular visual loss are the most common presenting symptoms (Matthews *et al.*, 1985). Vertigo, diplopia, dysarthria, and urinary frequency, urgency, and incontinence are also frequent symptoms. Severe fatigue, particularly during the active phase of the illness, is common.

Demyelinated axons are subject to manifestations resulting from axonal hyperexcitability (Raminsky, 1981). This is believed to be the underlying pathophysiology responsible for the positive symptoms in MS, namely, Lhermitte's sign, trigeminal neuralgia, facial myokymia, spasms, and a variety of sensory symptoms.

A number of environmental factors and changes in the internal body milieau are either known, or suspected, to affect the clinical status of patients with MS. Temperature increments of as little as 0.5°C *in vitro* in experimentally demyelinated fibers results in a block of conduction (Raminsky, 1973). This may explain the clinical worsening of patients induced by increased body temperature secondary to exercise, hot baths, or fever (Uthoff's phenomenon).

The relationship between trauma and the appearance or exacerbation of MS has been the subject of intense debate and controversy, and remains unresolved. Arnason (1983) has shown that in experimental allergic encephalomyelitis (EAE), lesions have a predilection for sites of previous trauma, although this may not be the case in humans (Bamford *et al.*, 1981). In a retrospective, controlled study, Bamford and co-workers found no causative relationship between trauma and the emergence or exacerbation of MS.

The influence of stress on the immune system is well-known (Dorian and Garfinkel, 1987). However, there is no current evidence to indicate a cause and/or effect relationship in MS (Foley *et al.*, 1988).

Cognitive impairment, which has not previously been recognized as a major feature of MS, has become increasingly demonstrated with the availability of sophisticated neuropsychologic testing techniques (Foley *et al.*, 1988). Petersen and Kokmen (1989) in their review of the cognitive and psychiatric abnormalities in MS, found no consistent relationship between the number and extent of observed cerebral demyelinating lesions seen on MRI, and the degree and characteristics of the associated cognitive abnormalities. Baumhefner and co-workers (1990) reported that in MS patients with the major plaque burden in the cerebrum, as seen on MRI, there was a strong correlation with neuropsychologic functioning.

The cognitive changes seem to occur gradually. There is no correlation with duration of the illness or the degree of the disability. The most consistent defect is in retrieval processes, possibly as a result of slowed information processing (Litvan *et al.*, 1988). Patients with MS have also been shown to have attention deficits and impaired visio-spatial skills, and have a clinical picture consistent with a subcortical dementia.

At present, we do not know the prevalence of mental changes in patients with MS, or the long-term course of these changes. In a study of 21 patients with definite or probable MS, and nine patients with isolated optic neuritis, Lyon-Caen and co-workers (1986) found mild to moderate impairment of cognitive function in 60% of patients within two years of the onset of the disease, despite the absence of subjective complaints by the patients themselves.

EVALUATION AND RATING

At the time of the initial evaluation, the patient should be scored using the scales developed by the International Federation of Multiple Sclerosis Societies, available from the National Multiple Sclerosis Society as the minimal record of disability (MRD); it includes first the disability status scale or expanded disability status scale (EDSS), which is actually an impairment scale developed by Kurtzke (1961), and is based on the standard neurological examination, scoring the functional systems usually involved in MS (pyramidal, cerebellar, brainstem, sensory, bowel, bladder, visual, and mental) from 0–5 (with 0 being normal and 5 being inability to perform functions within this system). After these are scored, together with an ambulation index, the EDSS is derived. In this, 0 is normal neurological examination, 6 is ambulatory with unilateral assistance, 8 is restricted to bed or wheelchair with effective use of arms, and 10 is death caused by MS. This EDSS is the evaluation used in most current clinical trials, and is useful for record keeping to monitor the clinical course, especially in rehabilitation.

The second part of the MRD is the incapacity status scale (ISS), which is actually a 'disability' scale based on the activities of daily living or Barthel index. It is scored in a similar fashion to the functional systems, with 0 being normal function in the activity and 5 being total inability to perform.

The last part of the MRD is the environmental status scale (ESS), which is 'handicap' in the terminology of the International Classification of Impairments, Disabilities and Handicaps of the WHO. On standard neurological assessment, the clinician may find no change in the impairment or EDSS whereas the patient will report progression. This is often projected by the patient in the ISS. EDSS is usually based on the neurological examination, but it can be performed by self-reporting, and the ISS and ESS are usually self reported with confirmation by family members or others.

IMMUNOSUPPRESSIVE TREATMENT OF MULTIPLE SCLEROSIS

Since MS is thought to be an immunologically mediated disease in which the immune system is overactive, immunosuppressive therapy may be important. Numerous diverse and even dangerous therapies have been attempted, most of which have been ineffective and no curative treatment is available.

The mainstay of therapy for acute MS exacerbations is adrenocorticotrophic hormone (ACTH) through an anti-inflammatory action, as well as a direct action on T and B lymphocytes (Lyon-Caen *et al.*, 1986). Several reports have described superior results with high dose intravenous methylprednisolone (Durelli *et al.*, 1986; Carter and Rodriguez, 1989). Although corticosteroids hasten recovery from acute exacerbations of MS, there is no evidence that they alter the course of the disease.

Treatment of chronic, progressive MS is controversial and has been extensively reviewed (Waksman, Reingold, and Reynolds, 1987; Sibley, 1988; Carter and Rodriguez, 1989). Current therapies include cyclophosphamide, azathioprine, plasmapheresis, interferon-B, total lymphoid irradiation, cyclosporin A, and monoclonal antibodies, none of which have had any significant impact on progression of the disease.

While alteration of impairment is not feasible, disabilities may be altered by rehabilitation. Symptomatic management of primary symptoms, such as spasticity and bowel and bladder dysfunction, combined with measures to restore the patient to the greatest possible level of function provide the most successful therapeutic approach.

PRIMARY SYMPTOMS

Gait abnormalities

Gait disturbance is one of the most frequent primary symptoms in patients with MS and may be caused by weakness, spasticity, ataxia, or a combination of these. The most commonly affected muscle groups in the lower extremities are the hip flexors, thigh abductors, and dorsiflexors and evertors of the foot.

Exercise will improve endurance and well-being, but it is not clear whether muscle strength is increased. Specific exercises minimize complications of reduced mobility in patients at risk, and these include active range of motion exercise and resistive exercise, both isometric and isotonic (Rosenthal and Scheinberg, 1990).

Orthotics are frequently indicated when weakness interferes with gait. The orthosis should meet individual requirements, be comfortable, simple to use, and cosmetically acceptable. Foot drop is a frequent manifestation of upper motorneuron lesions, resulting from the relative weakness of foot dorsiflexors and evertors. The readily available polypropylene ankle-foot orthosis (PAFO) is a useful device in this situation. Several types are available, all are worn inside the shoe and are secured by a strap around the calf. They differ in degree of rigidity and ankle support and once fitted, they should be checked to ensure that the calf band does not impinge on the peroneal nerve and to ensure that undue pressure is not placed on any part of the skin. Any ankle movement should closely approximate the location of the anatomic joint axis so the patient shows good function during ambulation.

Spasticity and spasms, both flexor and extensor, respond well to the gamma-amino butyric acid (GABA) agonist, baclofen (Davidoff, 1985). Reduction in spasticity improves endurance as well as gait efficiency. The response to baclofen varies, and careful dose-titration is recommended to achieve maximal symptom relief and avoidance of side-effects, such as drowsiness or weakness. Penn and co-workers (1989) reported the use of intrathecal baclofen in 20 patients with severe disabling spasticity that was not controlled with oral antispastic agents. All 20 patients responded to intrathecal infusion of baclofen into the lumbar area. The results are promising, but future trials are necessary to assess long-term effectiveness and risks of this form of treatment.

Diazepam is also an effective antispastic drug. Side-effects are similar to baclofen, but sedation is more prominent and dependence may be a problem. It is best reserved for those patients who do not respond to, or are unable to tolerate, baclofen. A combination of these two drugs may produce excellent relief of symptoms.

Dantrolene sodium weakens spastic muscles by interfering with the intramuscular contractible process. It can cause serious hepatotoxicity and use should be limited to patients in whom severe spasticity is refractory to other, less hazardous treatment.

Passive stretching through full range of movement should be performed several times daily on all spastic limbs. Regular repetition relieves the stiffness of spasticity and prevents fibrous contracture of muscles, and joint ankylosis.

Ataxia may result from disease in the cerebellum, its connections to the brainstem, or may follow significant dorsal column disease. Regardless of the etiology, ataxia does not respond to medication, but some patients will improve with specific exercise programs. Sensory information can be enhanced by visual cues (e.g. watching movement carefully) or by general sensory cues (e.g. by placing weight on the limbs). Frenkel's exercises, which are a series of exercises designed to improve lower extremity proprioceptive control, have been suggested for treatment of ataxia. Their greatest value is in compensating for loss of proprioception by enhancing visual cues, and success in cerebellar ataxia is therefore limited.

Gait aids should be selected only to provide assistance, and the patient will usually need training in how to use the aid as effectively as possible. Canes provide the least support and walkers the most. Crutches may be either axillary or non-axillary; non-axillary crutches are most commonly prescribed for patients with paraparesis who have adequate axial balance. The Lofstrand crutch has a padded hand bar and forearm cuff, which helps to stabilize the arm and wrist, and makes walking safer and easier. The Canadian crutch has both a forearm and an arm cuff, and can be used when there is triceps weakness.

Walkers provide maximal support at the cost of a slow and awkward gait. They are of particular use in patients with poor balance. Walkers with wheels are appealing to patients with upper extremity weakness or incoordination, but they introduce a measure of instability that can be dangerous.

Since many gait aids transfer weight-bearing capacity from lower to upper extremities, adequate upper extremity strength and mobility are mandatory in gait training. In addition, adequate truncal stability is necessary to maintain balance and correct posture.

Once the appropriate gait aid is prescribed, training by an experienced physiotherapist is essential. This should include techniques to negotiate stairs, inclines, and curbs.

When assisted walking is unsafe or impossible, or as a supplementary means of transportation, a wheelchair is indicated, which often allows for greater independence for the patient. Motorized chairs or scooters are available for patients with severe upper extremity weakness. The wheelchair should be individually fitted, and the patient trained in its correct use, including the proper methods of transferring to and from the wheelchair.

Bladder symptoms

Second to gait, bladder dysfunction is the most disabling symptom. This is dealt with in Chapter 11.

Bowel disorders

Constipation is the primary problem; it is caused by loss of the normal postprandial increase in colonic motility in patients with MS. Other neurologic factors contributing to constipation include immobility, inadequate dietary fiber and hydration, and side-effects of medications, particularly those atropine-like ones used to control irritable bladder symptoms. Adequate oral fluid intake, high fiber foods, and stool softners may be sufficient to ensure regular bowel movements. If constipation persists, a laxative or enema may be required.

Fecal incontinence is much less frequent in MS patients and may arise as a result of fecal impaction accompanied by spurious diarrhea. A rectal examination will reveal the presence of impaction. Patients who are not impacted may respond to daily use of suppositories to ensure predictable bowel movements or to anticholinergic medications such as propantheline bromide.

Sexual dysfunction

Sexual symptoms are a common source of disability in MS and may result from the primary effect of MS plaques, tertiary psychological problems, or frequently, both (Kirkeby *et al.*, 1988).

Treatment depends on the cause. Psychological problems are best managed by professional counselling. For impotence, intracavernous papavarine is beneficial and has largely obviated the need for penile implants. For those with anorgasmia, directing the partner to a pleasurable sexual practice may lower the threshold to climax; the use of stimulators, such as vibrators, may be helpful.

Dysphagia

This is an infrequent complaint and is usually associated with more severe disease. Difficulties may arise at any point in the normal swallowing mechanism (Larson, 1985). Coughing and choking indicate aspiration into the airway, which may be confirmed radiologically by means of a 'modified barium swallow'.

When dysphagia is severe, a percutaneous gastrostomy is simple to perform and well accepted by patient and carer.

Speech disorders

Dysarthria, although common in MS, is less frequently a source of major disability and generally parallels the severity of neurologic impairment (Darley, Brown, and Goldstein, 1972).

Patients with defective articulation should first be taught to slow their rate of speech and to make more time available for the tongue to compensate for the loss of control. When severe, exercises with specific speech muscles may be required. When these measures fail, alternatives to speech including picture, word phrase, and alphabet boards can be selected depending on the degree of motor, visual, and intellectual impairment.

Fatigue

This is one of the most disabling primary symptoms of MS. The pathogenesis is unknown. It is greater in the afternoon and late morning and is aggravated by physical activity and high ambient temperature.

Amantadine and pemoline have been reported to ameliorate fatigue in MS (Murry, 1985). The patient should organize the day around the times when fatigue is worse, to permit rest when needed. An on-site assessment of the home or workplace by an occupational therapist may be indicated to devise optimal solutions for each individual patient.

SECONDARY SYMPTOMS

Except for pressure sores, the above sections have already addressed the most common secondary symptoms. About 15% of patients with MS will develop pressure sores at some time during their illness and adequate preventive measures can reduce this incidence. Pressure is of paramount importance in initiating sores (see Chapter 11). The most common sites are legs, the ischeal tuberosities, sacrum, the greater trochanters, the heels, and malleoli of the ankles.

A reddened area that does not blanche on pressure is the first sign of tissue destruction. Tissue loss confined to the epidermis is referred to as a grade I sore. A grade II sore extends through the dermis to the subcutaneous fat. Both grade I and grade II sores can be successfully treated non-surgically with use of antiseptic washes and saline dressings.

A grade III sore extends through the subcutaneous fat and a grade IV sore extends to underlying muscle and bone. A direct consequence of this extension may result in osteomyelitis or pyoarthrosis. Surgical treatment is usually indicated with aggressive debridement of devitalized tissue and myocutaneous flaps. Patients should be prepared for surgery; a high protein diet is recommended to promote wound healing.

Patients at risk must be identified (e.g. those with lower extremity weakness, sensory loss, incontinence, and intellectual impairment), and the skin should be regularly examined for signs of compromise. Patients who are wheelchair bound need to be taught appropriate pressure relieving exercises and provided with a custom designed wheelchair cushion. Bedridden patients should, if possible, learn to turn themselves, and if not, should be turned every two hours. Eggcrate foam pads on regular mattresses help to distribute weight; specialized mattresses containing air, water, hydrophilic gels, or fluidized silicon beads are also options.

Aggressive treatment of spasticity with medication, daily passive range of motion exercises, prevention of incontinence, and meticulous perineal hygiene will further reduce the risk of pressure sores.

CONCLUSION

As with any disease of unknown etiology, many treatments have been proposed, although none have had significant impact on the disease. Based on current research, anti-inflammatory, antiviral, and immunosuppressive agents may be useful.

The physician can, however, do much to alleviate the troublesome symptoms of MS. This entails careful assessment of symptoms, both neurologic and non-neurologic, as well as knowledge of the intellectual, emotional, and social impacts of the illness, and the available support network. The physician is required to work closely with rehabilitation specialists including speech, physical, and occupational therapists, and social workers.

Using this multidisciplinary approach, the physician is rewarded with patients who, in spite of their severe and disabling disease, are able to contribute in a meaningful way to their families, friends, and communities.

References

Arnason BGW (1983) Relevance of experimental allergic encephalomyelitis, In Antel JP, ed, *Neurologic Clinics*, Vol. 1, No. 3, August 1983. Symposium on Multiple Sclerosis, Philadelphia, WB Saunders, 765–82

Bamford CR, Sibley WA, Thies C *et al*. (1981) Trauma as an etiologic and aggravating factor in multiple sclerosis, *Neurology*, **31**, 1229–34

Barnes MP, Bateman DE, Cleland PG *et al*. (1985) Intravenous methylprednisolone for multiple sclerosis in relapse, *J Neurol Neurosurg Psychiatry*, **48**, 157–9

Baumhefner RW, Tourtellotte WW, Syndulko K *et al*. (1990) Quantitative multiple sclerosis plaque assessment with magnetic resonance imaging, *Arch Neurol*, **47**, 19–26

Bloom BR (1980) Immunological changes in multiple sclerosis, *Nature*, **287**, 275

Carter JL and Rodriguez M (1989) Immunosuppressive treatment of multiple sclerosis, *Mayo Clin Proc*, **64**, 664–9

Charcot JM (1868) Histologie de la sclerose en plaques, *Gaz Hop (Paris)*, **41**, 554–66

Darley FL, Brown JR, and Goldstein NP (1972) Dysarthria in multiple sclerosis, *J Speech Hear Res*, **15**, 229–45

Davidoff RA (1985) Antispasticity drugs: mechanisms of action, *Ann Neurol*, **17**, 107–16

Dorian B and Garfinkel PE (1987) Stress, immunity and illness – a review, *Psychol Med*, **17**, 393–407

Durelli L, Cocito D, Riccio A *et al*. (1986) High-dose intravenous methylprednisone in the treatment of multiple sclerosis: clinical-immunologic correlations, *Neurology*, **36**, 238–43

Foley FW, Miller AH, Traugott U, LaRocca NG *et al*. (1988) Psychoimmunological dysregulation in multiple sclerosis, *Psychosomatics*, **29**(4), 398–403

Glick ME, Meshkinpoor H, and Haldeman S (1982) Colonic Dysfunction in multiple sclerosis, *Gastroenterology*, **83**, 1002–7

Johnson RT (1982) *Viral Infections of the Nervous System*, New York, Raven

Kirkeby HJ, Paulsen ZV, Peterson T *et al*. (1988) Erectile dysfunction in multiple sclerosis, *Neurology*, **38**, 1366–71

Kurtzke JF (1961) On the evaluation of disability in multiple sclerosis, *Neurology*, **11**, 686–94

Larson C (1985) Neurophysiology of speech and swallowing, In Logemann JA, ed, *Relationship of Speech and Swallowing*, New York, Thieme Stratton

Litvan I, Grafman J, Vendrell P, and Martinez JM (1988) Slowed information processing in multiple sclerosis, *Arch Neurol*, **45**, 281–5

Lyon-Caen O, Jouvert R, Hauser S *et al*. (1986) Cognitive function in recent onset demyelinating diseases, *Arch Neurol*, **43**, 1138–41

Matthews WB, Acherson EO, Batchelor JR, and Weller RO (1985) *McAlpine's Multiple Sclerosis*, New York, Churchill Livingstone

Murry TJ (1985) Amantadine therapy for fatigue in multiple sclerosis, *Can J Neurol Sci* **12**, 251–4

Oger J, Roos R, and Antel JP (1983) Immunology of multiple sclerosis, In Antel JP, ed, *Neurologic Clinics*, Vol. 1, No. 3, August 1983. Symposium on Multiple Sclerosis, Philadelphia, WB Saunders, 655–79

Penn RD, Savoy SM, Corcos D *et al*. (1989) Intrathecal baclofen for severe spinal spasticity, *N Engl J Med*, **320**, 1517–21

Peterson RC and Kokmen E (1989) Cognitive and psychiatric abnormalities in multiple sclerosis, *Mayo Clin Proc*, **64**, 657–63

Powell HC and Lampert PW (1983) Pathology of multiple sclerosis, In Antel JP, ed, *Neurologic Clinics*, Vol. 1, No. 3, August 1983, Symposium on Multiple Sclerosis, Philadelphia, WB Saunders, 631–44

Prineas JW (1985) The neuropathology of multiple sclerosis, In Vinken PJ, Bruyn GW, Klawans HL, and Koetsier JC, eds, *Handbook of Clinical Neurology*, Vol. 47: Demyelinating Diseases, New York, Elsevier, 213–57

Raminsky M (1973) The effects of temperature on conduction in demyelinated single nerve fibers, *Arch Neurol*, **28**, 287–92

Raminsky M (1981) Hyperexcitability of pathologically demyelinated axons and positive symptoms in multiple sclerosis. In Waxman SG and Ritchie JM, eds, *Demyelinating Diseases. Basic and Clinical Electrophysiology*, New York, Raven

Reder AT and Antel J (1983) Clinical spectrum of multiple sclerosis, In Antel JP, ed, *Neurologic Clinics*, Vol. 1, No. 3, August 1983. Symposium on Multiple Sclerosis, Philadelphia, WB Saunders, 573–99

Rodriguez M (1989) Multiple sclerosis: basic concepts and hypothesis, *Mayo Clin Proc*, **64**, 570–6

Rosenthal BJ and Scheinberg LC (1990) Exercise for multiple sclerosis patients, In Basmajian JV, ed, *Therapeutic Exercise*, Baltimore, Williams and Wilkins, 241–50

Sibley WA (1988), ed, *Therapeutic Claims in Multiple Sclerosis*, 2nd Edn, New York, Demos

Waksman BH, Reingold SC, and Reynolds WE (1987), eds, *Research on Multiple Sclerosis*, 3rd Edn, New York, Demos

13
Microsurgical DREZ-tomy for the treatment of pain and spasticity

M. Sindou

Chronic pain and disabling spasticity may be, at least partially, considered the result of persistent imbalance(s) in the modulatory systems regulating sensory functions and muscular tone. When the causative disorders cannot be properly corrected and if medical treatments, physical therapies, or both, are ineffective, functional neuro-surgery may be attempted.

Conservative methods, like neurostimulation or intrathecal pharmacotherapy, must of course be considered first. But not all pain syndromes correspond to logical indications for neurostimulation techniques. These methods can also fail, because of the lack of a sufficient number of inhibitory pathways to stimulate. Not all spastic states justify chronic intrathecal infusion of baclofen delivered by implantable pumps, especially when the handicapping disturbances are particularly focal in the limb(s). Therefore, ablative procedures aiming at selectively suppressing the excitatory afferents and at liberating the inhibitory systems, can be useful in a number of selected circumstances and under precise conditions.

Microsurgical DREZ-tomy (MDT) (Sindou, 1972), which is directed to the dorsal root entry zone, a very important area for spinal cord modulation, is a good example of an ablative method, aiming at correcting functional imbalances in the fields of pain and spasticity.

DORSAL ROOT ENTRY ZONE AS A TARGET FOR SURGERY OF PAIN

Rationale

During the 1960s, a large number of anatomical and physiological works on the spinal cord, particularly as expressed in the 'gate control theory' (Melzach and Wall, 1965), drew attention to the dorsal root entry zone (DREZ) as the first level of modulation for pain sensation. These works convinced the author to consider DREZ as a possible target for pain surgery, and in 1972 to undertake anatomical studies and preliminary surgical trials in humans in order to determine whether a destructive procedure at this level was feasible.

In our medical thesis (Sindou, 1972), DREZ was defined as an anatomical entity, which includes the central portion of the dorsal roots, the tract of Lissauer and the dorsal-most layers of the dorsal horn where the afferent fibers articulate with the cells from which the ascending extra-lemniscal pathways originate.

The dorsal root divides into 4–10 rootlets, of 0.25–1.50 millimetres in diameter according to the level. Each rootlet can be considered an anatomical–functional entity (a root in miniature) (Sindou, Fischer, and Mansuy, 1976; Sindou and Goutelle, 1983).

Our anatomical studies revealed the existence in the DREZ of a spatial segregation of afferent fibers according to their size and destination (Fig. 13.1). Upper part: each rootlet can be divided, thanks to the transition of its glial support, into a peripheral and a central segment. The transition between the two segments is at the pial ring (PR), which is located approximately one millimeter outside the penetration of the rootlet into the dorso-lateral sulcus. Peripherally, the fibers are mixed together. As they approach the PR, the fine fibers move towards the rootlet's surfaces. In the central segment, they group in the ventrolateral portion of the DREZ, to enter the dorsal horn (DH) through the tract of Lissauer (TL). The large myotatic fibers (myot) are situated centrally in the DREZ, whereas the large lemniscal fibers are located dorsomedially. MDT, represented by the large white arrowhead, cuts most of the fine and myotatic fibers and enters the medial (excitatory) portion of LT, and the apex of the dorsal horn. It should preserve most lemniscal presynaptic fibers, the lateral (inhibitory) portion of TL, and most of the DH. Lower part: selected and schematic data on DH connectivity. Note the monosynaptic excitatory arc reflex, the lemniscal influence on a DH cell and an interneuron (IN), the fine fiber excitatory input onto DH cells, and the IN, the origins in layer I and layers IV to VII of the anterolateral pathways (ALP), and the projection of the IN onto the motorneuron (MN). DC, dorsal column. Rexed laminae are marked from I to VII. The lateral regrouping of the small fibers allows them to be preferentially interrupted without disturbing most of the large ones.

The tract of Lissauer (TL), which is situated dorso-laterally to the dorsal horn, is composed of:

(1) a medial part, which the small afferents enter and where they trifurcate to reach the dorsal horn, either directly or through a two metamere ascending or descending pathway, and
(2) a lateral part through which a large number of longitudinal endogenous proprio-spinal fibers interconnect different levels of the substantia gelatinosa (SG).

According to Denny-Brown, Kirk, and Yanagisawa (1973), the TL plays an important role in the intersegmental modulation of the nociceptive afferents, because its medial part would transmit the excitatory effects of each dorsal root to the adjacent segments, and its lateral part would convey the inhibitory influences of the SG into the neighbouring metameres. Thus, a selective destruction of the medial part of the TL can cause a reduction in the regional excitability of the nociceptive afferents.

Most of the fine nociceptive afferents enter the dorsal horn through the TL medial part and the dorsal aspect of the SG; the recurrent collaterals of the large lemniscal fibers (Ramon y Cajal, 1901) approach the dorsal horn through the ventral aspect of SG (Szentagothai, 1964). Because the dendrites of some of the spino-reticulo-thalamic (SRT) cells make synaptic connections with the primary afferents inside the SG layers, the SG exerts a strong segmental modulating effect on the nociceptive input. When the large lemniscal afferents within peripheral nerves or dorsal roots are altered, there is a reduction in the inhibitory control that they exert on dorsal horn

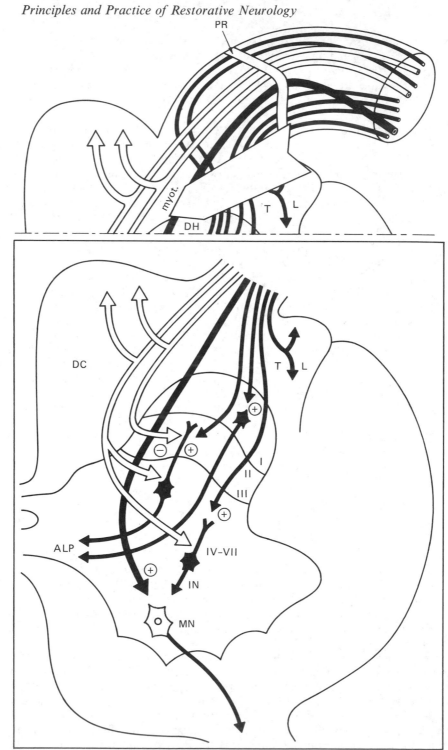

Figure 13.1 Segmental organization of primary dorsal root afferent fibers in man.

mechanisms (Melzach and Wall, 1965). This situation presumably results in excessive firing of the dorsal horn neurons. This phenomenon, thought to be at the origin of deafferentation pain, has been identified in some patients by electrophysiological recordings (Loeser, Ward, and White, 1968; Jeanmonod *et al.*, 1989) and reproduced in animal experiments (Loeser and Ward, 1967; Albe-Fessard and Lombard, 1983). Destruction of these hyperactive neurons can suppress the nociceptive impulses generated in the SRT pathways.

Surgical method

Based on these anatomical and physiological studies, we introduced in 1972, the concept of surgery in the DREZ (Sindou, 1972; Sindou, Quoex, and Baleydier, 1974) and began to make selective lesions in this target, using microsurgical techniques (Sindou *et al.*, 1974a).

The procedure, which has been detailed in several publications (Sindou *et al.*, 1986; Sindou and Jeanmonod, 1989), consists of microsurgical incisions and bipolar coagulations, performed ventro-laterally at the entrance of the rootlets, into the dorso-lateral sulcus, along all the spinal cord segments selected for surgery. The lesion, which penetrates the lateral part of the DREZ and the medial part of TL, extends down to the apex of the dorsal horn. The latter is recognized by its brown grey color. The lesions are two millimetres deep and made at a 45° angle medially and ventrally.

The procedure is presumed to preferentially destroy the pain pathways, which are the small nociceptive fibers grouped in the lateral bundle of the dorsal rootlets when entering the DREZ, as well as the excitatory medial part of the TL; the upper layers of the dorsal horn are also destroyed if microbipolar coagulations are made inside the grey matter of the dorsal horn apex. The procedure is also presumed to preserve, at least partially, the inhibitory structures of the DREZ (the lemniscal fibers reaching the dorsal column), as well as their recurrent collaterals to the dorsal horn and the SG proprio-spinal interconnecting fibers running through the lateral part of the TL. The method, called microsurgical DREZ-tomy (MDT) was conceived with a view to preventing complete abolition of tactile and proprioceptive sensations and avoiding deafferentation phenomena.

Indications and results

The indications and results of microsurgical DREZ-tomy have been discussed in detail elsewhere (Sindou and Daher, 1988). Our first attempt at surgery in the DREZ was in March 1972 for pain caused by the Pancoast-Tobias syndrome. Several other patients with cancer were operated on soon after. As the first results in malignant pain were encouraging, we decided the same year to attempt the procedure in patients with chronic non-cancerous pain syndromes, namely, painful paraplegia, amputation stump pain, and brachial plexus injury (performing microcoagulations of the dorsal horn apex with sharp bipolar forceps at the avulsed root levels and selective ventro-lateral DREZ lesions in the remaining rootlets).

In cancer pain, an effective result was obtained in 87.5% and 78.5% of the 38 and 32 patients respectively, at the cervical (or cervico-thoracic) and at the lumbar and/or sacral levels. These patients had topographically limited pains caused by well-localized lesions. Their survival time ranged from one month to four years (13 months on average). Surgery was complicated with wound infection in two cases, and was considered as having precipitated death in two cases.

Of 87 patients with pure neurogenic pain followed over a period of one to 16 years, 87% benefited from surgery. Long lasting good results (more than 75% relief) were especially achieved in the painful states caused by: 1. spinal cord lesions in which pain had a 'radiculo-metameric' distribution corresponding to or situated just below the level of the lesion; 2. brachial plexus injuries, and to a lesser degree, post-radiation plexopathies; 3. peripheral nerve injuries, especially causalgic syndromes, and after amputation; and 4. less constantly, in herpetic neuralgias. In the latter etiologies, relief was more pronounced when the predominant component of pain was of the paroxysmal type (electrical shooting crises) or corresponded to a superficial provoked hyperalgesia (allodynia), or both. In this group of pure neurogenic pain, there were no vital or significant neurological complications, especially as far as the dorsal column and the pyramidal tract were concerned.

Discussion

The advantage of MDT over the more recently introduced DREZ lesioning procedures using radiofrequency current (Nashold, Urban, and Zorub, 1976; Nashold and Ostdahl, 1979) or laser (Levy *et al.*, 1983; Powers *et al.*, 1984), is that when there is no marked pre-operative sensory deficit, the procedure allows tactile and proprioceptive sensory capacities of a significant degree to be retained, avoiding complete functional loss in the operated area. But because extensive operations at the lumbar-sacral segments would inevitably result in leg hypotonia, for pain below the waist in ambulatory patients, the procedure must be restricted to the treatment of topographically limited painful states.

DORSAL ROOT ENTRY ZONE AS A TARGET FOR SURGERY OF SPASTICITY

Rationale

The idea to treat severe spasticity by the MDT procedure arose from an observation made after performing selective microsurgical lesions in the DREZ for pain relief. It was noticed that muscular tone was diminished and myotatic reflexes were abolished in the territories corresponding to the operated painful areas (Sindou,1972). This may be explained by the fact that MDT 1. interrupts the afferent components of the myotatic mono, and polysynaptic reflexes, which had been cut off from suprasegmental inhibitory control by pathological conditions; 2. deprives the somatosensory relays of the dorsal horn of most of their excitatory inputs, while preserving their inhibitory segmental (lemniscal), intersegmental (lateral part of Lissauer's tract), and supra-segmental influences.

On these bases, MDT was applied, as early as 1973, for the treatment of disabling spasticity in the lower limb(s) of paraplegic patients or in the upper limb of hemiplegic patients (Sindou *et al.*, 1974b).

Surgical method

For paraplegia, the L2–S5 segments are approached through a T10–L2 laminectomy, whereas for the hemiplegic upper limb, a C4–C7 hemilaminectomy with conservation of the spinous processes is sufficient to reach the C5–T1 segments. Identification of the metameric levels selected as supporting the harmful tonic mechanisms (and/or corresponding to the painful territories) is achieved by studying the muscle responses to bipolar electrical stimulation of the anterior and/or posterior roots. Then, the ventro-lateral aspect of the DREZ is exposed to perform the microsurgical lesions, two millimetres in depth and at a 45° angle obliquely in the dorso-lateral sulcus, along all the selected segments of the spinal cord.

Indications and results

Indications and results of MDT for spasticity have been discussed in more detail elsewhere (Sindou *et al.*, 1986; Sindou and Jeanmonod, 1989). MDT was applied in 53 bedridden patients with serious spasticity in one (six cases) or both (47 cases) lower limb(s). Forty-nine patients had abnormal postures in flexion and three in hyper-extension; 37 had additional pain. Both spasticity and spasms were significantly decreased or suppressed in 75% and 88.2% respectively. When present, pain was relieved without total loss of sensation in 91.6% of patients. These benefits, combined with complementary orthopedic surgery in 23 patients, resulted in either disappearance or marked reduction of the abnormal postures in 85.3% and restriction of joint movement in 96.8%. Mild to severe complications occurred in 25 patients, which precipitated, or were responsible, for death in five patients with advanced multiple sclerosis. MDT enabled most patients to sit and lie comfortably and allowed them to achieve a significantly improved quality of life.

MDT was also applied in 16 hemiplegic patients with severe spasticity in the upper limb. There were no deaths and general complications; loss of motility in the leg ipsilateral to the procedure occurred once. The excess spasticity was slightly diminished (two cases), markedly reduced (nine cases), or totally abolished (five cases), making possible an improvement in voluntary movements in eight patients and at least a good passive mobilization in seven more. In one only, a marked tendency for spasticity to return was observed. Of the 12 patients with pain, nine were relieved and three improved. MDT led to a gain in functional status in 93%. This was achieved without impairing sensation in the upper limb in eight, and with its diminution only, in the eight others.

Follow-up for these two groups of patients ranged from 2 to 15 years (average, five years). There was rarely long-term significant loss of effectiveness.

Discussion

The long-term efficacy of MDT might be related to its specific modulatory action on tone regulation structures. This procedure indeed suppresses the majority of excitatory input to spinal cord segments as a result of a section of the large Ia myotatic fibers participating in the monosynaptic stretch reflex, and perhaps more significantly, through an interruption of the so-called 'flexor reflex afferents' (Eccles, Eccles, and Magni, 1961; Lundberg, 1979). MDT maintains most inhibitory ones, thus biasing the tone regulation towards inhibition.

CONCLUSIONS

Provided that selection of patients is rigorous, MDT can be effective in relieving pain and suppressing the excess spasticity. Originality of MDT lies in the fact that the procedure is performed at the junction between the peripheral and central parts of the somatosensory system, a position in which to destroy specific components of this system as a result of their spatial segregation and to act upon gating mechanisms by influencing their modulatory activity regarding inhibition. Electrophysiological evidence of the selective effects of MDT has been determined by intraoperative recordings of the spinal cord evoked surface potentials and comparison of pre- and post-operative somesthetic evoked potentials (Jeanmonod *et al.*, 1989).

References

Albe-Fessard D and Lombard MC (1983) Use of an animal model to evaluate the origin of and protection against deafferentation pain. In Bonica JJ *et al.*, eds, *Advances in Pain Research and Therapy*, Vol 5, New York, Raven, 691–700

Denny-Brown D, Kirk EJ and Yanagisawa N (1973) The tract of Lissauer in relation to sensory transmission in the dorsal horn of spinal cord in the macaque monkey, *J Comp Neurol*, **151**, 175–200

Eccles J, Eccles R, and Magni F (1961) Central inhibitory action attributable to presynaptic depolarization produced by muscle afferent volleys, *J Physiol*, **159**, 147–66

Jeanmonod D, Sindou M, and Mauguiere F (1989) Intra-operative spinal cord evoked potentials during cervical and lumbo-sacral microsurgical DREZ-tomy (MDT) for chronic pain and spasticity (preliminary data), *Acta Neurochir*, suppl, **46**, 58–61

Jeanmonod D, Sindou M, Magnin M, and Boudet M (1989) Intraoperative unit recordings in the human dorsal horn with a simplified floating microelectrode, *Electroencephalogr Clin Neurophysiol*, **72**, 450–4

Levy WJ, Nutkiewicz A, Ditmore M, and Watts C (1983) Laser-induced dorsal root entry zone lesions for pain control: Report of three cases, *J Neurosurg*, **59**, 884–6

Loeser JD and Ward AA (1967) Some effects of deafferentation of neurons of the cat spinal cord, *Arch Neurol*, **17**, 629–36

Loeser JD, Ward AA, and White LE (1968) Chronic deafferentation of human spinal cord neurons, *J Neurosurg*, **29**, 48–50

Lundberg A (1979) Multisensory control of spinal reflex pathways. In Granit R and Pompeiano O, eds, *Reflex control of posture and movement, Progress in Brain Research*, Vol 50, Amsterdam, Elsevier, 11–28

Melzack R and Wall PD (1965) Pain mechanism. A new theory, *Science*, **150**, 971–9

Nashold BS and Ostdahl PH (1979) Dorsal root entry zone lesions for pain relief, *J Neurosurg*, **51**, 59–69

Nashold BS, Urban B, and Zorub DS (1976) Phantom relief by focal destruction of substantia gelatinosa of Rolando. In Bonica JJ, Albe-Fessard D, eds, *Advances in Pain Research and Therapy*, vol 1, New York, Raven, 959–63

Powers SK, Adams JE, Edwards MSB, Boggan JE, and Hosobuchi Y (1984) Pain relief from dorsal root entry zone lesions made with argon and carbon dioxide microsurgical lasers, *J Neurosurg*, **61**, 841–7

Ramon y Cajal S (1901) *Histologie du système nerveux*, Vol 1, Paris, Maloine, 986

Sindou M (1972) *Etude de la Jonction Radiculo-Médullaire Postérieure: La Radicellotomie Postérieure Sélective dans la Chirurgie de la Douleur*, Medical Thesis, Lyon

Sindou M and Daher A (1988) Spinal cord ablation procedures for pain, In Dubner R, Gebhart GF, and Bond MR, eds, *Proceedings of the Fifth World Congress on Pain, Pain Research and Clinical Management*, Vol 3, Amsterdam, Elsevier, 477–95

Sindou M and Goutelle A (1983) Surgical posterior rhizotomies for the treatment of pain, In Krayenbühl H, ed, *Advances and Technical Standards in Neurosurgery*, Vol 10, Wien, Springer Verlag, 147–85

Sindou M and Jeanmonod D (1989) Microsurgical DREZ-otomy for the treatment of spasticity and pain in the lower limbs, *Neurosurgery*, **24**, 655–70

Sindou M, Quoex C, and Baleydier C (1974) Fiber organization at the posterior spinal cord-rootlet junction in man, *J Comp Neurol*, **153**, 15–26

Sindou M, Fischer G, and Mansuy L (1976) Posterior spinal rhizotomy and selective posterior rhizidiotomy, *Prog Neurol Surg*, **7**, 201–50

Sindou M, Fischer G, Goutelle A, and Mansuy L (1974a) La radicellotomie postérieure sélective. Premiers résultats dans la chirurgie de la douleur, *Neurochirurgie*, **20**, 391–408

Sindou M, Fischer G, Goutelle A, Schott B, and Mansuy L (1974b) La radicellotomie postérieure sélective dans le traitement des spasticités, *Rev Neurol*, **130**, 201–15

Sindou M, Mifsud JJ, Boisson D, and Goutelle A (1986) Selective posterior rhizotomy in the dorsal root entry zone for treatment of hyperspasticity and pain in the hemiplegic upper limb, *Neurosurgery*, **18**, 587–95

Szentagothai J (1964) Neuronal and synaptic arrangement in the substantia gelatinosa, *J Comp Neurol*, **122**, 219–39

14
Rehabilitation in Parkinson's disease, day care programs for demented patients, and aids for living and home modifications for patients with neurologic physical disability

F. H. McDowell

REHABILITATION IN PARKINSON'S DISEASE

The major symptoms of Parkinson's disease, bradykinesia, tremor, and rigidity, lead to increasing physical inactivity as the disease progresses. This problem, coupled with increasing loss of automatic associated postural movements, which cause postural instability, make rehabilitation programs important in dealing with an individual with advancing Parkinson's disease. The tendency for a patient with Parkinson's disease to become increasingly inactive leads to major problems with physical deconditioning. It is often impossible in this situation to determine whether a patient's complaints of inability to carry out daily activities or fatigue are caused by progression of the disease or to a poor physical condition.

Programs of rehabilitation involve keeping patients as physically active as possible through exercise programs, insistence on maximal physical activity, and insistence on making certain that patients do as much as possible for themselves, no matter how much time it takes.

Exercise and rehabilitation programs have been recommended for the past 50 to 100 years, because this was in many instances the only therapy available. With the advent of levodopa treatment, the belief in the need for continued exercise, physical activity, and rehabilitation programs was largely forgotten. Before the introduction of levodopa treatment, the literature contained a number of recommendations for exercise programs; but unfortunately there were no data indicating the exact effect of exercise programs (Rabiner and Hand, 1941; Bilowit, 1956; Knott, 1957; Doshay and Boshes, 1960; Doshay, 1962; Erickson et al., 1962; Boshes and Doshay, 1964).

Programs for physical activity included stretching exercises to avoid leg contractures, general improvement in strength of the upper extremities, encouragement of walking increasing distances, and general measures to keep patients in fairly good physical condition. When levodopa became available, and the results were so strikingly good at first, it was believed that the increasing normal physical activity made possible with levodopa treatment would be all that was needed in the way of rehabilitation. Some patients, after treatment with levodopa, although they did improve, were left with many of the difficulties associated with inactivity resulting from long-standing Parkinson's disease. These included hamstring contractures, which prevented patients from standing erect and locking their knees, which needed to be corrected with stretching exercises before patients could regain a normal gait. It was soon clear that it was necessary, despite a good response to levodopa, to keep patients as physically active as possible and in good physical shape so that they could manage for themselves as much as possible and delay the time when dependency almost inevitably appeared (Stern *et al.*, 1970; Wroe and Greer, 1973).

During the past decade, there has been a renewed interest in the value of physical therapy and rehabilitation techniques in improving function in patients with Parkinson's disease (Stefaniwsky and Bilowit, 1973). Reports indicate that regular physical therapy, as often as twice a week, may produce some moderate improvement (Franklyn *et al.*, 1981; Gibberd *et al.*, 1981a, 1981b). In the few controlled trials of rehabilitation so far conducted, there is often minimal evidence that patients improve more than the controls.

In one study to test the value of exercise, 14 patients were selected to have three one-hour sessions of exercise per week (Palmer *et al.*, 1984). One-half were used as controls, and the other half for the program. Patients were evaluated by a battery of tests of motor function, including the degree of bradykinesia on forearm pronation and supination, the number of seconds required to walk 30 feet, rigidity tested by torque forces, pursuit time in tracking a moving object, and the degree of tremor. Exercise was performed while sitting; one group performed routine stretching exercises and the other karate exercises. There was improvement in both groups in walking speed, arm tremor, and bradykinesia. Rigidity was unchanged, and time pursuit tasks were worse. Both groups reported that they felt better and were more confident in performing daily activities. The explanation for improvement was not clear but is believed to result from an improved sense of well-being and renewed motivation.

In another study of a small number of patients with stage II and III Parkinson's disease, a 13 week trial of exercises using the APDA home exercise program was used. Patients improved in such things as step length, walking speed, and the number of times they could sit up and down in one minute. There was no improvement in balance, posture, writing, or general daily activities. Patients reported being less depressed (Szekely, Kosanovich, and Sheppard, 1982).

Rehabilitation programs largely consist of stretching exercises for the upper and lower extremities, walking, and exercise programs such as cycling to increase leg strength. For several years, patients with severe gait problems with festination, freezing, and falling have been admitted to The Burke Rehabilitation Center. The program has consisted of exercise several times per day to improve physical conditioning, walking, training to reduce festination and freezing, and occupational therapy to improve conduct of daily activities. In the program, patients have improved; they walk better, walk more rapidly, are more stable on their feet, fall less, and generally look better and report feeling better. Improvement was attributed to the program but other factors, such as lessened depression, being out of the home, and contact with other patients, contribute to improvement. To date, although these programs have improved function in some patients, they have not improved postural stability, which has become a serious problem for a great number. Loss of automatic associated arm and leg movements, and decreased speed of application of balancing movements when balance is perturbed, is common in Parkinson's disease. When slightly off balance, they are prone to falling, because patients cannot correctly or quickly restore their center of gravity.

There are a number of specific situations in which patients are very likely to become posturally unstable and generally most episodes of falling or instability can be traced to these events. These include:

(1) Instead of getting up from a chair, standing in an upright position with feet firmly planted on the floor before beginning to walk, and then striding out with long steps, patients tend to rise from the chair, with a stooped forward posture, begin to walk with short steps, and then tend to bend forward and chase their center of gravity until they either fall down or run into something.

(2) Similarly, when patients back up, they may find that the upper portion of their body moves backward sooner than their legs, and they tend to take short rapid backward steps, either falling down or running into something.

(3) Patients may also have great difficulty in changing rate and direction of movements in close quarters. Patients who suddenly turn while walking may find that their upper body turns, but their legs do not follow as rapidly, and then they are off balance and fall.

(4) Patients also tend to freeze and festinate when approaching an object they intend to reach for and pick up. By not getting close enough to the object to stand up straight and reach, they bend forward. They may bend so far forward that they cannot straighten up and may fall over the object.

(5) When patients approach a chair, they may festinate and try to sit down before they are fully and safely placed over the seat of the chair; when sitting down, patients often miss the seat of the chair and fall.

Patients with postural instability have also noted that they cannot walk and keep their mind on anything else. They cannot answer questions from friends and family; they cannot adjust pocketbooks or clothing while walking, because this can be so distracting that even the slightest perturbation of balance may result in a fall. Educating patients about these particular events is sometimes helpful in avoiding falls; but if patients get up, back up, or turn on impulse, they often forget the problems and fall. At times patients appear to fall without provocation, and without any of the above activities taking place. This is not wholly explained by any studies that have been undertaken so far.

It is extremely desirable for patients to wear protective clothing if they tend to fall on particular parts. Patients who fall forward on their knees can be protected to some extent by using knee pads with sponge rubber covering the patella. This tends to reduce the chances of major knee damage. The same protection can be applied to avoid damage to elbows if patients tend to fall and injure their arms. Head injury is common for patients with Parkinson's disease, but to date encouraging patients to wear protective helmets to prevent head injury has not been well received.

A major problem in standing is the development of hamstring contracture, which prevents patients from being able to lock their knees when standing. Locking knees when standing reduces the muscular effort needed to keep the patient upright. Patients who have slight hamstring contractures tend to stand with their knees slightly flexed, which requires muscular effort to keep them upright. After a few minutes of standing in this position, the quadriceps muscle fatigues, and patients tend to fall or sag to the floor. When sitting, it is important to have legs outstretched and elevated slightly to avoid hamstring contracture and pedal edema. Sitting for long periods with the legs flexed on the thigh, with minimal change in posture, leads to hamstring contracture, which must be avoided if a patient is to have reasonably normal gait.

A significant problem for a patient with advancing Parkinson's disease is disturbance of speech, usually a decline in voice volume and difficulty with enunciation, rate of speech, and prosody. The most frequent complaint is a decline in voice volume; friends and family have difficulty in hearing what the patient says, and frequently have to ask for a repetition. The patient is usually unaware of the decline in voice volume, because for themselves they seem to be talking loudly enough. Reminding a patient to speak up generally will correct the problem for a few moments; but as patients continue to speak, their voice volume again tends to drop off and they cannot be heard. Correcting this problem has not been very successful. Asking patients to record their speech may give some insight into the difficulty that others might have in hearing them. Speech therapy has been extensively tried in this situation and has produced some improvement, but unfortunately it is not long-lasting. While the patient is with the speech therapist, the voice volume tends to be quite adequate, but a few moments or half an hour after therapy is finished, voice volume declines. Reports of studies on speech therapy generally indicate improvement lasting three to six months. Often there is little difference between those treated and those acting as controls (Scott and Caird, 1981, 1983). It is possible that any improvement may result from interest of the staff in the patient and improved motivation. Voice amplifiers have been used, but generally patients either forget to apply them, or use them inadequately.

Patients also have problems with articulation. Speech becomes more rapid, poorly enunciated, and with little emphasis on pronunciation. This, coupled with a declining voice volume, may make speech totally inaudible and not understandable. Speech therapy for this problem is often helpful in reducing speed of speaking and improving word pronunciation, but the improvement tends to be short lived.

Patients with Parkinson's disease usually develop a stooped posture. This is especially prominent with progression of the disease, and can cause considerable concern for the patient and family. When encouraged to stand up straight, patients can virtually always do so, indicating that there is no structural problem in the spine. Patients tend to forget to stand up straight, and after a few moments assume a stooped posture again. They will stay that way until reminded to straighten up. Back and trunk exercises have helped improve this problem somewhat, which is probably largely the result of reminding patients of their postural state. If patients do not constantly keep their minds on this problem of posture, they tend to resume a stooped posture. Evidence from our own program suggests that exercises that tend to strengthen trunk muscles, and especially back muscles, may be of some help in reducing the abnormal posture.

Occupational therapy is largely directed towards helping patients cope with everyday problems. Studies by occupational therapists on home health needs indicate that two thirds of the patients in a community are helped by equipment to aid in bathing, using the toilet, and eating (Beattie and Caird, 1980). Patients are observed performing daily activities such as dressing, eating, bathing, and getting in and out of bed. The therapist may be able to teach the patient better ways of performing these activities and usually can provide home health aides or home modification, which will enable the patients to do more for themselves and increase independence.

DAY CARE PROGRAMS FOR DEMENTED PATIENTS

The concept of rehabilitation, used correctly, means restoring something to its previous condition. This is not possible for patients with dementing disorders such as

Alzheimer's disease. These conditions are relentlessly progressive and patients become increasingly less adaptable and able to function in their usual environment. The result of this for the patient is often social isolation, boredom, and depression, and an exhausting experience for the care giver responsible for an individual patient with declining intellect.

Day care programs for severely intellectually impaired patients can at least relieve the care giver for brief periods of the responsibility of looking after the individual. In these programs, an individual with dementia may take part in physical and intellectual activities, which appear to restore some interest in personal care, outside activities, and other people, and can relieve boredom and reduce social isolation. Such day care programs have been started in many places in the USA and Europe, and provide for continued human contact for someone with marked intellectual loss.

A daily program at the Burke Rehabilitation Center was started about 10 years ago (Panella, 1987). It provides patients with severe intellectual loss a group of activities. These are conducted over a seven-hour period, and include orientation exercises to time, place, and person; general exercises; dance, music, and art therapy; group discussion; lunch; and outdoor exercise when possible. Patients generally come to the program twice a week, but some come four or five days per week. Initially, study of the response of those attending the program, using rating scales for assaying the behavior of the demented patient, showed that patients improved (Haycox, 1984). They became more interested in other people, more interested in how they looked, more conscious of proper social behavior, and had less trouble with urinary and bowel incontinence. This period of improvement was observed only for about four to six months, and then it became clear that the inexorable progression of the dementia gradually reversed any gains in function and performance.

Intellectual loss continued and patients became progressively less able to adjust and deal with their environment, to be socially acceptable, and to interact with people. These programs are limited in their scope; they require that patients are ambulatory and reasonably continent of bowel and bladder. Severely demented patients are unable, generally, to take part, and mildly demented patients do not tolerate such programs because they do not see themselves as becoming demented or suitable.

Patients have remained in these programs for as long as two years. The general time of participation is six to nine months. These patient populations make an ideal study group for testing therapeutic claims, which are believed to either slow the progression of Alzheimer's disease or reverse it. Patients are closely observed by a number of individuals on a daily or twice-weekly basis, and this gives a great opportunity to obtain accurate evidence of improvement or decline of intellect.

Space requirements for the program depend on how large a group can be handled and the number of staff available. Staff requirements are large, often one for every three patients. Generally, it is advisable to have several rooms so that when patients become restless, they can move from one room to another. Attention spans are generally short, so that several short programs, with exercise in between, are desirable. Adequate toileting facilities are needed and programs must be developed to provide for regular toileting to avoid incontinence.

Similar programs can be established in almost any community, and often depend on volunteer help. There should be one full-time paid director who can organize and keep the program going. Professional help in art, music, and dance therapy is desirable, but often volunteers with these talents can be found.

Day care programs for demented patients are not paid for by Medicare or private insurance. Expenses can be high depending on how many paid staff are used. A full-time salaried staff can increase daily rates to the point beyond the reach of most families. Community support or the help of volunteers are essential for reasonable daily rates.

While such programs do not in any way change the progression of the dementing process, they do relieve depression and restore, for the patient, some sense of being a person able to interact with others. As such, programs are a humane form of care for patients, and nearly vital for care givers.

AIDS FOR LIVING AND HOME MODIFICATION FOR PATIENTS WITH NEUROLOGIC PHYSICAL DISABILITY

Virtually all neurological disorders cause some degree of impairment in motor function, which can lead to inability to carry out usual activities and loss of independence. The problems that are most frequently encountered are those of weakness, paralysis, ataxia, intention tremor, bradykinesia, and involuntary movements. Currently there are very few adequate ways to resolve these impairments in motor function; if patients are going to remain independent, it is necessary to modify their environment so that they can continue to function as independently as possible. This means, for most patients, that some program of home modification is necessary.

The areas where home modifications are most needed are the bathroom, bedroom, and kitchen. Being able to dress and remain independent in performing usual daily hygienic routines are essential for patients to retain their self-respect and ability to live with others.

The bathroom is the most common area where patients are likely to have difficulty. Modern bathrooms, even for able people, are often unsafe because of slippery surfaces, crowded conditions, and unstable supports attached to the wall. Patients who have difficulty using bathing and toileting facilities are often greatly helped by a number of simple modifications. These include changing the bathtub into a safe area for bathing, which requires the purchase of a shower or bath chair that sits in the tub allowing the patient to sit down, slide across into the tub, and be centrally placed so that they can shower themselves (Fig. 14.1). Usually a flexible extension of the showerhead is necessary so that the patient can sit and be able to wash thoroughly. The area around the bathtub or shower stall should be provided with several sturdy supports so that patients can balance themselves, pull themselves upright, or hold on securely while bathing. Hand grips attached to the side of a bathtub are often very helpful in allowing patients to steady themselves while they are stepping in and out of the tub, or in getting up from a shower chair. The toilet is often a major source of difficulty because most modern toilets are set too low for patients with a physical disability, and an elevation of the toilet seat is often very helpful (Fig. 14.2), which greatly facilitates getting up. Around the toilet there should be grab bars, which allow patients to pull themselves up from the toilet or to steady themselves while sitting down.

All of these mentioned modifications, or pieces of apparatus, can be purchased in most health supply stores or drug stores in the USA, or they can be purchased by catalog from a number of organizations, such as Sears Roebuck. They should always be securely fastened to the wall of the bathroom so they can bear the full weight of a patient of any size. Patients confined to wheelchairs may have considerable difficulty with bathrooms because of the door width. Most bathroom doors are not wide enough to allow the passage of a wheelchair or, once in the bathroom, much room to

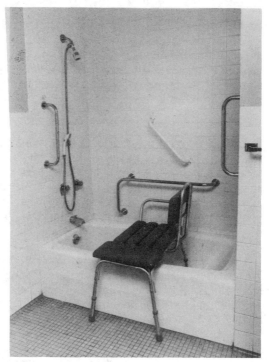

Figure 14.1 Modified shower and bath area.

maneuver a wheelchair. Enlarging doors is rather expensive and at times prohibitively so because bathroom doors are not only small but the bathrooms are too small to be functional for a disabled person in a wheelchair. It is generally extremely expensive to modify a bathroom, and when conditions arise when patients in wheelchairs cannot get into a bathroom, other adaptations must be considered. These involve the purchase of a commode, which can be placed near the wheelchair to allow the patient to move from the chair to the commode. Commodes are purchasable in almost any health supply store.

Getting in and out of bed, and turning over in bed, is often extremely difficult for patients with neurologically-induced disability. The use of a trapeze fastened to the head of the bed, and hanging over the bed, allows patients to use their arm strength, in addition to trunk and leg strength, to maneuver in and out of bed and to turn over in bed (Fig. 14.3). Beds should not be so high that the patient, when sitting on the edge, cannot plant the feet firmly to the floor before getting up. A side rail on the bed is often useful, giving the patient something to pull on as they stand up. Chairs in bedrooms should be sturdy armchairs. The arms must reach far enough forward so that the patient can easily slide forward in the chair and push themselves up with their arms.

Clothing for patients with physical disability should be adapted to meet their needs. Generally, it is advisable not to have clothing with small buttons or small zippers. It is now possible that all clothing could be adapted to Velcro fasteners, enabling the patient to easily put them together when dressing and pull them apart when undressing. Velcro fasteners are available for almost any portion of attire that

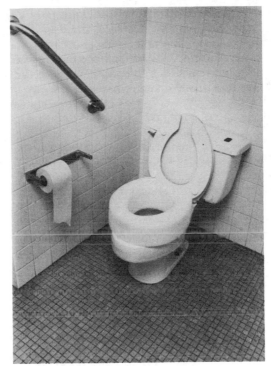

Figure 14.2 An elevated toilet seat in position.

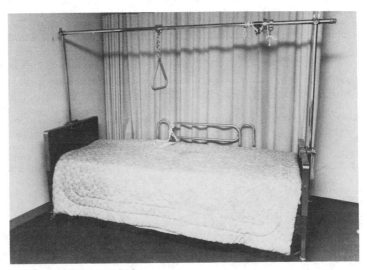

Figure 14.3 A trapeze in position over a bed.

requires closing, including shirts, pants, dresses, and shoes. Clothing that opens down the front rather than the back is preferable, because most patients with physical disability cannot manage clothing that closes in the back.

Kitchen modifications are usually beyond the means of most patients. For those who wish to use a kitchen and can afford it, lowering the counters to wheelchair height, as well as the cabinets and sink, can make it possible for someone with good arm function to carry on with cooking. For patients with hemiplegia, cerebellar dysfunction and advanced Parkinson's disease, it is unlikely that function in the kitchen is possible, and for some, should be avoided because of the danger of falling.

There are a number of companies that specialize in home health aids and a wide variety of aids for the bathroom, bedroom, and kitchen can be purchased. Catalogues are available from:

1. North Coast Medical Inc.; ADL catalogue 1989; 450 Salmar Ave., Campbell CA 95008, USA.

2. Professional Health Care Catalogue; Fred Sammons Inc. Box 32, Brookfield, IL 60513, USA.

References

Beattie A, Caird FT (1980) The occupational therapist and the patient with Parkinson's disease, *Br Med J*, **280**, 1354–5

Bilowit DS (1956) Establishing objectives in rehabilitation of patients with Parkinson's disease, *Phys Ther Rev*, **36**, 176–8

Boshes LD and Doshay LJ (1964) Practical management of Parkinson's disease, *Geriatrics*, **19**, 644–53

Doshay LJ (1962) Method and value of exercise in Parkinson's disease, *N Engl J Med*, **267**, 644–53

Doshay LJ and Boshes L (1960) Three essentials in therapy of Parkinson's disease, *Postgrad Med*, **27**, 602–10

Erickson DJ, Clark EC, Mulder DW *et al.* (1956) Therapeutic exercise in management of paralysis agitans, *JAMA*, **162**, 1041–3

Franklyn S, Kohout LJ, Stern GM, and Dunning M (1981) Physiotherapy in Parkinson's disease, In Rose FC and Capildeo R, eds, *Research Progress in Parkinson's Disease*, Turnbridge Wells, Pitman

Gibberd FB, Page NGR, Spencer KM, Kinnear E, and Hawksworth JB (1981a) Controlled trial of physiotherapy and occupational therapy for Parkinson's disease, *Br Med J*, **282**, 1196

Gibberd FB, Page NGR, Spencer KM, Kinnear E, and Williams JB (1981b) A controlled trial of physiotherapy and occupational therapy for Parkinson's disease, In Rose FC and Capildeo R, eds, *Research Progress in Parkinson's Disease*, Turnbridge Wells, Pitman

Haycox JA (1984) A simple reliable clinical behavioral scale for assessing demented patients, *J Clin Psychiatry*, **45**, 23–4

Knott M (1957) Report of a case of Parkinsonism treated with proprioceptive facilitation techniques, *Phys Ther Rev*, **37**, 229

Palmer SS, Mortimer JA, Webster DD, Bistevins R, and Dickinson GL (1984) A comparison of stretch exercises and karate training as therapy for Parkinson's Disease, *Arch Phys Med Rehabil*, **65**, 626

Panella J (1987) *Day Care Programs for Alzheimer's Disease and Related Disorders*, New York, Demos

Rabiner AM and Hand M (1941) Activity as a therapeutic agent in the Parkinsonian syndrome, *Trans Am Neurol Ass*, **67**, 234–6

Scott S and Caird FT (1981) Speech therapy for patients with Parkinson's disease, *Br Med J*, **283**, 1088

Scott S and Caird FT (1983) Speech therapy for Parkinson's disease, *J Neuro Neurosurg Psychiatry*, **46**, 140–4

Stefaniwsky L and Bilowit DS (1973) Parkinsonism: facilitation of motion by sensory stimulation, *Arch Phys Med Rehabil*, **54**, 75–7

Stern PH, McDowell F, Miller JM, and Robinson M (1970) Levo-dopa and physical therapy in treatment of patients with Parkinson's disease, *Arch Phys Med Rehabil*, **51**, 273–7

Szekely BC, Kosanovich NN, and Sheppard W (1982) Adjunctive treatment in Parkinson's disease, *Rehabil Lit*, 43, 72–6

Wroe M and Greer M (1973) Parkinson's disease and physical therapy management, *Phys Ther*, **53**, 849–55

15
Thalamotomy in parkinsonism

H. Narabayashi

Tremor and rigidity are two positive motor symptoms in parkinsonism. Pharmacological therapy, consisting of levodopa, dopamine (DA) agonists, anticholinergics, and others, is obviously the routine, first choice treatment. However, when the medical therapy has failed to produce satisfactory improvement, the possibility of surgical treatment is still worth considering. Patients with severe tremor, hemiparkinsonism, or markedly asymmetric symptoms may be suitable for unilateral thalamotomy using the microelectrode recording technique. Use of the microelectrode recording technique (Albe-Fessard, Arfel, and Guiot, 1963) is the most essential part of this operation to permit highly precise targetting of the surgical lesion.

TREMOR MECHANISM

Tremor of parkinsonism is completely and permanently relieved by a small surgical lesion within the ventral intermediate nucleus (VIM) of the thalamus (Fig. 15.1). The VIM is located posteriorly to the vental lateral nucleus (VL) and anteriorly to the ventral posterior nucleus (VP). The VIM is differentiated from the VL by its difference in cytoarchitechtonics and fiber connections (Hassler, 1959); the VL receives pallidal afferents as opposed to the VIM. A surgical lesion confined to the VL relieves rigidity but does not produce sustained alleviation of tremor. Therefore, in contrast to rigidity, which will be described later, tremor seems to be related neither to the pallidal efferent pathway nor to the nigrostriatum.

Through the 5–7 µm semimicroelectrode at the tip of the insertion-needle, unitary activity of neurons in the depth of the thalamus is recorded. The VIM usually has rhythmic burst discharges synchronous with peripheral tremor. The VIM is found to receive proprioceptive afferents from muscles and joints of the contralateral side of the body through the medial lemniscus, therefore producing the rhythmic discharges when the extremity is involved in tremor. Proprioceptive neurons usually occupy the ventral half of the VIM, and are delicately somatotopically organized, similarly as in the VP. High frequency electrical stimulation of such a neuronal area immediately inhibits tremor in the corresponding part of extremities, and an electrocoagulative lesion of the area abolishes tremor completely (Narabayashi, 1982, 1986, 1989).

Pre-operative   Post-operative

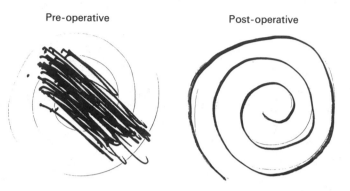

Figure 15.1 Immediate and almost complete alleviation on the operating table of severe tremor after a thalamic lesion shown by handwriting in a hemiparkinsonian (male, 66 years of age). a. Pre-operative. b. Post-operative, two minutes after placing a 4 mm diameter lesion in the left VIM thalamus.
(Cited from *Eur Neurol* (1989), **29**(Suppl 1) by courtesy of S Karger AG, Basel)

MECHANISMS OF RIGIDITY

Rigidity is abolished by a small circumscribed lesion in either the medial pallidum (Narabayashi and Okuma, 1953; Narabayashi, Okuma, and Shikiba, 1956) or the VL thalamus (Narabayashi, 1988). This suggests that the rigidity-producing mechanism is conveyed by the pallidothalamic projection, because the VL is the termination of the pallidal efferents. High frequency electrical stimulation of the medial pallidum increases muscle tone and the amount of tonic stretch reflex (Narabayashi, 1962).

Presently it is explained that rigidity in parkinsonism is the result of DA deficiency within the nigrostriatal system. The DA deficiency affects the underlying pallidal neurons to produce rigidity. Yoshida reported that unitary discharges of pallidal neurons are facilitated tonically by application of MPTP to the animal, which is the toxic agent depleting the nigrostriatal DA (Yoshida and Fujimoto, 1987; Yoshida, 1991).

RECOVERY OF NORMAL FUNCTION AFTER THALAMOTOMY

As explained above, neural networks underlying rigidity and tremor are considered to be different, anatomically and physiologically, although the detailed neuronal mechanisms of each symptom still remain to be fully investigated.

Both rigidity and tremor are routinely and completely abolished in about 98% of cases (Narabayashi, 1988), without producing any side-effects in motor, speech, and psychological functions, by placing a three to four millimeter diameter electrocoagulation lesion in the base of the thalamus, which involves neurons and fibers of two subnuclei, the VL and VIM.

With abolition of these symptoms on the operating table within a few seconds after placing a lesion, immediate recovery of delicate voluntary movements on the operating table is routinely observed and is usually quite remarkable. Rotation of hand, separating and counting of fingers, and repeated flexion and extension of wrist and elbow become almost normal in skill and speed, together with clearing up of articulation and increase in speech volume. Repeated flexion and extension movements at ankle and knee are also normalized. These dramatic changes with immediate recovery of voluntary skills are a common observation even in the extremely rigid and tremulous parkinsonian patients.

These marked and immediate improvements are still very impressive to neurologists standing beside the operating table. They therefore strongly believe that the extrapyramidal symptoms disturb proper performance of voluntary actions and skill and that, when such disturbances are satisfactorily removed, the original neuronal activity governing normal movement and skill starts to reappear and recovers promptly.

Therefore, thalamotomy works only for removal of disturbing factors, rigidity and tremor, without damaging the proper function or smooth performance of normal movement. In other words, in parkinsonism there might be no irreversible damage or loss of the mechanisms responsible for performance of normal movement due to the disease itself or to surgery.

AKINESIA IN PARKINSONISM

A long-term follow-up study of unilaterally or bilaterally operated cases has been published elsewhere (Narabayashi, 1990). The effects on rigidity and tremor with improvement in ADL (activities of daily life) are sustained for many years, when the patients are relatively young (e.g. below 50 years of age) at the time of surgery.

With the introduction of the microelectrode technique, bilateral surgery remains exceptional and should be performed with extreme care, with a greater than one year interval between operations; in relatively young patients, bilateral surgery is possible without changes in speech and psychic function (Narabayashi, 1990).

In parkinsonian symptomatology, akinesia has been considered as the third major symptom after rigidity and tremor (Barbeau, 1972; Narabayashi, 1983). When the patient with bilateral parkinsonism is operated on the more severe side, the former two symptoms may completely disappear and be accompanied by recovery of skilled movement on that side, but often the patient still remains akinetic (reduced initiation and poverty of movement with remaining rigidity and tremor on the unoperated side).

Levodopa therapy improves rigidity and akinesia efficiently, even in these unilaterally operated cases. Therefore, it is concluded that akinesia is a third symptom that still remains even after unilateral elimination of rigidity. Bilateral surgery was not recommended using the classical thalamotomy because of the possible danger of side-effects, and these observations were not further analysed. Notably, Hughes and co-workers described that the effect of levodopa was the same on both the operated and unoperated side (Hughes *et al.*, 1974).

With accumulation of bilaterally operated young cases (average, two cases each year), it has become apparent that these patients are almost normal in social activities and home life without akinesia, under a minimum dose, if any, of medicine. There is almost no, or minimum, akinesia.

Therefore, the question arises, whether akinesia in these relatively younger cases, bilaterally operated, is a third motor symptom or not. It is highly probable that akinesia in these cases is only secondary to rigidity, at least in the younger cases.

DISCUSSION

Patients with classical parkinsonism starting around 60 years of age often tend to become progressively akinetic, even after the same surgical treatment. Similar progression is also observed with long-term pharmacotherapy in younger cases and classical later starting cases with parkinsonism, which were compared in their long-term course with a similarly successful pharmacological treatment. Younger starting cases (Narabayashi *et al.*, 1986a) stay in the highly improved state, often with nearly normalized ADL, for many (i.e. 10–20) years; the later starting group tend to show progressive deterioration in postural balancing, freezing in gait, emotional deterioration, loss of motivation, and tendency to inertia, which may constitute a part of akinesia in a broad sense (Narabayashi *et al.*, 1986b; Narabayashi and Kondo, 1987).

These observations and clinical experiences also suggest that the nature of akinesia in the later starting cases might be different from that of the younger starting cases, and is more complicated. Such differences in long-term observations of clinical pictures between two groups seems to indicate that the age difference is an important factor in accounting of symptoms. This also suggests that the older brains with parkinsonism may have more widespread, and more severe, morphological and chemical pathology than the younger brains. The author estimates that the damage involves mostly the nigrostriatal DA system in the younger group, but in the older age group involves both DA and norepinephrine (NE) systems (Narabayashi *et al.*, 1986b; Narabayashi and Kondo, 1987).

References

Albe-Fessard D, Arfel G, and Guiot G (1963) Activités électriques caractéristiques structures cérébrales chez l'homme, *Ann Chir*, **17**, 1185–214

Barbeau A (1972) Contribution of levodopa therapy to the neuropharmacology of akinesia. In Siegfried J, ed, *Parkinson's Disease*, Vol 1, Bern, Hans Huber, 151–75

Hassler R (1959) Anatomy of the thalamus. In Schaltenbrand G and Bailey P, eds, *Introduction to Stereotaxis with Atlas of the Human Brain*, Stuttgart, Thieme, 230–90

Hughes RC, Polgar JG, Weightman D, and Walton JN (1974) L-dopa in parkinsonism and the influence of previous thalamotomy, *Br Med J*, **I**, 7–13

Narabayashi H (1962) Neurophysiological ideas on pallidotomy and ventrolateral thalamotomy for hyperkinesis, *Confin Neurol*, **22**, 291–303

Narabayashi H (1982) Tremor mechanisms, In Schaltenbrand G and Walker AE, eds, *Stereotaxy of the Human Brain*, 2nd Edn, Stuttgart, Thieme, 510–4

Narabayashi H (1983) Pharmacological basis of akinesia in Parkinson's disease, *J Neural Trans*, **Suppl 19**, 143–51

Narabayashi H (1986) Tremor: its generating mechanism and treatment, In Vinken PJ, Bruyn GW, and Klawans HL, eds, *Extrapyramidal Disorders, Handbook of Clinical Neurology*, 5, Amsterdam, Elsevier, 597–607

Narabayashi H (1988) Lessons from stereotaxic surgery using microelectode techniques in understanding parkinsonism, *Mt Sinai J Med*, **55**, 50–7

Narabayashi H (1989) Stereotaxic Vim thalamotomy for treatment of tremor, *Eur Neurol* **29**(Suppl 1), 29–32

Narabayashi H (1990) Surgical treatment in the levodopa era, In Stern G, ed, *Parkinson's Disease*, London, Chapman & Hall, 597–646

Narabayashi H and Kondo T (1987) Results of a double-blind study of L-threo-DOPS in parkinsonism. In Fahn S, Marsden CD, Calne D *et al.*, eds, *Recent Developments in Parkinson's Disease*, 2, New Jersey, Macmillan, 270–91

Narabayashi H and Okuma T (1953) Procaine oil blocking of the globus pallidus for the treatment of rigidity and tremor of parkinsonism, *Proc Japan Acad*, **29**, 134–7

Narabayashi H, Okuma T, and Shikiba S (1956) Procaine oil blocking of the globus pallidus, *Arch Neurol Psychiatry*, **75**, 36–48

Narabayashi, H, Yokochi M, Iizuka R, and Nagatsu T (1986a) Juvenile parkinsonism. In Vinken PJ, Bruyn GW, and Klawans HL, eds, *Extrapyramidal Disorders, Handbook of Clinical Neurology*, 5, Amsterdam, Elsevier, 153–65

Narabayashi H, Kondo T, Yokochi F, and Nagatsu T (1986b) Clinical effects of L-threo-3,4-dihydroxy-phenylserine in cases of parkinsonism and pure akinesia. In Yahr MD and Bergmann KJ, eds, *Parkinson's Disease, Advances in Neurology*, 45, New York, Raven, 593–602

Yoshida M and Fujimoto K (1987) Neuronal activities of the basal ganglia in normal as well as in parkinsonian animals, In Benecke R, Conrad B, and Marsden CD, eds, *Motor Disturbances*, **1**, London, Academic, 111–8

Yoshida M (1991) The neuronal mechanism underlying parkinsonism and dyskinesia: differential roles of the putamen and caudate nucleus, *Neurosci Res*, **12**, 31–40

16
Neurostimulation methods for correcting functional imbalances

J. Siegfried

Functional electrical stimulation is a neural prosthetic technique that utilizes stimulation of neural tissue (Hambrecht and Reswick, 1977). The advent of implantable electronic stimulators led to a dramatic change in functional neurosurgery whereas previously, the only procedures providing long-term effective therapy were those that produced lesions to ablate a structure or interrupt a pathway. It is safer to apply chronic stimulation, which can be discontinued at any time, than to perform an irreversible, destructive, or ablative procedure.

Whether an electrode is destined for the spinal epidural space or the deep gray matter of the brain, there are some universally desired characteristics. These include lack of toxicity after long-term stimulation, positional stability, and easy insertion and removal. In attempting to achieve these general characteristics, some specific alterations according to placement site have also been made (Siegfried and Rea, 1988). There have been two areas of stimulator improvement in the past decade. These are in programmability and internalization. The ability to vary all parameters non-invasively increases the potential patterns of stimulations, which therefore increases the likelihood that the physician and patient can find a therapeutic combination of stimulation characteristics. The capability to totally internalize the unit (neuropacemaker) has several advantages, such as the patient need not apply the external apparatus, there are no external devices to break, and the physician can have complete control of the parameters used.

Stimulation techniques have been employed for the treatment of many disorders including pain, movement disorders, respiratory disorders, disturbances of micturition, blindness, deafness, and epilepsy.

CHRONIC INTRACTABLE PAIN

Surgery to relieve pain by electrical stimulation was first performed on a peripheral nerve by Sweet and Wall in 1965 (see Sweet and Wespic, 1968). This followed publication of the gate control theory of pain by Melzack and Wall (1965), which postulated that activation of large myelinated nerve fibers might block the transmission of pain impulses in the spinal cord. Despite some inconsistencies in this theory, it provided a theoretical framework for new pain treatments. Many other hypotheses have been suggested to explain the favorable effect of neurostimulation in pain relief including antidromic activation of large-diameter afferents in the posterior columns, blockade of conduction of pain pathways in the spino-thalamic tract, activation of descending inhibitory systems, coding at supraspinal levels, liberation or activation of opioid substances, or a combination of these.

Classification of chronic pain into two categories has been of great importance for a rational approach to treatment, whether medical or neurosurgical. Neurogenic pain and somatogenic pain are such distinct entities that a subjective description and clinical examination allow them to be clearly differentiated. Somatogenic pain is deep, dull pain varying in intensity at different times and localized in a region without any sensory disorder. It follows excitation of nociceptive receptors as a result of irritation, tension, or compression, causes of which may be physiological as well as chemical. The major feature of somatogenic pain is that it is generally responsive to opioids. Neurogenic pain, also called deafferentation pain, is generally of the burning type and is localized in a region having sensory disturbances. Its substrate is a neurological lesion of afferent sensory pathways. Neurogenic pain is one of the most distressing pains, and one of the most difficult to treat. It is practically unaffected by opioids, but electrical stimulation has its best indication in the control of pain due to direct involvement of nervous tissues.

Transcutaneous electrical neurostimulation

Because of the experimental and clinical evidence that peripheral input can significantly alter the perception of nociceptive impulses, input modulation, either by transcutaneous electrical nerve stimulation (TENS) or by counter-irritant measures, which probably activate the lower threshold nociceptive afferents, is an appropriate therapeutic approach (Casey, 1988). The transcutaneous method consists of stimulating, by means of electrodes fixed on the skin, the peripheral nerves responsible for sensory innervation of the painful area. Electrodes are considered to be in good position when stimulation at low intensity evokes paresthesias or vibrations in the entire sensory territory of the stimulated nerve. When direct stimulation of the nerve is impossible, because it is too deep, the electrodes are placed on or across the painful area itself. Results of large series suggest that TENS is most useful when the following four conditions are present (Keravel and Sindou, 1983): pain is secondary to deafferentation; pain is precisely localized; TENS is applied close to the nervous structures innervating the painful area; and there is a sufficient preservation of lemniscal fibers so that impulses produced by stimulation can be transmitted to the brain.

Peripheral nerve stimulation

Stimulation of a peripheral nerve requires its exposure with application of ring electrodes. This technique is rarely used now despite the good results obtained with it in neurogenic pain following peripheral nerve lesions. It has been replaced by stimulation of the posterior spinal root corresponding to the injured nerve, a less traumatic method.

Stimulation of dorsal spinal roots

When neurogenic pain is restricted to the area supplied by one to three peripheral nerves, the posterior spinal roots involved should be directly stimulated either by puncture of the intervertebral space and introduction of a flexible electrode into the dorsal lateral epidural space via the needle or by making a small opening into this intervertebral space and inserting a multicontact electrode mounted on plastic. Stimulation must be accompanied by tingling (paresthesia) in the painful area. The electrode is initially connected to an external stimulator and if short, repetitive stimulation suppresses or attenuates the pain for a brief period, the electrode is then, after three to four days, connected to a programmable pacemaker implanted into a subcutaneous pocket, generally in the abdomen. This pacemaker is then programmed. On average, it requires a 30-second stimulation every two minutes to obtain satisfactory control of the pain. If the pain is not significantly improved during the trial period, the electrode is withdrawn. We obtain beneficial to excellent results in 80% of patients with neurogenic pain caused by peripheral nerve lesions (Siegfried, 1991).

Stimulation of the dorsal cord

When neurogenic pain involves an area greater than that supplied by one to three peripheral nerves, the dorsal columns should be stimulated, because the greatest concentration of afferent tactile sensory fibers is found in this tract. The technique is the same as that of dorsal spinal root stimulation, but with an electrode placed more medially along the posterior column on the painful side. Although the technique seems simple, it requires considerable experience and special apparatus. It is the only method that controls neurogenic pain when the nerve lesion is postganglionic. Favorable long-term results are obtained in 60% of cases (Siegfried, 1991).

Stimulation of thalamic sensory nuclei

Spinal stimulation is ineffective when the nerve lesion extends to the preganglionic portion, such as with traumatic brachial plexus avulsion, or when pain is of spinal or cerebral origin. In these cases, good results can be obtained by stimulation of the thalamic sensory nuclei somatotopically related to the painful area. This involves stereotactic introduction of an electrode into the thalamic sensory nucleus corresponding to the pain localization (ventroposteromedian nucleus for facial pain, the median part of the ventroposterolateral nucleus for the upper limbs, and the lateral part of this nucleus for the lower limbs). After electrode placement, when electrical stimulation evokes paresthesias precisely located in the painful region, the electrode is fixed to the bone and connected to a temporary external cable allowing it to be tested for several days. In over 90% of cases, the improvement in pain is such that a programmable pacemaker is then implanted into an infraclavicular subcutaneous pouch a few days later. Beneficial long-term results are maintained in almost 80% of the cases (Siegfried, 1989). Failures occur when pain has been present for more than three years before the operation; perhaps degeneration of the sensory pathways up to the thalamic nuclei has occurred. In central post-stroke pain, success appears to depend on the location of the lesion (thalamic or parathalamic) as demonstrated by computerized tomography or magnetic resonance imaging. Little change is needed in the stimulation parameters over the long term; this suggests that the method may be safe with little modification of brain tissue over the years.

Electrical stimulation has its best indication in the control of pain caused by direct involvement of nervous tissues. Our own experience of 18 years in more than 700 patients has shown that the proper site for stimulation depends on the level of lesion. We believe that stimulation of dorsal roots, dorsal cord, and sensory thalamus for neurogenic pain is useful, particularly in patients resistant to more conservative treatment.

PERIPHERAL VASCULAR DISEASE

Spinal cord electrostimulation is proposed as an alternative method of managing patients with peripheral vascular disease whose problems cannot be solved by conventional methods. Vasodilator fibers in the dorsal spinal cord roots have been known for many years. Cook and Weinstein (1973) described autonomic changes in the legs of patients with multiple sclerosis during dorsal cord stimulation. These included regional increases in blood flow such as elevated skin temperature, changes in skin color, and improved tissue integrity. Based on this experience, Cook used direct stimulation of the posterior columns of spinal cord in patients with obstructive arteriosclerotic peripheral vascular disease unresponsive to sympathectomy and arterial bypass (Cook, 1976; Cook and Weinstein, 1976). He described relief of pain associated with increased skin temperature, improved plethysmographic blood flow, and improved tissue integrity. He considered these changes in circulation to be beyond that achieved by sympathectomy, and postulated that the benefits resulted from activation of vasodilator fibers. He thought persistent spinal cord stimulation might avoid the need for amputation in some patients. Large series of patients treated by this method showed that 93% had clinically significant control of their ischemic pain, 94% showed improvement in walking distance, and significant increase in blood flow was demonstrated in some patients by toe pressure, skin temperature, and ^{133}Xe measurements (Groth, 1985).

MOVEMENT DISORDERS

The use of chronic therapeutic stimulation for movement disorders was introduced by Cooper, who placed surface electrodes directly on the anterior cerebellar cortex (Cooper, 1973), by Bechtereva with stimulation of the diencephalon (Bechtereva *et al.*, 1975), and by Cook with dorsal cord stimulation (Cook and Weinstein, 1973). Control of involuntary movements and improvement in spasticity were the goals for neurostimulation of different targets in the central nervous system.

Stimulation of the dorsal cord

Following the pioneer observations of Cook and Weinstein (1973) who noted improvements in the motor function of patients receiving spinal cord stimulation for pain caused by demyelinating disease, many groups examined the effect of chronic spinal cord stimulation on abnormal motor function in a variety of upper motor-neuron dysfunctions. Reduction of spasticity, improvement of coordination, and diminution of dystonia and hyperkinesia have been reported.

INVOLUNTARY MOVEMENTS

Gildenberg (1978) was the first to use spinal cord stimulation in torticollis patients hoping to alter the abnormal pattern of the tonic neck reflexes. He noted that the best results were obtained with a stimulation frequency of 1100 Hz. In 63 patients, Waltz, Scozzari, and Hunt (1985) reported 36.5% with marked improvement (characterized by loss of evidence of torticollis, full range of motility of the head and neck, and no pain) and moderate improvement in 31%. In our experience, general improvement may be seen in some patients with moderate or slight spasmodic torticollis, but the major improvement is reduction in the distressing pulling and painful sensations in the muscles, even though the position of the head might not return to normal.

The use of cervical cord stimulation in the treatment of other involuntary movements, such as cerebral palsy, is controversial and even though improvements have been reported, more in the control of dystonia than in the improvement of dyskinesias, we feel that, for these indications, this method has little to recommend it (Siegfried and Lazorthes, 1985).

SPASTICITY

Cook (1976) reported good results in 90% of 70 multiple sclerosis patients treated with spinal cord stimulation. He recommended its use for patients with proven multiple sclerosis and moderate impairment, and mentioned improvements in peripheral circulation, respiration, and micturition. He observed effects that extended far beyond the immediate area of application, such as improved arm function with stimulation at the midthoracic level. In a cooperative study at three different clinics (Siegfried, Lazorthes, and Broggi, 1981), we analysed 53 patients with different spastic movement disorders treated with permanent implantation of a spinal cord stimulation system from a series of 164 patients tested transiently. In 36 with multiple sclerosis with a post-operative follow-up of one to five years, four showed very good improvement of their spasticity, 18 had good improvement, 12 had fair improvement, and two patients were unchanged. In a series of seven with familial spastic paraplegia (Strümpell-Lorrain), spasticity was clearly improved clinically and quantitatively, using measurements of stretch and H-reflexes, in five. On the contrary, spasticity with cerebral palsy (six patients treated transiently) and myelopathy (11 patients tested transiently) was not improved and permanent implantation was not performed. Although Gybels and Van Roost (1987) disagree, we are of the opinion that spinal cord stimulation for moderate spasticity is useful. It is reversible and, after correct selection with a trial period of stimulation, one third of the patients show an improvement in motor disability for at least a few years. However, with cerebral palsy, results are not satisfactory. In cases of demyelinating and degenerative disease of the spinal cord, some integrity of the afferent and efferent pathways must be present. With these restrictions, a therapeutic approach with spinal cord stimulation is justified, because it is non-destructive and devoid of stress, although intrathecal application of baclofen may be, in the majority of cases, the treatment of choice.

Cerebellar stimulation

The first extensive report of the results from cerebellar stimulation in patients with movement disorders was published in 1976 by Cooper and co-workers, which included 50 patients with cerebral palsy (Cooper *et al.*, 1976). This group was enlarged to 141 patients in a subsequent report in 1979. In the later group, 41% of the patients were rated as having moderate to marked improvement, 32% demonstrated mild improvement, and 24% had no clinical change. Other similar favorable results were reported initially from other centers. However, as more neurosurgeons adopted the technique, papers began to report that the effects of cerebellar stimulation were unpredictable, and later papers expressed doubt about the usefulness of chronic cerebellar stimulation for reduction of spasticity.

Chronic stimulation of the dentate nucleus was applied successfully by Schvarcz, Sica, and Morita (1980) to relieve spasticity and to improve motor function in patients with cerebral palsy. All four of their cases were relieved of spasticity, and were able to perform complex voluntary movements that were impossible prior to stimulation; additionally, the quality of their speech, posture, balance, and gait were improved. No other experiences with chronic stimulation of the dentate nucleus have been reported.

There is no doubt that the primary function of the cerebellum is the regulation of control of movements, posture, and tone. It may be that it exerts some control of many other functions of the nervous system because it has extensive fiber connections with other parts of the brain and spinal cord. The rationale for increasing the inhibitory effect of the cerebellum by electrical stimulation can be understood; however, the clinical results are disputed, and its application has progressively decreased. Better clinical evaluation, better studies of different stimulation parameters, and more precise indications could renew interest in this method.

Cerebral stimulation

The first modern study of chronic therapeutic deep brain stimulation in human movement disorders appeared in several articles by Bechtereva and colleagues between 1972 and 1975. They reported that chronic stimulation had favorable effects in patients who had tremor associated with Parkinson's disease, Wilson's disease, and dystonia musculorum deformans. Unfortunately, information regarding the number of patients, the techniques for electrode placement, and the proposed target was not divulged. Mundinger (1982) was the first to report the implantation of chronic electrodes in the thalamus for movement disorders. Good results in facial dyskinesias in a series of torsion dystonia, double athetosis, and arm dystonia in a case of traumatic spasticity are reported, apparently with stimulation of the ventrolateral part of the thalamus, the zona inserta, or both. He also emphasized the importance of stimulation-induced paresthesias overlying the affected area, so that the sensory thalamic nuclei were certainly involved. Mazars, who first stimulated sensory thalamic nuclei to alleviate neurogenic pain, also found that associated abnormal movements were controlled (Mazars, Mcrienne, and Cioloca, 1980). He stressed the importance of stimulation paresthesias over the affected part of the body. He also felt that for stimulation to be successful, the dyskinesias had to be associated with a sensory deafferentation, and that stimulation acted as a substitute for sensory information delivered to nucleus ventroposterolateralis. Effects on spasticity of these patients, suffering from thalamic or central post-stroke pain syndrome with sensory and motor deficit, was not mentioned. The largest series of patients with involuntary movement disorders being treated by deep brain stimulation is the one of Cooper, Upton, and Amin (1980). To improve the efficacy, thalamic somato-sensory responses were recorded to aid in electrode placement and in obtaining optimal stimulation parameters; effects on related spasticity are not reported.

In 1982 we implanted two sensory thalamic nuclei electrodes, one on each side, in a patient 41 years of age suffering with neurogenic pain in the legs after traumatic paraplegia, associated with severe spasticity. There was virtually immediate control of pain and clonus with bilateral ventroposterolateral thalamic stimulation. After stimulation was stopped, the clonus reappeared within two minutes. An additional case, a couple of years later, produced the same effect. We also observed, in four cases of central post-stroke pain syndrome, who had received thalamic stimulation for neurogenic pain, that stimulation, given satisfactory paresthesias in the painful area with impulses of 1–2 mA, 200 microseconds, and 33 Hz, suppressed almost instantly the choreoathetotic movements associated with the thalamic syndrome. As long as stimulation continued, the involuntary movements were controlled, but at its completion, the dyskinesias reappeared slowly over one to two minutes. Using this knowledge, the neuropacemaker was programmed with a period of stimulation of one minute every two minutes. Long follow-up confirmed the continued effectiveness of stimulation (Siegfried, 1986). It has been argued that somatosensory inputs of a specific and restricted nature may be used to control or monitor movements. Clinical examples of cutaneous input modifying motor activity include the 'geste antagoniste' (putting the index finger on the chin), which is, in some cases, sufficient to control spasmodic torticollis, and the inability of athetosic patients to control their movements without the help of sensory input. The theory that the stimulation of sensory thalamic nuclei supplies absent or decreased 'sensory input' is therefore very attractive.

Electrical stimulation of deep brain structures has been practised since the introduction of stereotactic brain operations in humans in 1947, particularly for localization during stereotactic thalamotomies in patients with extrapyramidal movement disorders. The many sensations that were reported, depended on the electrode site and the stimulation parameters. Hassler and co-workers found that stimulation of the basal parts of nucleus ventrolateralis of the thalamus, site of high-frequency coagulation in the treatment of tremor, caused some increase in tremor amplitudes followed by a pause (Hassler *et al.*, 1960). The increase in amplitude depended upon the phase of the tremor when the stimulation occurred. Even in its absence, tremor may be evoked by stimulus rate of four to eight per second. Stimulation with higher frequencies mostly reduces the intensity of tremor, and may even lead to its complete arrest, in addition to synergy of flexion. Benabid (1987) reported his first series with Parkinsonian tremor well controlled by chronic stimulation of the nucleus intermedius thalami through implanted stimulators. We have confirmed these favorable results and have emphasized the value of the method as an alternative therapeutic approach when serious side effects from classical high-frequency coagulation can be anticipated as with bilateral operations (Blond and Siegfried, 1991).

RESPIRATORY DISORDERS

Glenn, Holcomb, and Shaw (1976) reported the results of chronic stimulation of the phrenic nerve for treatment of hypoventilation arising from suprasegmental denervation. This method is widely used, the main indications being respiratory paralysis after cervical-medullary injury above the origin of the phrenic motor neurons and the chronic central hypoventilation syndrome (sleep apnea or Ondine's curse). The method has also been tried in chronic obstructive pulmonary disease and chronic hiccup. Stimulation of the phrenic nerve in patients requiring diaphragm pacing is accomplished by a radiofrequency system consisting of four components, transmitter, antenna, receiver capsule, and nerve cuff. The transmitter is a small battery-powered unit; energy is delivered to the surgically-implanted receiver capsule by an antenna. Energy from the transmitter is magnetically coupled to the receiver circuit in a form of pulses of radiofrequency currents. A pulse duration modulation technique is used to code the transmitted pulse with the desired current amplitude to be applied to the nerve.

In all series reported in the literature, the implantation of electrophrenic stimulators has been of significant benefit to the majority of the patients. The reason for this is probably careful patient selection as well as adequate pre-operative investigations and post-operative controls.

Another approach in the treatment of respiratory disorders by electrostimulation has been developed by Mugica and co-workers (1985). It consists of a direct non-phrenic muscular diaphragm pacing system with multiple electrodes, placed along the margin of a hemidiaphragm, with delayed start of stimuli from front to back.

MICTURITION DISORDERS

Electrical stimulation in the control of micturition disorders can be applied at different levels, pelvic floor (perineal muscles, sphincters), detrusors sacral roots, conus medullaris, and dorsal columns. The last two levels, which are of real value in micturition disorders of neurological origin, will be reported. Physiological experimentation in animals and man has revealed a dual system of innervation for the bladder and sphincter. It consists of an intrinsic innervation for the bladder wall of ganglion cells, which are incapable of initiating an effective contraction of the bladder but are under the control of more proximal nerve centers. The extrinsic innervation is centered in the conus medullaris in the so-called micturition center extending from S2 through S4. Efferent motor neurons in this center, in the intermediolateral cell column, send axons via the sacral roots S2, S3, and S4. The physiological center is capable of controlling bladder function in an automatic way through a sensorimotor reflex arc. Two types of motor innervation have been delineated, a parasympathetic and a somatic element. The micturition reflex is parasympathetic, and normally the vesicospinal center is under control of higher cortical and subcortical centers. Spinal cord lesions above the T12 vertebral level isolate the micturition center, releasing it from suprasegmental control and leaving a reflex bladder. Where reflex activity is inefficient in emptying the bladder, neural stimulation of the conus medullaris can activate the reflex mechanisms (Friedman, Nashold, and Grimes, 1977). The neuro-prothesis consists of two parts, the external radiofrequency stimulator and the implantable subcutaneous radiofrequency receiver attached to two platinum bipolar stimulating electrodes, which are inserted into the conus medullaris at the S1–S1 level. Very satisfactory results has been reported so far with repeated daily bladder contraction with voiding, low urinary residuals, reduced bladder infections, increased bladder capacity, and freedom from catheterization.

It was soon shown that spinal dorsal cord stimulation in patients with multiple sclerosis improves bladder disturbances more than motor dysfunction in a higher percentage of patients. Illis (1982) reported that bladder function improved in 75% of patients with multiple sclerosis. The improvements included regaining normal bladder function after a long lasting regime of permanent catheterization. The same percentage of improvement was published by Hawkes, Fawcett, and Coke (1981), supported by urodynamic evaluations; they documented improved urinary flow and reduced external sphincter pressure as judged from urethral pressure profiles. In patients with spinal cord disease or injury, Meglio, Cioni, and D'Amico (1980) demonstrated a decrease of basal bladder pressure, an increase in bladder capacity, and reduction of residual urine.

EPILEPSY

Chronic electrical stimulation of the cerebellum was introduced more than 15 years ago by Cooper (Cooper *et al.*, 1978a, 1978b) for epilepsy patients who were not controlled by antiepileptic medication, and were either not candidates for surgical ablation of epileptic foci, or as a non-destructive alternative. Despite initial encouraging results, when the method was used widely, it produced equivocal results and was abandoned. It has been suggested that the cerebellar cortex in humans is too large to be adequately stimulated by electric current delivered through relatively small surface electrodes. Stimulation of smaller structures, which could have inhibitory influences, has been undertaken. Electrical stimulation with chronically implanted electrodes in the caudate nucleus (Drlickova, Sramka, and Nadvornik, 1984) and of the centro-median thalamic nucleus (Velasco *et al.*, 1978) and recently of the vagus nerve have been described.

OTHER APPLICATIONS

Chronic electrical stimulation with implantation of prosthetic devices in other fields such as the treatment of blindness and deafness are discussed elsewhere in this book (see Chapter 7). Stimulation of centrum medianum in cases of prolonged post-traumatic unconsciousness has shown, in some cases, a clear improvement of the overall situation with rapid improvements of vegetative functions (oral feeding became possible, bronchial hypersecretion was reduced, and pulmonary infection resolved) as well as a progressive improvement of consciousness (Cohadon *et al.*, 1985). Many tentative experiments with electrical stimulation have been performed, such as for intractable behavioral disorders, unfortunately without any rationale.

CONCLUSION

A most remarkable contribution to the neurosurgical treatment of functional disorders in recent years has been not only the creation of non-destructive methods and their constant improvements, but also the successive codification of the choice of intervention according to the type of disturbance. This approach has only just started and requires refinement in the years to come. Only an increasingly greater understanding of the mechanisms of neurological disorders with functional impairment will lead to increasingly more specific therapies. Neurostimulation devices must also be improved and developed. We need more quantitative, objective, and controlled studies over a long period of time of patients treated by chronic electrical stimulation to assess critically the benefits of this non-destructive and reversible therapeutic method.

References

Benabid AL, Pollack P, Louveau A, Henry S, and de Rougemont J (1987) Combined (thalamotomy and stimulation) stereotactic surgery of the VIM thalamic nucleus for bilateral Parkinson disease, *Appl Neurophysiol*, **50**, 344–6

Bechtereva NP, Bondartchuk AN, Smirnov VM, Mcliutcheva LA, and Shandurina AN (1975) Method of electrostimulation of the deep brain structures in treatment of some chronic disease, *Confinia neurologica*, **37**, 136–40

Blond S and Siegfried J (1991) Thalamic stimulation for the treatment of tremor and other movement disorders, *Acta Neurochir*, **52** (Suppl.), 109–11.

Casey KL (1988) Toward a rationale for the treatment of painful neuropathies, In Dubner R, Gebhart GF, and Bond MR, eds, *Proceedings of the Vth World Congress on Pain*, Amsterdam, Elsevier, 165–74

Cohadon F, Richer R, Bougier A, Deliac P, and Loiseau H (1985) Deep brain stimulation in cases of prolonged post-traumatic unconsciousness, In Lazorthes Y and Upton ARM, eds, *Neurostimulation*, New York, Futura, 247–50

Cook AW (1976) Electrical stimulation in multiple sclerosis, *Hosp Pract*, **11**, 51–8

Cook AW and Weinstein S (1973) Chronic dorsal column stimulation in multiple sclerosis, *NY State J Med*, **73**, 2868–72

Cook AW and Weinstein S (1976) Vascular disease of extremities. Electrical stimulation of spinal cord and posterior roots. *NY State J Med*, **76**, 366–8

Cooper IS (1973) Effect of chronic stimulation of anterior cerebellum on neurological disease, *Lancet*, **i**, 1321

Cooper IS, Riklan M, Amin I, Waltz JM, and Cullinan T (1976) Chronic cerebellum stimulation in cerebral palsy, *Neurology*, **26**, 744–53

Cooper IS, Riklan M, Amin I, and Cullinan T (1978a) A long-term follow-up study of cerebellar stimulation for the control of epilepsy, In Cooper IS, ed, *Cerebellar Stimulation in Man*, New York, Raven, 19–38

Cooper IS, Riklan M, Tabaddor K, Cullinan T, Amin I, and Watkins ES (1978b) A long-term follow-up of chronic cerebellar stimulation for cerebral palsy, In Cooper IS, ed, *Cerebellar Stimulation in Man*, New York, Raven, 55–99

Cooper IS, Upton ARM, and Amin I (1980) Reversibility of chronic neuralgic deficits: Some effects of electrical stimulation of the thalamus and internal capsule in man, *Appl Neurophysiol*, **43**, 244–58

Drlickova V, Sramka M, and Nadvornik P (1984) Caudate nucleus stimulation during epilepsy treatment, *Acta Neurochir*, **Suppl 33**, 155–9

Friedman H, Nashold BS, and Grimes J (1977) Electrical stimulation of the conus medullaris in the paraplegic, In Hambrecht FT and Reswick JB, eds, *Functional Electrical Stimulation*, New York, Marcel Dekker, 173–83

Gildenberg PL (1978) Treatment of spasmodic torticollis by dorsal column stimulation, *Appl Neurophysiol*, **41**, 113–21

Glenn ZL, Holcomb WG, and Shaw RK (1976) Long-term ventilatory support by diaphragm pacing in quadriplegia, *Ann Surg*, **113**, 566–77

Groth KE (1985) Spinal cord stimulation for the treatment of peripheral vascular disease, In Fields HL *et al.*, eds, *Advances in Pain Research and Therapy*, Vol 9, New York, Raven, 861–70

Gybels J and Van Roost D (1987) Spinal cord stimulation for spasticity, In Symon L *et al.*, eds, *Advances and Technical Standards in Neurosurgery*, Vol 15, Wien, Springer, 63–96

Hambrecht FT and Reswick JB (1977) eds, *Functional Electrical Stimulation*, New York, Marcel Dekker

Hassler R, Riechert T, Mundinger F, Umbach W, and Ganglberger JA (1960) Physiological observations in stereotaxic operations in extrapyramidal motor disturbances, *Brain*, **83**, 337–50

Hawkes CH, Fawcett D, and Coke ED (1981) Dorsal column stimulation in multiple sclerosis: effects on bladder leg blood flow and peptides, *Appl Neurophysiol*, **44**, 62–70

Illis LS and Sedgwick EM (1982) Stimulation procedures, In Illis LS, Sedgwick EM, and Glanville HJ, eds, *Rehabilitation of the Neurological Patient*, Oxford, Blackwell, 384–410

Keravel Y and Sindou M (1983) Anatomical conditions of efficiency of transcutaneous electrical neurostimulation in deafferentation pain, In Bonica JJ, Lindblom U, Iggo A, eds, *Advances in Pain Research and Therapy*, Vol 5, New York, Raven, 763–7

Mazars G, Merienne L, and Cioloca G (1980) Control of dyskinesias due to sensory deafferentation by means of thalamic stimulation, *Acta Neurochir*, **30**(Suppl), 239–93

Meglio M, Cioni B, and D'Amico E (1980) Epidural spinal cord stimulation for the treatment of neurogenic bladder, *Acta Neurochir*, **54**, 191–9

Melzack R and Wall PD (1965) Pain mechanisms. A new theory, *Science*, **150**, 971–9

Mugica J, Bisson A, Dejean D, Bourgeois I, Martel-Bertrand S, and Smits K (1985) Preliminary test of a muscular diaphragm pacing system on human patients, In Lazorthes Y and Upton ARM, eds, *Neurostimulation*, New York, Futura, 263–79

Mundinger F and Neumüller H (1982) Programmed stimulation for control of chronic pain and motor disease, *Appl Neurophysiol*, **45**, 102–11

Schvarcz JR, Sica R, and Morita E (1980) Chronic self-stimulation of the dentate nucleus for the relief of spasticity, *Acta Neurochir*, **30**(Suppl), 351–9

Siegfried J (1986) Effets de la stimulation du noyau sensitif du thalamus sur les dyskinesies et la spasticité, *Rev Neurol*, **142**, 380–3

Siegfried J (1988) Neurostimulation zur Behandlung von chronischen Schmerzen durch Schädigung peripherer Nerven, In Lücking CH, Thoden U, and Zimmermann M, eds, *Nervenschmerz*, Stuttgart, Gustav Fischer, 292–6

Siegfried J (1989) Neurosurgical treatment of neurogenic pain, In *Advances in Pain Research and Therapy*. Third International Symposium, The Pain Clinic, Florence, September 10–14, 1988, New York, Raven

Siegfried J (1991) Therapeutical neurostimulation – Indications reconsidered, *Acta Neurochir*, **52** (Suppl.), 112–17

Siegfried J and Lazorthes Y (1985) La neurochirurgie fonctionnelle de l'infirmité motrice d'origine cérébrale, *Neurochirurgie*, **31**(Suppl 1), 1–118

Siegfried J, Lazorthes Y, and Broggi G (1981) Electrical spinal cord stimulation for spastic movement disorders, *Appl Neurophysiol*, **44**, 77–92

Siegfried J and Rea G (1988) Advances in neurostimulation devices, In Pluchino F and Broggi G, eds, *Advanced Technology in Neurosurgery*, Berlin, Springer, 199–207

Sweet WH and Wepsic J (1968) Treatment of chronic pain by stimulation of fibers of primary afferent neurons, *Trans Am Neurol Ass*, **93**, 103–5

Velasco F, Velasco M, Ogarrio C, and Fanghanel G (1987) Electrical stimulation of the centromedian thalamic nucleus in the treatment of convulsive seizures: a preliminary report, *Epilepsia*, **28**, 421–30

Waltz JM, Scozzari CA, and Hunt DP (1985) Spinal cord stimulation in the treatment of spasmodic torticollis, *Appl Neurophysiol*, **48**, 324–38

17
Surgical treatment of epilepsy

J. M. Oxbury

Surgical treatment should be considered in any patient whose epilepsy cannot be controlled by doses of medication which are free from unacceptable side-effects. The purpose of surgery is to relieve patients of their epilepsy, with its life threatening and disabling social consequences, and the unpleasant side-effects of heavy drug doses, and if possible to restore them to normality. Relief from the epilepsy can set the scene for social rehabilitation following what for most has been a severe disability lasting many years.

Operations fall into 4 main categories (see Table 17.1 after Engel, 1987a): temporal lobe excisions which account for around 70% of operations and are performed by virtually all centres offering an epilepsy surgery service; extratemporal cortical excisions – 25% of operations; hemispherectomy and callosal section which are less frequently performed. All but callostomy are effective only as a treatment for focal (partial) seizures. Temporal lobe excisions and hemispherectomy are the most successful operations, the former restoring up to 50% of those operated to complete normality.

Certain general criteria should be fulfilled before seriously considering surgery:
1. The patient's disability must be due to epilepsy rather than other conditions such as psychogenic seizures or hyperventilation (Fenwick, 1987, 1991).
2. The disability must be sufficient to justify the risks associated with pre-operative assessment and surgery, bearing in mind that not all patients who are assessed will be operated upon and not all patients operated upon will have a successful outcome.

Table 17.1 Relative frequency of surgical operations for epilepsy: data from 40 centres contributing to 1986 Palm Desert Conference (after Engel, 1987a)

	Centres	Patients	Seizure-free (%)
Anterior temporal lobectomy	40	2336	55.5
Extratemporal excision	32	825	43.2
Hemispherectomy	17	88	77.3
Callosotomy	16	197	5.0

3. There should be good evidence that the epilepsy is resistant to all drugs currently available and is not of a form that is usually self-limiting (e.g. benign focal epilepsy of childhood).
4. The patients should accept at the outset that overall there is only a 50% chance of long-lasting complete freedom from seizures post-operatively, and at most a 25% chance of maintaining such freedom off all medication, although there should be an additional 25–30% chance of a marked reduction in seizure frequency.

An accurate prediction of outcome can be made most easily when the nature of the pathology underlying the epilepsy can be specified pre-operatively. Data from centres using surgical techniques which permit adequate histopathological examination of the excised material indicate that the chances of an entirely successful outcome are considerably reduced when the specimen does not include an unequivocal abnormality (Oxbury and Adams, 1989). Predicting outcome is much more speculative when the decision to operate is based on neurophysiological findings alone without a good appreciation of the likely pathology.

The idea behind the use of cortical excisions is that focal seizures arise from an overactivity, or hypersynchrony, in localizable groups of neurones followed by propagation of abnormal electrical activity to other brain areas (Engel, 1987b; Robitaille, 1987). Many believe that these electrical foci are associated with histologically definable pathology. Discreet excisions of focal pathology, or of cortical areas from which a patient's aura may be elicited by electrical stimulation, however, often fail to produce lasting relief from seizures (Rasmussen, 1974). So, it seems necessary also to excise contiguous cortical areas where neurones are recruited during development of the seizure (Rasmussen, 1983). Most epilepsy surgery services render 50–60% patients seizure-free post-operatively and an additional 20–30% have a post-operative seizure frequency less than 10% of the pre-operative rate (Engel, 1987a).

TEMPORAL LOBE EXCISIONS

An excision from one temporal lobe is the most commonly performed operation to treat epilepsy. Patients whose predominant seizure type is an automatism, often preceded by an aura incorporating an abdominal sensation, are the most likely to benefit (Duncan and Sagar, 1987; Oxbury and Adams, 1989). The first electrical components of many of these seizures is localized in one hippocampus or amygdala (Wieser, 1986, 1987, 1988; Maldonado et al., 1988). Neuronal depletion in the hippocampus and/or amygdala, with gliosis, and indolent glioma or dysembryoplastic epithelioma (Daumas-Duport et al., 1988), are the two most common pathological findings (Bruton, 1988). Both forms of pathology are associated with a particularly good prognosis for relief of the epilepsy (Falconer, 1971a; Oxbury and Adams, 1989). Other pathology, found less frequently, includes: calcified cavernous angioma; old abscess cavity; cortical malformation (Sellier et al., 1987; Janota and Polkey, 1992); other tumours such as epidermoid; a small traumatic scar or area of infarction; arteriovenous malformation and tuberous sclerosis.

Surgery must be unilateral because bilateral excisions cause a permanent severe global amnesia (Scoville and Milner, 1957). Care must be taken during pre-operative assessment to ensure that surgery is not carried out contralateral to pre-existing severe medial temporal lobe damage or a similar severe amnesia may ensue (Penfield and Mathieson, 1974).

Operative procedures

The *en bloc* anterior temporal lobectomy, devised by Murray Falconer (Falconer, 1953, 1971b; Polkey, 1987) removes, in a single piece, the anterior 5.5–6.5 cm of temporal lobe (proportionately less in children), the lateral and basal parts of the amygdala, and the anterior 2.0–2.5 cm of hippocampus and hippocampal gyrus. The excised specimen usually has a fixed weight of 35–45 g and is available for detailed histological examination. The operation has not only been very effective as a treatment but also it has led to major contributions to understanding the genesis of temporal lobe epilepsy. Dominant hemisphere excisions tend to be slightly smaller than those from the non-dominant hemisphere and often spare the superior temporal gyrus. The operation can be used for both adults and children (Falconer, 1972; Davidson and Falconer, 1975; Hopkins and King, 1991). The chances of good outcome and of possible deleterious effects are well documented (Oxbury and Adams, 1989; Adams *et al.*, 1990).

Other 'tailor-made' operations excise variable portions of anterior temporal neocortex *en bloc* in one piece, and then amygdala, hippocampus and parahippocampal gyrus *en bloc* in a second piece (Olivier, 1988a). Alternatively, the removal, especially of the medial structures, may be piecemeal by suction (Awad *et al.*, 1989; Estes *et al.*, 1989) which makes histological analysis difficult or impossible. The precise extent of such removals varies according to a number of factors (Rasmussen, 1975; Olivier, 1987, 1988a) including: findings at pre- and intra-operative depth electrode and electrocorticographic recordings, the estimated memory capacity of the contralateral temporal lobe, whether removal is from the language dominant or non-dominant side, and the patient's response to electrical brain stimulation if the operation is conducted under local anaesthesia.

Limited removals include removal of the amygdala alone, removal of the amygdala with the anterior pes hippocampus (Feindel, 1989) and selective amygdalo-hippocampectomy. The first two of these procedures do not, in general, produce as good seizure control as the more extensive removals. Selective amygdalohippocampectomy (Yasargil and Wieser, 1987; Wieser, 1988) has been defined by Yasargil *et al.* (1985) as a unilateral excision of the amygdaloid body, hippocampal body and parahippocampus extending from the hippocampal fimbria to the collateral sulcus. Other parts of the anterior temporal lobe are not excised. The fixed weight of the excised portion is 3–5 g in contrast to the 35–45 g of an *en bloc* temporal lobectomy specimen. The approach to the mesiobasal structures as described by Professor Yasargil is via the floor of the sylvian fissure. An alternative approach is to enter the temporal horn of the lateral ventricle through a longitudinal incision in the middle temporal gyrus (Olivier, 1988b).

The rationale for selective amygdalohippocampectomy is that many temporal lobe seizures commence in the hippocampus and/or amygdala, and so control might be obtained by removing these structures alone (Wieser, 1988). If so, the control would be achieved by a removal much smaller than the standard *en bloc* excision and perhaps, therefore, with a greater saving of cognitive function and/or memory. There is a distinct possibility that the extent of any such savings could depend on which surgical approach is used since each must produce damage to neighbouring structures en route to the hippocampus and amygdala, although which precise structures will differ for the two approaches. Ideally the operation should be performed only when pre-operative EEG recordings have demonstrated consistent seizure onset from hippocampus and/or amygdala (Wieser, 1988) or, perhaps, when unequivocal hippo-campal abnormality has been demonstrated by volumetric MRI. These structures are, of course, the major site of pathology in many patients and, although the precise relationship between pathology and electrical manifestations of seizure onset has yet to be demonstrated, it may be pertinent that patients who benefit from anterior temporal lobectomy may have a greater degree of sclerosis in anterior hippocampus than in posterior parts (Babb *et al.*, 1984).

Spencer *et al.* (1984) have described a surgical technique giving access to the posterior part of the temporal horn to resect posteromedial temporal lobe structures in patients with posterior hippocampal foci.

Outcome

Any consideration of the outcome from surgery must take into account changes in seizure frequency, in the level of social disability, and in cognitive and memory function. It must also consider any overtly unwanted effects of operation such as hemianopia or hemiplegia since these could constitute an even greater disability than the epilepsy which may or may not have been cured. Furthermore, the complications which may develop during pre-operative investigation, especially with invasive techniques such as intracranial EEG recording, should be borne in mind. A number of factors influence outcome including the nature of the pathology underlying the epilepsy, the patient's age at operation, the side of the operation, the type of operation and particularly whether or not the hippocampus is included in the excision and whether the patient's IQ is within the normal range or below. To these may be added, when pre-operative investigation does not show definite unilateral temporal lobe pathology, the degree of certainty, based on EEG data, that seizure onset is consistently from one temporal lobe.

Pathology

Falconer and his group at the Maudsley Hospital in London clearly recognized that there was a particularly good outcome in terms of seizure relief amongst patients whose temporal lobe excision specimens contained either what the group termed mesial temporal sclerosis or a small cryptic tumour or glial malformation (Falconer *et al.*, 1964; Falconer, 1971a). This has been confirmed subsequently by many others.

The term mesial temporal sclerosis (MTS) was introduced by Falconer *et al.* (1964) to describe all degrees of hippocampal neurone loss and gliosis, from very mild to very severe, and to acknowledge that this pathology may involve other medial temporal lobe structures in addition to the hippocampus. MTS is the commonest pathological finding in temporal lobectomy specimens. It was the sole pathology in 47 of 100 such specimens described by Falconer (1971a) and 92% of the 47 operations had a successful outcome; it is clear from the clinical description of the cases that most of those with MTS had it in the severe form.

Ammon's horn sclerosis (AHS) is a variety of MTS in which there is a particularly severe degree of hippocampal neurone loss and gliosis. It was defined by Margerison and Corsellis (1966), in an autopsy study of the brains of people who had suffered from epilepsy, as pyramidal neurone loss and gliosis in the H_1 sector of the hippocampus, and in the endofolium, with granule cell loss from the dentate gyrus.

They found that the condition was unilateral in 82% of cases, although approximately half of these had lesser degrees of sclerosis in the contralateral hippocampus, and there was a strong correlation with the clinical features of temporal lobe epilepsy. Ounsted *et al.* (1966) suggested that Ammon's horn sclerosis is the consequence of a complicated convulsion* in early childhood and becomes the cause of the subsequent habitual temporal lobe epilepsy. Sagar and Oxbury (1987), in a study of 32 temporal lobectomy excision specimens, found a highly significant correlation between AHS and a history of a complicated convulsion in early childhood.

A history of a complicated convulsion in early childhood acts as an excellent marker to AHS. Establishing the side of unilateral pathology depends upon the clinical history, EEG data, MRI findings, and the outcome of neuropsychological assessment including intracarotid sodium amytal tests. Documentary evidence of focal features in an early childhood complicated convulsion is a strong, but not absolute, pointer to contralateral hippocampal sclerosis. The diagnosis is supported by: unilateral hippocampal volume loss seen on MRI (Jack *et al.*, 1990; Berkovic *et al.*, 1991); ipsilateral, or very predominantly ipsilateral, sphenoidal and/or anterior temporal interictal spikes on sphenoidal EEG recording (Morris *et al.*, 1989); specific verbal memory impairment when the sclerosis involves the hippocampus of the dominant hemisphere (Oxbury and Oxbury, 1989); and sometimes by transient memory impairment following amytal administered to the contralateral, but not ipsilateral, internal carotid artery or, occasionally, posterior cerebral artery (Jack *et al.*, 1988). Further evidence may be derived from ictal recordings with sphenoidal electrodes during the course of prolonged video/EEG monitoring. Only a small number of cases require EEG recordings with intracranial electrodes (foramen ovale, subdural, or depth).

AHS was the sole pathology in 39 of the excision specimens from 100 consecutive temporal lobectomies described by Oxbury and Adams (1989). Complete freedom from seizures was achieved post-operatively by 65% of these cases, and another 24% had their seizure frequency reduced to less than 10% of the pre-operative rate. The habitual epilepsy of these patients usually begins during the first decade of their life and operation no later than adolescence has a very good chance of producing an excellent outcome. Patients with left dominant hemisphere AHS usually have poor verbal memory pre-operatively, and temporal lobectomy causes little change (Oxbury and Oxbury, 1989; Dodrill *et al.*, 1992); it is even more difficult to detect a pre- *vs* post-operative difference in neuropsychological parameters for those undergoing right-sided excisions.

The term indolent glioma has been applied to the focal lesions of variable size which have some histological features of either astrocytoma or oligodendroglioma but seem to be extremely benign (small cryptic tumour of Falconer *et al.* (1964) and Falconer (1971a); dysembryoplastic neuroepithelial tumour of Daumas-Duport *et al.* (1988); and see Bruton (1988) for a detailed discussion). This pathology accounted for approximately 20% of Falconer's cases and 30% of the cases of Oxbury and Adams (1989). The prognosis for seizure relief after *en bloc* temporal lobectomy is excellent. Falconer (1971a) reported that 92% had a successful outcome and 68% of the cases of Oxbury and Adams (1989) became completely seizure-free. The diagnosis depends upon high quality neuroimaging. There is often calcification which can be detected by the use of appropriate CT techniques (Adams *et al.*, 1987) and MRI is particularly

---

*A complicated convulsion (Aicardi and Chevrie, 1976) is one which is prolonged beyond a half hour, recurs during 24 hours, or shows focal features including lateralized post-ictal weakness.

Table 17.2 Seizure frequency 5 years after temporal lobectomy. 24 consecutive children (aged < 16 years) operated upon by Adams in Oxford during 1983–1986

| | No.[1] | Side | | Age at operation (years) | | Preop. seizure frequency (seizures/year) | |
		Left	Right	Median	Range	Median	Range
Seizure free[2]							
off medication[3]	14	1	13	12	2–14	275	55–1000+
on medication	6	3	3	13	8–15	360	100–700
Occasional seizures (minor disability)	2	1	1	12	12–13	1000+	150–1000+
Frequent seizures (major disability)	2	2	0				

[1] Pathology: 10 indolent glioma, 9 Ammon's horn sclerosis and one less severe hippocampal sclerosis, 3 other alien tissue, one unspecified degenerative condition.
[2] Seizure Free = no seizures of any sort (including isolated auras) for at least 2 years at 5 years post-operative.
[3] The probability of becoming seizure-free off medication following right-side-operation is significantly higher than after left operation ($p < 0.01$, Fisher exact probability test).

useful when there is no calcification. Complex EEG investigation is not necessary once the diagnosis has been established beyond reasonable doubt by neuroimaging.

Age at operation

Both Davidson and Falconer (1975) and Rasmussen (1977) reported large series of temporal lobe excisions carried out on children aged 15 years or under. More recent reports of operations in childhood include those of Meyer *et al.* (1986), Drake *et al.* (1987), Hopkins and Klug (1991), and Adams *et al.* (1990). The pathology underlying the epilepsy in most of these children was either hippocampal sclerosis (MTS or AHS) or indolent glioma. The outcome in terms of seizure relief can be at least as good as that achieved in adults, and possibly better. The Oxford experience is that a large proportion of those operated upon in childhood remain seizure free post-operatively off all medication (Table 17.2). The post-operative cognitive and memory changes in children are similar to those seen in adults (Adams *et al.*, 1990). The social outcome, in terms of improved life quality, is probably best when the surgery is carried out during or before adolescence (Jensen, 1976; Jensen and Vaernet, 1977) so that the person can enter employment and permanent personal relationships without the encumberance of epilepsy.

Patients with intractable seizures of the sort characteristic of temporal lobe epilepsy who have unequivocal neuroimaging evidence of temporal lobe alien tissue, usually an indolent glioma, should undergo surgery as soon as the diagnosis is established. The Oxford experience is that the outcome from surgery is usually excellent in those aged less than 10 years, and children as young as 2 years have been operated upon very successfully. With those who have Ammon's horn sclerosis, there may be some grounds for waiting until the age of 12–14 years.

Side of operation

In general, right-sided operations are more successful than left-sided operations. Olivier (1988b) reported that 67% of patients who had a right temporal lobectomy including hippocampus became seizure free, or almost so, compared to 49% of those who had a similar, but slightly smaller, operation on the left. Table 17.2 shows that 94% of children having a right temporal lobectomy at the Radcliffe Infirmary are seizure-free 5 years later compared to 57% of those having left-sided operations, and the proportion who are off medication is considerably higher after right-sided operations.

Both children and adults run the risk that their verbal memory capacity will deteriorate after a left temporal lobe operation (Oxbury and Oxbury, 1989; Rausch, 1991; Adams *et al.*, 1990; Dodrill *et al.*, 1992), but the risk is lower for those with established left hippocampal pathology whose verbal memory is already poor. The extent of any verbal memory deterioration may correlate with the extent of the left medial temporal lobe excision (Katz *et al.*, 1989), although Ojemann and Dodrill (1985) argued that it depended more on the extent of the neocortical excision and the data of Milner (1967) suggested that it depended on both. The situation after right temporal lobectomy is less clear, but certainly those with well preserved non-verbal memory are at risk that it will deteriorate after an excision including normal, or relatively normal, hippocampus.

Type of operation

Temporal lobe excisions which spare the hippocampus are less likely to achieve freedom from seizures than those which include the anterior 1–3 cm of hippocampus. The proportion of patients in the series of Olivier (1988b) who became seizure-free, or virtually so, after temporal lobectomy including the hippocampus has been mentioned above. When the hippocampus was spared, only 60% of right-sided and 34% of left-sided operations achieved the same degree of success. The reason for sparing the hippocampus is usually concern that its inclusion in the excision will precipitate a serious deterioration of memory.

Wieser (1988) reported freedom from seizures, at a mean of 5 years after operation, in 61% of patients who underwent selective amygdalohippocampectomy and who did not have pre-operative evidence of pathology other than hippocampal sclerosis. This success rate is comparable to that of temporal lobectomy. The rationale for the operation is that the smaller excision is more sparing of cognitive and memory function. It has yet to be established whether the pre- *vs* post-operative memory changes are different, with patients matched for pathology, according to whether their operation was a selective amygdalohippocampectomy or a standard temporal lobectomy.

Unwanted effects of temporal lobe surgery

The main unwanted effects and their frequency of occurrence are listed in Table 17.3. Death is rare but must be considered as a potential risk of any brain operation. Persistent hemiparesis, and dysphasia if the operation is on the dominant hemisphere, may occur from infarction or haemorrhage as an operative complication but occasionally happens without any clear explanation. The liability to a symptomatic visual field defect increases with increasing excision size (Katz *et al.*, 1989).

Some patients feel that their memory improves post-operatively, especially if the epilepsy ceases and medication is withdrawn. Others, particularly those operated on when older than 25 years, comment that their memory is a little worse and this is

Table 17.3 Unwanted effects of temporal lobe excisions

Death	<0.5%
Visual field defect	
asymptomatic homonymous upper $\frac{1}{4}$	Common
symptomatic > upper $\frac{1}{4}$ defect	10–15%
Transient diplopia	Common
Persistent hemiparesis	1–2%
Persistent dysphasia	1%
Memory	
verbal memory impairment	
minor global memory decline	Common
severe amnesic syndrome	Rare
Behavioural	
personality change	
overt psychosis	1–2%
transient depression	Common
Wound infection	

particularly so if the epilepsy does not cease. Material specific memory deficits, for verbal material after left-sided excisions and non-verbal material after right-sided excisions, have been mentioned above (see also Rausch, 1991; Dodrill *et al.*, 1992). The severe global amnesic syndrome is much feared but fortunately rare. Much attention has been given to trying to define the pre-operative routine neuropsychological and carotid (and selective) amytal test criteria for concluding reliably that the contralateral hemisphere, which will remain unoperated, has adequate memory capabilities (Rausch, 1991). Nevertheless, uncertainties remain and considerable caution is necessary.

EXTRATEMPORAL EXCISIONS

Extratemporal cortical excisions are overall less successful than temporal lobe excisions at producing complete, or virtually complete, elimination of seizures.

Rasmussen (1989a) reported that only 26% of patients having frontal excisions became seizure-free, or virtually so, although another 30% had a markedly reduced seizure frequency. Analogous figures for parieto-occipital excisions were 34% and 23% (Rasmussen, 1989b). As with temporal lobe excisions, however, outcome from extratemporal excisions is considerably improved when the epilepsy is associated with definite structural pathology which can be completely excised (Awad *et al.*, 1991). Excision of pathology rather than of an electrical focus is the most important factor. Blume *et al.* (1991) reported 32% of patients becoming seizure-free, and another 42% having a significant reduction in seizure frequency, from posterior hemisphere excisions; most of the patients had definite structural pathology such as porencephaly or indolent glioma.

Clearly, the successful surgical treatment of epilepsy by extratemporal excision is heavily dependent upon defining structural pathology in a cortical area where excision can be effected without producing a permanent unacceptable neurological deficit.

HEMISPHERECTOMY

Hemispherectomy was introduced in the mid-1940s by Krynauw (1950) and proved very effective in giving seizure relief to children with severe epilepsy associated with an infantile hemiplegia. Unfortunately the operation had to be abandoned because up to one third of those operated developed morbidity/mortality from delayed haemorrhagic complications leading to obstructive hydrocephalus, superficial siderosis, and intracranial haematomata (Adams, 1983). Modified surgical techniques have, however, been introduced (Adams, 1983; Rasmussen, 1987) which allow the operation to be carried out very successfully without, at least as yet, producing serious late sequelae.

The main indications for hemispherectomy are: severe intractable epilepsy associated with the congenital hemiplegia syndrome or as part of the hemiconvulsions–hemiplegia–epilepsy syndrome of Gastaut; in Rasmussen's syndrome; and in Sturge–Weber syndrome. Hemispherectomy is predominantly an operation for children who already have a hemiplegia. Most of them, other than those in the early stages of Rasmussen's syndrome, are to some extent mentally retarded and many are severely retarded. Many also have a severe behaviour disturbance, often with aggression, which causes great disruption to the lives of their families. Hemispherectomy not only stops the epilepsy in 75–80%, it usually also produces a marked improvement of behaviour and some gain of cognitive ability. There is little change in the severity of the already established hemiparesis.

CALLOSOTOMY

The place of callosotomy in the treatment of epilepsy remains unestablished (Taylor, 1990). Very few patients are rendered seizure-free by the operation but drop attacks may be dramatically reduced in frequency and there may be a moderate reduction in the frequency of generalized tonic-clonic convulsions. Unwanted effects of the operation include: memory impairment, transient mutism, aphasia especially in children with atypical language dominance, and features of hemispheric disconnection including symptoms indicative of antagonism between the hemispheres. The unwanted effects are less likely to occur if the posterior callosum is spared or at least sectioned only as a second stage procedure.

References

Adams CBT (1983) Hemispherectomy – a modification. *J Neurol Neurosurg Psychiat*, **46**, 617–9

Adams CBT, Anslow P, Molyneux A, and Oxbury J (1987) Radiological detection of surgically treatable pathology, In Engel J, ed, *Surgical Treatment of the Epilepsies*, New York, Raven, 213–33

Adams CBT, Beardsworth ED, Oxbury SM, Oxbury JM, and Fenwick PBC (1990) Temporal lobectomy in 44 children: outcome and neuropsychological follow up, *J Epilepsy*, **3** (Suppl), 157–68

Aicardi J and Chevrie J-J (1976) Febrile convulsions: neurological sequelae and mental retardation, In Brazier MAB, Coceani F, eds, *Brain Dysfunction in Infantile Febrile Convulsions*, New York, Raven, 247–77

Awad IA, Katz A, Hahn JF, Kong AK, Ahl J, and Lüders H (1989) Extent of resection in temporal lobectomy for epilepsy—I. Interobserver analysis and correlation with seizure outcome, *Epilepsia*, **30**, 756–62

Awad IA, Rosenfeld J, Ahl J, Hahn JF, and Luders H (1991) Intractable epilepsy and structural lesions of the brain: mapping resection strategies, and seizure outcome, *Epilepsia*, **32**, 179–86

Babb TL, Brown WJ, Pretorius J, Davenport C, Lieb JP, and Crandall PH (1984) Temporal lobe volumetric cell densities in temporal lobe epilepsy, *Epilepsia*, **25**, 729–40

Berkovic SF, Andermann F, Olivier A, Ethier R, Melanson D, Robitaille Y, Kuzniecky R, Peters T, and Feindel W (1991) Hippocampal sclerosis in temporal lobe epilepsy demonstrated by magnetic resonance imaging, *Ann Neurol*, **29**, 175–82

Blume WT, Whiting SE, and Girvin JP (1991) Epilepsy surgery in the posterior cortex, *Ann Neurol*, **29**, 638–45

Bruton CJ (1988) *The Neuropathology of Temporal Lobe Epilepsy*. Maudsley Monographs 31, Oxford, Oxford University Press

Daumas-Duport C, Scheithauer BW, Chodkiewicz J-P, Laws ER, and Vedrenne C (1988) Dysembryoplastic neuroepithelial tumor: a surgically curable tumor of young patients with intractable partial seizures. Report of thirty-nine cases, *Neurosurgery*, **23**, 545–56

Davidson S and Falconer MA (1975) Outcome of surgery in 40 children with temporal-lobe epilepsy, *Lancet*, **i**, 1260–3

Dodrill CB, Hermann BP, Raush R, Chelune G, and Oxbury S (1992) Use of neuropsychological tests for assessing prognosis following surgery for epilepsy. Proceedings of Second Palm Desert International Conference on the Surgical Treatment of the Epilepsies. Palm Desert, California, 20–24 February 1992

Drake J, Hoffman HJ, Kobayashi J, Hwang P, and Becker LE (1987) Surgical management of children with temporal lobe epilepsy and mass lesions, *Neurosurgery*, **21**, 792–7

Duncan JS and Sagar HJ (1987) Characteristics, pathology and outcome after temporal lobectomy, *Neurology*, **37**, 405–9

Engel J (1987a) Outcome with respect to epileptic seizures, In Engel J, ed, *Surgical Treatment of the Epilepsies*, New York, Raven, 553–71

Engel J (1987b) New concepts of the epileptic focus, In Wieser HG, Speckmann E-J, Engel J, eds, *The Epileptic Focus*, London, John Libbey, 83–94

Estes ML, Morris HH, Lüders H, Dudley AW, Lesser RP, Dinner DS, Friedman D, Hahn JF, and Wyllie E (1989) Surgery for intractable epilepsy. Clinicopathologic correlates in 60 cases, *Cleve Clin J Med*, **55**, 441–7

Falconer MA (1953) Discussion on the surgery of temporal lobe epilepsy: surgical and pathological aspects, *Proc Roy Soc Med*, **46**, 971–5

Falconer MA (1971a) Genetic and related aetiological factors in temporal lobe epilepsy: a review, *Epilepsia*, **12**, 13–31

Falconer MA (1971b) Anterior temporal lobectomy for epilepsy, In Robb C, Smith R, eds, *Operative Surgery*, Vol 14. Neurosurgery, London, Butterworths, 142–9

Falconer MA (1972) Place of surgery of temporal lobe epilepsy during childhood, *Br Med J*, **2**, 631–5

Falconer MA, Serafetinides EA, and Corsellis JA (1964) Etiology and pathogenesis of temporal lobe epilepsy, *Arch Neurol*, **10**, 233–48

Feindel W (1989) Temporal lobectomy with amygdalectomy and small hippocampal resection: review of 100 cases. Paper given at Montreal Neurological Institute EEG Department 50th Anniversary (1939–1989) Meeting. Symposium on Presurgical Evaluation and Surgical Therapy. 26–27 January 1989

Fenwick P (1987) Epilepsy and psychiatric disorders, In Hopkins A, ed, *Epilepsy*, London, Chapman and Hall, 511–52

Fenwick P (1991) Psychiatric disorders in epilepsy, In Swash M, Oxbury J, eds, *Clinical Neurology*, Vol 1, Edinburgh, Churchill Livingstone, 255–76

Hopkins IJ and Klug GL (1991) Temporal lobectomy for the treatment of intractable complex partial seizures of temporal lobe origin in early childhood, *Dev Med Child Neurol*, **33**, 26–31

Jack CR, Nichols DA, Scharbrough FW, Marsh WR, and Petersen RC (1988) Selective posterior cerebral artery amytal test for evaluating memory function before surgery for temporal lobe seizure, *Neuroradiol*, **168**, 787–893

Jack CR, Sharbrough FW, Twomey CK, Cascino GD, Hirschorn KA, Marsh WR, Zinsmeister AR, and Scheithauer B (1990) Temporal lobe seizures: lateralisation with MR volume measurements of the hippocampal formation, *Radiol*, **175**, 423–9

Janota I and Polkey CE (1992) Cortical dysplasia in epilepsy – a study of material from surgical resections in intractable epilepsy, In Pedley TE, Meldrum BS, eds, *Recent Advances in Epilepsy 5*, Edinburgh, Churchill Livingstone, 37–49

Jensen I (1976) Temporal lobe epilepsy: social conditions and rehabilitation after surgery, *Acta Neurol Scand*, **54**, 22–44

Jensen I and Vaernet K (1977) Temporal lobe epilepsy: follow-up investigation of 74 temporal lobe resected patients, *Acta Neurochirurg*, **37**, 173–200

Krynauw RA (1950) Infantile hemiplegia treated by removing one cerebral hemisphere, *J Neurol Neurosurg Psych*, **13**, 243–67

Katz A, Awad IA, Kong AK, Chelune GJ, Naugle RI, Wyllie E, Beauchamp G, and Lüders H (1989) Extent of resection in temporal lobectomy for epilepsy – II. Memory changes and neurologic complications, *Epilepsia*, **30**, 763–71

Maldonado HM, Delgado-Escueta AV, Walsh GO, Swartz BE, and Rand RW (1988) Complex partial seizures of hippocampal and amygdalar origin, *Epilepsia*, **29**, 420–33

Margerison JH and Corsellis JAN (1966) Epilepsy and the temporal lobes. A clinical electroencephalographic and neuropathologic study of the brain in epilepsy, with particular reference to the temporal lobes, *Brain*, **89**, 499–530

Meyer FB, Marsh WR, Laws ER, and Sharbrough FW (1986) Temporal lobectomy in children with epilepsy, *J Neurosurg*, **64**, 371–6

Milner B (1967) Brain mechanisms suggested by studies of temporal lobes, In Darley FC, ed, *Brain Mechanisms Underlying Speech and Language*, New York, Grune and Stratton, 122–45

Morris HH, Kanner A, Lüders H, Murphy D, Dinner DS, Wyllie E, and Kotagel P (1989) Can sharp waves localised at the sphenoidal electrode accurately identify a mesio-temporal epileptogenic focus, *Epilepsia*, **30**, 532–9

Ojemann GA and Dodrill CB (1985) Verbal memory deficits after temporal lobectomy for epilepsy, *J Neurosurg*, **62**, 101–7

Olivier A (1987) Commentary: Cortical Resections, In Engel J, ed, *Surgical Treatment of the Epilepsies*, New York, Raven, 405–16

Olivier A (1988a) Surgery of Epilepsy: methods, *Acta Neurolog Scand*, **78** (suppl 117), 103–13

Olivier A (1988b) Risk and benefit in the surgery of epilepsy: complications and positive results on seizures tendency and intellectual function, *Acta Neurol Scand*, **78** (suppl 117), 114–21

Ounsted C, Lindsay J, and Norman R (1966) Biological Factors in Temporal Lobe Epilepsy. Clinics in Development Medicine No 22. London, The Spastics Society Medical Education and Information Unit in association with William Heinemann Medical Books Ltd

Oxbury JM and Adams CBT (1989) Neurosurgery for epilepsy, *Br J Hosp Med*, **41**, 372–7

Oxbury JM and Oxbury SM (1989) Neuropsychology: memory and hippocampal pathology, In Reynolds EH, Trimble MR, eds, *The Bridge Between Neurology and Psychiatry*, Edinburgh, Churchill Livingstone, 135–50

Penfield W, Mathieson G (1974) An autopsy and a discussion of the role of the hippocampus in experiential recall, *Arch Neurol*, **31**, 145–54

Polkey CE (1987) Anterior temporal lobectomy at the Maudsley Hospital, London, In Engel J, ed, *Surgical Treatment of the Epilepsies*, New York, Raven, 641–5

Rasmussen T (1974) Cortical excision for medically refractory focal epilepsy, In Harris P, Maudsley C, eds, *Epilepsy*, Edinburgh, Livingstone, 227–39

Rasmussen T (1975) Surgical treatment of patients with complex partial seizures, In Penry JK, Daly DD, eds, *Advances in Neurology 11*, New York, Raven, 415–42

Rasmussen T (1977) Surgical aspects, In Blaw ME, Rapin I, Kingsbourne M, eds, *Topics in Child Neurology*, Spectrum Publications, 143–57

Rasmussen TB (1983) Surgical treatment of complex partial seizures: results, lessons and problems, *Epilepsia*, **24** (suppl. 1), S65–S76

Rasmussen T (1987) Extratemporal cortical excisions and hemispherectomy, In Engel J, ed, *Surgical Treatment of the Epilepsies*, New York, Raven, 417–24

Rasmussen T (1989a) Tailoring of cortical excisions for frontal lobe epilepsy. Paper given at Montreal Neurological Institute EEG Department 50th Anniversary (1939–1989) Meeting. Symposium on Presurgical Evaluation and Surgical Therapy. 26–27 January 1989

Rasmussen T (1989b) Surgery for parietal and occipital seizures. Paper given at Montreal Neurological Institute EEG Department 50th Anniversary (1939–1989) Meeting. Symposium on Presurgical Evaluation and Surgical Therapy. 26–27 January 1989

Rausch R (1991) Effects of temporal lobe surgery on behavior, In Smith D, Treiman D, Trimble M, eds, *Advances in Neurology*, New York, Raven, 279–92

Robitaille Y (1987) Neuropathological findings in epileptic foci, In Wieser HG, Speckmann E-J, Engel J, eds, *The Epileptic Focus*, London, John Libbey, 95–112

Sagar HJ and Oxbury JM (1987) Hippocampal neuron loss in temporal lobe epilepsy: correlation with early childhood convulsions, *Ann Neurol*, **22**, 334–40

Scoville WB and Milner B (1957) Loss of recent memory after bilateral hippocampal lesions, *J Neurol Neurosurg Psych*, **20**, 11–21

Sellier N, Kalifa G, Lalande G, Demange P, Ponsot G, Dulac O, and Robain O (1987) Focal cortical dysplasia. A rare cause of epilepsy, *Ann Radiol*, **30**, 439–45

Spencer DD, Spencer SS, Mattson RH, Williamson PD, and Novelly RA (1984) Access to the posterior medial temporal lobe structures in the surgical treatment of temporal lobe epilepsy, *Neurosurg*, **15**, 667–71

Taylor D (1990) Collosal section for epilepsy and the avoidance of doing everything possible, *Developmental Medicine and Child Neurology*, **32**, 267–70

Van Buren JN (1987) Complications of surgical procedures in the diagnosis and treatment of epilepsy, In Engel J, ed, *Surgical Treatment of the Epilepsies*, New York, Raven, 465–75

Wieser HG (1986) Selective amygdalohippocampectomy: indications, investigative techniques and results, *Adv Tech Stand Neurosurg*, **13**, 39–133

Wieser HG (1987) The phenomenology of limbic seizures, In Wieser HG, Speckmann E-J, Engel J, eds, *The Epileptic Focus*, London, John Libbey, 113–36

Wieser HG (1988) Selective amygdalohippocampectomy for temporal lobe epilepsy, *Epilepsia*, **29** (suppl 2); S100–S113

Yasargil MG and Wieser HG (1987) Selective amygdalohippocampectomy at the University Hospital, Zurich, In Engel J, ed, *Surgical Treatment of the Epilepsies*, New York, Raven, 653–8

Yasargil MG, Teddy PJ, and Roth P (1985) Selective amygdalohippocampectomy. Operative anatomy and surgical technique, *Adv Tech Stand Neurosurg*, **12**, 93–123

18
Applications of molecular genetics to restorative neurology

Joseph B. Martin

Advances in the application of molecular genetic techniques to the clinical neurosciences have occurred at an astonishing pace over the past decade. Questions that once seemed unanswerable are now approachable with definitive strategies. The use of DNA probes that exhibit restriction fragment length polymorphisms (RFLPs) combined with linkage analysis in pedigrees affected with either autosomal dominant or recessive disorders has resulted in the chromosomal localization of the mutant gene in over 25 diseases (Gusella et al., 1984; Martin 1987, 1989) (Table 18.1). The actual gene defect has been identified in Duchenne muscular dystrophy, neurofibromatosis type 1, myotonic dystrophy and retinoblastoma. These developments offer exciting opportunities to define the precise pathogenesis of inherited diseases and develop rational treatments, which is a goal of restorative neurology. Selected aspects of these advances are reviewed in this chapter.

GENETIC LINKAGE ANALYSIS

Two types of DNA variations provide the molecular basis for RFLPs. Polymorphic heterozygous DNA segments cloned from anonymous regions, or those within or adjacent to individual genes, can serve as markers to study chromosomal localization of disease-causing genes (Gusella et al., 1984). Single base-pair changes on one chromosome provide the specificity of distinguishing segments of DNA cut by restriction enzymes and displayed according to size on Southern blots. Repeated sequences on DNA (unexpressed) can also serve as polymorphic markers (Caskey, 1987). The likelihood of a linkage between the probe and the disease gene is expressed quantitatively as a ratio of the probability of linkage, or logarithm of the odds (LOD score). By conventional criteria, a LOD score greater than three establishes linkage and a LOD score of two excludes linkage (Gusella et al., 1984).

The application of spaced markers at intervals of 10 centimorgans (10 cM) would require a total of about 300 probes (to cover 3×10^9 base pairs) (Martin, 1989). To date more than 95% of the human genome has been covered, although the saturation of probes is uneven. Current speculations suggest that a 1 cM linkage map may be within reach in the next five years. The possibility of constructing a physical map of

Table 18.1 Chromosomal localization and gene abnormalities in selected neurological diseases

Genetic classification and disease	Chromosome	Gene defect	Comments on genetic heterogeneity
Autosomal dominant			
Charcot-Marie-Tooth disease (type 1)	1q2	Unknown	Unknown
Huntington's disease	4p16.3	Unknown	None demonstrated in over 50 pedigrees
Spinocerebellar atrophy	6-centromere	Unknown	Unknown
Von Recklinghausen's neurofibromatosis (NFI)	17q-centromere	Known	None demonstrated in over 25 pedigrees
Familial amyloidotic polyneuropathy	18q11.2–q12.1	Single-bp substitution in mRNA for transthyretin	Allelic heterogeneity
Myotonic dystrophy	19-centromere	Known	None demonstrated
Familial Alzheimer's disease	21q21	Unknown (in rare cases, β-amyloid)	Possible heterogeneity
Bilateral acoustic neurofibromatosis (NFII)	22q	Unknown	Unknown
Autosomal recessive			
Gaucher's disease	1q21	Amino acid substitution in glucocerebrosidase	Allelic heterogeneity
Friedreich's ataxia	9p22-centromere	Unknown	None found in 23 pedigrees
Ataxia-telangiectasia	11q22–23	Unknown	None found in 31 families
Wilson's disease	13q14–21	Unknown (not ceruloplasmin)	Unknown
G_{M2}-gangliosidosis Tay–Sachs disease (type 1)	15q22–q25	Mutation in gene encoding α-chain of hexosaminidase	Allelic heterogeneity
Sandhoff disease (type 2)	5q13	Mutation in gene encoding β-chain of hexosaminidase	Allelic heterogeneity
X-linked recessive			
Duchenne dystrophy	Xp21.21	Absence of dystrophin	Multi-allelic heterogeneity
Becker dystrophy	Xp21.21	Defect in dystrophin	Multi-allelic heterogeneity
Pelizaeus–Merzbacher disease	Xq21–q22	Defect in myelin proteolipid protein	Unknown
Adrenoleukodystrophy	Xq27–q28	Unknown	Unknown

Table 18.1 — continued

Genetic classification and disease	Chromosome	Gene defect	Comments on genetic heterogeneity
Lesch–Nyhan syndrome	Xq27	HPRT deficiency, variations	Multi-allelic heterogeneity
Emery–Dreifuss dystrophy	Xq28	Unknown	Unknown
Recessive with germinal chromosomal defect			
Central neurofibromatosis	22q11–q13	Unknown	Unknown
Retinoblastoma	13q14	Known	Allelic heterogeneity
Meningioma	22q12.3–qter	Unknown	Unknown
Von Hippel–Lindau disease	3p	Unknown	Unknown
Mitochondrial diseases with maternal transmission			
Mitochondrial myopathy		Deletion in mitochondrial DNA	
Leber's hereditary optic atrophy		Amino acid substitution in NADH dehydrogenase, subunit 4	

From Martin JB (1989) *Trends Neurosci*, **12**, 130.

DNA clones spaced at 1 to 5 × 10^6 base pair intervals within the next five to ten years is currently being debated as part of the feasibility of the human genome project.

DUCHENNE MUSCULAR DYSTROPHY

The application of 'reverse genetics', which is going from a gene to discover the cellular protein for which it encodes, has been used successfully in Duchenne muscular dystrophy (DMD). DMD is an X-linked recessive degenerative disorder of skeletal and cardiac muscles that affects males and is transmitted usually by asymptomatic females (Davies *et al.*, 1983). It is the most common form of the childhood-onset dystrophies. Becker described a more benign X-linked myopathy compatible with survival to mid-life, which is now known to be caused by a mutation in the same gene that causes DMD.

Molecular genetics

The gene causing DMD was localized to the mid-region of the short arm of the X-chromosome by cytogenetic techniques taking advantage of translocations and other mutations that caused Duchenne-like illness in females (Engel, 1986). In females with translocation, the finding that in every case the Xp21 region of the X chromosome was disrupted gave the first definitive clue to the chromosomal site of the mutation. The identification of the gene involved in DMD was made possible by analysis of a male subject with DMD, mental retardation, retinitis pigmentosa, and chronic granulomatosis (Hoffman *et al.*, 1988; Brown and Hoffman, 1988). Cytogenetic analysis showed a deletion of the Xp21 region. Seven DNA fragments from this region analysed by subtraction hybridization identified multiple intragenic and extragenic probes with RFLPs in the region of Xp21. Kunkel and co-workers identified one cloned segment, pERT87, which was shown to be deleted in 5–10% of DMD patients (Kunkel *et al.*, 1985; Monaco and Kunkel, 1987). Subclones of pERT87 were used to initiate chromosome walking. Extensive cloning of the gene showed that it was comprised of over 70 exons spanning more than 2300 kb (Koenig *et al.*, 1987, 1988). The gene encodes a protein of 440 kd, named dystrophin. The biochemical structure of dystrophin has analogies with other cytoskeletal proteins, particularly the actinins and spectrins (Mandel, 1989; Hoffman and Kunkel, 1989). Dystrophin has three major domains. The amino-terminal region has close homology to the actin-binding domain of α-actinin. The middle portion of dystrophin is comprised of 24 repeats (containing approximately 109 amino acids each) that has some structural analogy to the smaller number of repeats found in certain spectrins and in α-actinin. The carboxy-terminal domain has no known similarity to any other protein sequence.

Biology of dystrophin

The cellular location of dystrophin, which may be a latticework of dimers arranged in an anti-parallel array (Koenig *et al.*, 1989), suggests a function either to stabilize the plasma membrane during muscular contraction, or to anchor the cytoskeleton to the membrane. Dystrophin is tightly bound to membrane glycoproteins. It seems likely that absence of dystrophin results in membrane disintegration with leakage of intracellular components (enzymes like creatine phosphokinase, CK) from the muscle cell.

Clinical applications

A molecular and genetic analysis of the numerous mutations affecting the dystrophin gene has provided fascinating examples to explain the differences in Duchenne and Becker phenotypes (Gutmann and Fischbeck, 1989). Early work with cDNA probes showed that approximately two-thirds of both Duchenne and Becker patients had deletions in the dystrophin gene. The size of the deletion did not correlate with clinical severity. In an extensive study of 370 patients, Hoffman *et al.* (1988) concluded that the concentration rather than the size of dystrophin determined the disease severity. Duchenne patients all lacked dystrophin, patients with the severe form of Becker dystrophy had 3–10% of normal levels, and those with more than 20% had mild symptoms. Analysis of the disruptions of encoding for the protein caused by genetic deletions suggested that in-frame deletions (where remaining unaffected codons occur in correct order) may result in altered dystrophin, which is partially functional resulting in a lesser clinical severity, whereas frame-shift deletions give rise to no detectable dystrophin and a severe phenotype (Hoffman *et al.*, 1989; Fenner, Koenig, and Kunkel, 1989). In a series of 258 separate deletions, Koenig *et al.* (1989) showed that clinical severity in 92% of cases could be accounted for by this reading-frame model. Deficiency of dystrophin also causes dystrophy in the mouse; strikingly, however, the murine phenotype is much less severe and extensive regeneration of muscle cells is demonstrated. Multiple intragenic and extragenic probes with RFLPs in the region of Xp21 now permit great improvements in the prenatal and carrier status assessment of patients.

Some patients formerly classified as limb-girdle dystrophy are now known to have Becker dystrophy. Norman and co-workers (1989) found that four of 15 patients (27%) with a diagnosis of limb-girdle dystrophy had deletions in the dystrophin gene. These workers conclude 'all male patients with progressive muscular dystrophy of limb-girdle pattern should be routinely screened with . . . cDNA probes as a useful adjunct to their clinical diagnosis'.

Dystrophin is also found in cardiac muscle and in brain. In the brain, it primarily appears in neurons without any particular regional propensity. Its functions in neurons is unknown.

Treatment

The possibilities of treatment of DMD with genetically engineered cells is now under intense experimental study. It is possible to introduce the gene into cultured myoblasts from dystrophic mice and to reintroduce the primitive muscle cell precursors into the animal by direct injection. Such muscle cells have been shown to survive *in vivo* and to differentiate into mature muscle cells. The experimental approach is clear and the possibility that similar treatments may be therapeutically beneficial in patients with DMD is under investigation. Such therapy, although intriguing to envision, is not without its problems such as immune rejection, and need for multiple (and possibly repeated) injections. In Becker patients, it may be possible to enhance dystrophin production by pharmacologic agents that turn on gene expression.

HUNTINGTON'S DISEASE

Molecular genetics

Progress in isolating the gene for Huntington's disease (HD) has been unexpectedly difficult. The original probe, G8 (D4S10) linked to HD (Gusella *et al.*, 1983; Martin, 1984) is located approximately 5×10^6 bp from the telomere on the short arm of chromosome-4. The HD gene is located between D4S10 and the telomere. The identification of additional DNA markers telomeric to D4S10 (D4S43—Gilliam *et al.*, 1987; D4S95—Hayden *et al.*, 1988; Wasmuth *et al.*, 1988; D4S90—Robbins *et al.*, 1989) has permitted extensive genetic mapping of the region. Most pedigree analyses looking for recombinations between markers and the HD gene indicate that the HD gene lies within 500 000 to 1 million bp of the telomere. The proposed physical order of probes on chromosome-4 is D4S10-D4S95-D4S90-HD-telomere. However, several linkage studies leave some doubt about this conclusion, suggesting that the gene is more proximal (between D4S10 and D4S90 for example—Theilmann *et al.*, 1989; Snell *et al.*, 1989).

Because extensive pedigree analysis has shown all HD families to be linked to D4S10, and because the mutation rate in HD is very low (some would say that no new mutations have ever been proven), it was generally considered that most (perhaps all) cases of HD arose from the same mutation. The data suggesting that some cases of HD are caused by a defect more proximal on 4p, raise the possibility of non-allelic heterogeneity, that more than one site in the outer one to two million bp of chromosome-4p may be causative.

Because HD is dominant and a single chromosome mutation is sufficient to cause the full phenotype, it will be necessary to sequence both normal and abnormal chromosomes (normal and affected). Lacking any cytogenetic clues, it may be necessary to sequence the entire region and it is not completely clear what to look for. At the outset, genes identified by structure (promoter regions, start sites, TATA boxes, etc.) will need to be examined one-by-one, both for tissue localization and putative functions, and for evidence of mutations. Fortunately, the daunting task lying ahead is being shared in a collaborative initiative involving a number of laboratories.

Genetic studies in homozygotes confirm that the HD mutation is dominant. Whether this will indicate a 'gain of function' pathogenetic mechanism to explain the selectivity of cell death remains to be shown (Martin, 1984; Martin and Gusella, 1986). The therapeutic potential for altering an inappropriate or excessive cellular function (which might be held in check if the normal gene were present) might be more amenable to pharmacologic manipulation than would be the case if gene replacement was required (see below, under Therapeutic Strategies).

Presymptomatic testing

Presymptomatic diagnosis of the presence of the HD mutation has now been initiated in several centers (Meissen *et al.*, 1988; Hayden *et al.*, 1988; Brandt *et al.*, 1989). The earliest studies of predictive testing used D4S10, which was limited by a 4–5% recombination rate. More recently, 99% accuracy has been obtained with D4S95 and other probes in families of sufficient size. However, one-third to one-half of pedigrees remain of insufficient size for linkage analysis (Meissen *et al.*, 1988). Until the gene itself is found, it is unlikely that these limitations will be overcome.

The ethical issues surrounding presymptomatic testing for a fatal disease that has no treatment have been extensively aired (Wexler *et al.*, 1985; Meissen *et al.*, 1988; Brandt *et al.*, 1989). Despite early concerns about reactions of the subject to a positive test, experience in several centers now shows that patients cope well, at least in a setting where adequate psychologic, genetic, and neurologic counseling is provided.

ALZHEIMER'S DISEASE

Molecular genetic studies have advanced on several fronts since earlier reviews of the subject (Martin, 1987, 1989). These advances will be considered under two areas of study.
1) Localizing the gene in familial Alzheimer's disease (AD).
2) Molecular/cellular biological studies of the amyloid precursor protein (APP).

Familial Alzheimer's disease

The original pedigree analysis of four families with early onset familial Alzheimer's disease (FAD) indicated linkage to chromosome-21q (St. George-Hyslop *et al.*, 1987). Subsequent studies by this group and others permit the following conclusions.
1) It is very likely in a subset of patients with FAD (usually with early age of onset), the disease is caused by an abnormality on chromosome-21 (Gusella, 1989). This site has been confirmed by Goate *et al.* (1989).

2) It is also likely that some pedigrees, the best studied being the Volga-German family (Schellenberg *et al.*, 1989), are not due to a defect on the same region of chromosome-21 implicated in earlier studies. Moreover, studies in patients with later age of onset (Robbins *et al.*, 1989) also failed to confirm linkage with probes on the proximal long arm of chromosome-21. These authors suggest that non-allelic genetic heterogeneity may be confounding the results. As pointed out by Gusella (1989), the final proof of non-allelic heterogeneity will require positive identification of a second location. Progress in locating the gene responsible for FAD is likely to be even slower than for HD. The chromosomal region suspect for the gene in FAD remains large, and family studies are limited by the small numbers of available surviving affected members to compare with non-affected members.

Amyloid precursor protein

The extraordinary development in our understanding of the biology of the amyloid precursor protein (APP) has provided a series of hypotheses concerning its role in the pathogenesis of AD. These may be summarized as follows.

1) The β (A_4) protein is a 4.2 kDa peptide that is deposited in both neuritic plaques and the walls of small cerebral vessels in AD. Although the normal cellular locus of APP is primarily neuronal, extracellular deposition of APP in AD occurs both in brain and in other tissues.

2) There is no over-expression of the APP gene transcripts in the brain in either sporadic AD or in FAD, although over-expression does occur in some cases of Down's syndrome.

3) There are at least three alternative mRNA transcripts produced by alternative splicing of RNA from a single gene in brain. There is no evidence for more than one gene for APP, which is located telomeric to the FAD-linked markers on chromosome-21 and separated from them by 8 to 15 $\times$ 10^6 bp. The full-length complementary DNA (cDNA) for the β-amyloid protein encodes a protein of amino 695 acids (APP_{695}). The alternative larger forms have 751 (APP_{751}) and 770 (APP_{770}) amino acids, respectively.

4) These larger forms of APP are of particular interest because they contain domains recognized by structure to be serine proteinase inhibitors of the Kunitz type. Recent comparisons of the APP structure with other known proteins show that the secreted form of APP contains an amino-terminal portion identical to protease nexin–2 (PN–2). PN–2 is known to inhibit chymotrypsin and trypsin and to also inhibit proteases associated with the growth factors, epidermal growth factors (EGF), and nerve growth factor (NGF).

5) Despite tantalizing hypotheses concerning the role of Kunitz-type protease inhibitors in the pathogenesis of APP deposition in brain or other tissues, it remains only that, a hypothesis. There is no direct convincing evidence for abnormal metabolism of APP in brain to establish whether its deposition is a primary or secondary factor in the pathogenesis of AD (Abraham and Potter, 1989).

6) The source of APP in brain and other tissues remains problematic. APP cannot be readily detected in blood. The possibility that it arises from non-neural tissues and reaches the brain via altered blood vessels (altered blood–brain barrier) has not been proven or excluded.

7) An alternative mRNA for APP is described, in which the 208 amino acids in the carboxyl-terminal region are deleted and replaced by 20 amino acids with homology

to the Alu repeat family. It is speculated that this represents a fourth form of APP (it lacks the transmembrane domain of APP).

8) The biological effects of the β-amyloid peptide or secreted form of APP have been studied with conflicting results. Both neurite promoting (Yankner *et al.*, 1988) and neurotoxic effects have been shown to occur (Yankner *et al.*, 1989). Further studies of these important biologic effects will be required to determine whether these responses are physiologic or pathologic, and whether APP deposition in brain contributes to neuronal destruction in AD.

DISEASES OF MITOCHONDRIA

Certain neurological syndromes have now been shown to be associated with abnormalities in mitochondrial DNA. Diseases caused by mitochondrial abnormalities are inherited by maternal transmission, because mitochondrial DNA is exclusively of maternal origin. Mitochondrial DNA is 16.5 kb in length and encodes for 13 proteins, all components of the mitochondrial respiratory chain and oxidative phosphorylation system (Harding, 1989).

Mitochondrial myopathies

These are a heterogeneous group of disorders characterized by proximal muscle weakness, external ophthalmoplegia, dementia, seizures, and cardiac conduction defects. These disorders have several eponyms and other descriptive names that include: progressive external ophthalmoplegia; Kearns–Sayre syndrome; mitochondrial encephalopathies with lactic acidosis and stroke (MELAS); and myoclonus epilepsy with ragged-red fibers (MERRF). All share to one degree or another abnormalities in muscle, grouped together by the term 'ragged-red fibers'. An exception to the latter is Leigh syndrome, which consists of encephalopathy in childhood, psychomotor regression, brainstem dysfunction, and optic atrophy, without ragged-red fibers. In an updated report, Holt and co-workers showed that 30 of 72 patients with mitochondrial myopathy had major deletions of a variable portion of muscle mitochondrial DNA (Holt *et al.*, 1989). Each of the 30 patients with DNA deletions presented with progressive external ophthalmoplegia and limb weakness, and 8 had the additional features of the Kearns–Sayre syndrome (ophthalmoplegia plus pigmentary retinopathy, complete heart block, and cerebellar syndrome). Moraes and co-workers examined another series of 123 patients and found that 32 showed mitochondrial DNA deletions (Moraes *et al.*, 1989). Deletions ranged from 1.3 to 7.6 kb in size and were mapped to different sites in the mitochondrial DNA (mtDNA). Biochemical analysis showed decreased activities in several mitochondrial respiratory chain enzymes (NADH dehydrogenase, succinate-cytochrome c reductase, and cytochrome c oxidase). The molecular definition of the deletions in terms of actual base pair and protein mutation remains to be defined.

Leber's hereditary optic atrophy

This condition is a maternally transmitted form of optic nerve degeneration. It is now known to be the result of a single base error in the coding sequence for NADH dehydrogenase, subunit 4. This mutation correlated precisely with the clinical defect in nine of 11 pedigrees (Wallace *et al.*, 1988; Parker *et al.*, 1989; Singh, Lott, and

Wallace, 1989). Two pedigrees were discordant, however, suggesting the possibility of heterogeneity at the site of mutation.

SCRAPIE, PRIONS, CREUTZFELDT–JAKOB DISEASE, AND GERSTMANN-STRÄUSSLER DISORDER

A particularly informative example of the extraordinary power of molecular genetics is illustrated by the advances of Prusiner and colleagues in tracing the 'infectious' etiology of this group of diseases (Prusiner, 1982, 1989).

Scrapie, a disease of sheep, can be transmitted to hamsters and mice by intracerebral inoculation of brain tissue. The agents responsible, termed 'prions' for 'proteinaceous infectious particles, which resist inactivation by procedures that modify nucleic acids' (Prusiner, 1982), have since been shown to be transmissible pathogens that cause several degenerative diseases of the CNS in humans and animals. These diseases include, in humans, kuru, Creutzfeldt–Jakob disease (CJD), and Gerstmann-Sträussler syndrome (GSS). Several animal diseases reviewed by Prusiner are also prion-related (Prusiner, 1989). Although the precise form of the 'infective' material has not been defined in these disorders, there is now overwhelming evidence to support the hypothesis that a gene that regulates prion protein synthesis and regulation is involved in these disorders. These disorders are discussed in detail by Prusiner (1989).

Prion protein

Prion protein (PrP) has a molecular weight of 27–30 kd and is the product of a single gene located on chromosome-20. PrPs^c is believed to be an altered form of the normal cellular PrP (termed PrP^c) that gains capacity for infectivity by a post-translational modification, which has yet to be identified.

GSS and familial CJD are remarkable diseases in being both genetic and infectious. Recent studies in autosomal dominant GSS have shown that a single base pair change in codon 102 of the PrP gene (resulting in a mutation of Pro→Leu) is genetically linked to the disease (LOD score now greater than 7—Prusiner, personal communication). Additional studies in other pedigrees with GSS or familial CJD show that other mutations in PrP (codon 117: Met→Val; codon 200: Q→K) are also linked to the clinical disorder. Mutations have also been identified in some cases of sporadic CJD. These observations are compelling evidence that an alteration in the functions of PrP^c induced by a mutation is the cause of the disease.

These conclusions are supported by elegant concurrent studies in animals with scrapie-infected disorders. These can be summarized as follows. Host genetic control of scrapie incubation time can be modified by introduction of the foreign (susceptible) gene into a non-susceptible host. Two genes have been been identified that influence prion incubation periods in mice, Pid-1 and Prn-i. Pid-1 is located within the D subregion of the major histocompatibility complex (Prusiner, 1989). Prn-i is linked to the gene encoding PrP and influences incubation times by its interaction with the PrP gene. Transgenic mice (normally resistant to scrapie) bearing the syrian hamster (susceptible) PrP gene all expressed the hamster PrP gene in brain. Transgenic mice with the hamster PrP gene developed scrapie infection in about 75 days compared to non-transgenic control mice who failed to develop disease after more than 500 days (Scott *et al.*, 1989).

These observations provide the strongest evidence yet presented that the PrP gene alone is capable of both making the mouse susceptible, and of generating the full clinical and neuropathologic spectrum of scrapie. The remaining issue is to determine what structural change occurs in PrP^c to make it capable of producing disease, an event clearly related to PrP^{sc}. Studies of the structural relationships between PrP^c and PrP^{sc} show that the latter differ in sensitivity to proteinase k digestion and in solubility after detergent extraction (Oesch *et al.*, 1985; Meyer *et al.*, 1986).

The differences in PrP^c and PrP^{sc} are not caused by alternative mRNA splicing because a single exon contains the entire open reading frame of PrP. A number of post-translational modifications in PrP to form PrP^c and PrP^{sc} have been elucidated, but the precise changes that distinguish the two isoforms (and thereby might account for differences in pathogenicity) remain to be established.

In summary, the examples of disease mechanisms represented by this category of diseases illustrate the powerful utility of molecular biology, including clinical studies of linkage analysis, to push back the frontiers of knowledge.

HUMAN GENE THERAPY

It is apparent that scientific advances hold great promise for elucidating the biochemical basis of many of the devastating neurological diseases. What are the possibilities for definitive treatment, particularly for the genetic diseases, including gene therapy?

The topic has recently been lucidly reviewed by Friedmann (1989) and a portion of the following conclusions come from his analysis. The term 'gene therapy' includes several strategies, gene replacement, gene correction, and gene augmentation, progressing from the most technically difficult (and distant in applicability) to the most promising.

Gene replacement

The attractiveness of this approach is obvious; locate the defective (mutant) gene, remove it, thereby negating its adverse effects, and replace it with the correct (wild-type) gene. Unfortunately, this has never been accomplished, even in simpler organisms or species (*Escherichia coli*, nematodes, yeast, or mice), and the likelihood that it can be achieved in humans is small. As Friedmann states, 'There is little or no conceptual groundwork to suggest how that might be accomplished'.

Gene correction

The possibility of introducing genetic material (DNA specifically) into the right location to correct a gene dysfunction seemed equally unlikely, even two or three years ago. Now experimental studies have shown the feasibility of 'homologous recombination', in which targeted sequences can be introduced into cells and can take over the functions of the targeted genes. The eventual key to the success of this approach will be site-specific recombination. At the present time, DNA introduced by several conventional gene transfer methods, calcium phosphate-mediated transfection, electroporation, or direct microinjection, has been shown in several mammalian systems to function, as determined by expression of the encoded mRNA and protein.

In primitive cells, such as embryonal stem cells, DNA can be incorporated into the genome in a manner capable of replication with subsequent cell division.

The ethical implications of such an approach are profound. It is clear that the earlier the fertilized embryo is obtained, the more likely such an approach would be to correct the defect in a sufficient number of lineage cells to make the therapy effective. Such manipulations are unlikely to be acceptable in the treatment of human diseases in the foreseeable future.

Gene augmentation

The most promising therapeutic strategies for CNS disorders involve the introduction of gene sequences into cells *in vitro* and the replacement of those cells into the host to augment or enhance a deficient function. The first experiments involving correction of genetic defects in mammals were achieved in 'transgenic' mice. The success of this approach is illustrated by the hpg mouse, which is infertile as a result of an autosomal recessive mutation (deletion) in the gene that encodes for gonadotropin releasing hormone (GnRH, also called luteinizing hormone releasing hormone or LHRH). This autosomal recessive disorder was successfully corrected by introducing the complete gene sequence for GnRH, together with an appropriate promoter sequence, directly into the fertilized zygote, which had been removed from the pregnant female mouse. The 'transgenic' zygote was then reintroduced into the uterus. The developing embryo incorporated the transgene into its cells and, in a demonstration nothing short of miraculous, the adult transgenic mouse was shown to produce GnRH in appropriate cells in the hypothalamus, and to be fertile. The significance of this result is emphasized by the fact that despite 'random' insertion of the GnRH gene into genomic sites distant from the normal location of the gene, the transgene was expressed; that is, the protein GnRH was synthesized and released, and even more remarkably GnRH production occurred in the 'right' cells.

However, such dramatic genetic corrections are not acceptable forms of therapy for human diseases. What then can be done? There are other potentially useful alternatives in selected circumstances. The first is to remove autologous cells (fibroblasts or astroglia), introduce the gene required for the desired therapeutic effect, and reintroduce the genetically engineered cell back into the host. An example that is currently under study is the introduction of the NGF gene into fibroblasts. The modified cells are then introduced into the CNS to examine their ability to enhance survivability of cholinergic neurons that are known to be NGF dependent (or responsive). This approach will receive extensive investigation in the future for replacement of dopamine in experimental models of Parkinson's disease, of NGF in animals with cholinergic deficits—models of Alzheimer's disease, and perhaps for multiple neurotransmitter replacements in animal models of Huntington's disease.

A second approach to gene correction is the use of vectors to introduce genes into cells *in vivo*. This approach has used retroviral vectors successfully to introduce DNA into dividing cells (Geller and Breakefield, 1988). More problematic are neurons, which are in a post-mitotic state. In this case, herpes viruses have been advocated as potential vectors. Despite success *in vitro*, it remains to be shown that such an approach can be used safely and efficiently *in vivo*.

It would be a misrepresentation of the current studies in the field of molecular genetics, with implications for neurology, to not mention a note of concern about the future of this endeavor. The scientific techniques of locating genes, isolating their cellular products, and detecting the cellular biology of mutated genes (e.g. Duchenne dystrophy and cystic fibrosis) are rapidly outstripping the resources available to take advantage of them. There is at the moment more work to do than the people power or financial support available. Science has made discoveries feasible, which are likely to be missed because of these 'shortages'. It will be a challenge in the years ahead to address how best to proceed in taking maximum advantage of the potential discoveries available. Although advances in molecular engineering have not yet been shown to cure a genetic disease, they hold promise of elucidating the mechanisms of disease and of offering a rationale for approaching therapy.

References

Abraham CR and Potter H (1989) Alzheimer's disease: Recent advantages in understanding the brain amyloid deposits, *Biotechnology*, **7**, 147

Brandt J, Quaid KA, Folstein SA *et al.* (1989) Presymptomatic diagnosis of delayed-onset disease with linked DNA markers, *JAMA*, **261**, 3108

Brown RH and Hoffman EP (1988) Molecular biology of Duchenne muscular dystrophy, *Trends Neurosci*, **11**, 480

Caskey CT (1987) Disease diagnosis by recombinant DNA methods, *Science*, **236**, 1223

Davies KE *et al.* (1983) Nucleic acids, *Res*, **11**, 2303

Engel AC (1986) Duchenne Dystrophy, In Engel AG and Banker BD, eds, *Myology*, New York, McGraw-Hill, 1185

Fenner CA, Koenig M, and Kunkel LM (1989) Alternative splicing of human dystrophin mRNA generates isoforms at the carboxy terminus, *Nature*, **338**, 509

Friedmann T (1989) Progress toward human gene therapy, *Science*, **244**, 1275

Hayden MR, Robbins C, Allard D *et al.* (1988) Improved predictive testing for Huntington's disease by using three linked DNA markers, *Am J Hum Genet*, **43**, 689

Hoffman EP, Fischbeck KH, Brown RH *et al.* (1988) Characterization of dystrophin in muscle-biopsy specimens from patients with Duchenne or Becker muscular dystrophy, *N Engl J Med*, **318**, 1363

Hoffman EP and Kunkel LM (1989) Dystrophin abnormalities in Duchenne/Becker muscular dystrophy, *Neuron*, **2**, 1019

Hoffman EP, Kunkel LM, Angelini C *et al.* (1989) Improved diagnosis of Becker muscular dystrophy by dystrophin testing, *Neurology*, **39**, 1011

Holt IJ, Harding AE, Cooper JM *et al.* (1989) Mitochondrial myopathies: clinical and biochemical features of 30 patients with major deletions of muscle mitochondrial DNA, *Ann Neurol*, **26**, 699

Koenig M, Hoffman EP, Bertelson CJ *et al.* (1987) Complete cloning of the Duchenne muscular dystrophy (DMD) cDNA and preliminary genomic organisation of the DMD gene in normal and affected individuals, *Cell*, **52**, 509

Koenig M, Monaco AP, and Kunkel LM (1988) The complete sequence of dystrophin predicts a rod-shaped cytoskeletal protein, *Cell*, **53**, 219

Koenig M, Beggs AH, Moyer M *et al.* (1989) The molecular basis for Duchenne versus Becker muscular dystrophy: Correlation of severity with type of deletion, *Am J Hum Genet*, **45**, 498

Kunkel LM, Monaco AP, Middlesworth W *et al.* (1985) Specific cloning of DNA fragments absent from the DNA of a male patient with an X chromosome deletion, *Proc Natl Acad Sci USA*, **82**, 4778

Mandel JL (1989) News and Views: Dystrophin: the gene and its product, *Nature*, **339**, 584

Martin JB (1984) Huntington's disease: New approaches to an old problem, *Neurology*, **34**, 1059

Martin JB (1987) Molecular genetics: Applications to the clinical neurosciences, *Science*, **238**, 765

Martin JB (1989) Molecular genetic studies in the neuropsychiatric disorders, *Trends Neurosci*, **12**, 130

Martin JB and Gusella JF (1986) Huntington's disease, pathogenesis and management, *N Engl J Med*, **315**, 1267

Meissen GH, Meyers RH, Mastromauro CA *et al.* (1988) Predictive testing for Huntington's disease with use of a linked DNA marker, *N Engl J Med*, **318**, 535

Meyer RK, McKinley MP, Bowman KA *et al.* (1986) Separation and properties of cellular and scrapie prion proteins, *Proc Natl Acad Sci USA*, **83**, 2310

Monaco AP and Kunkel LM (1987) A giant locus for the Duchenne and Becker muscular dystrophy gene, *Trends Genet*, **3**, 33

Moraes CT, DiMauro S, Zeviani M *et al.* (1989) Mitochondrial DNA deletions in progressive external ophthalmoplegia and Kearns-Sayre syndrome, *N Engl J Med*, **320**, 1293

Norman AJ, Coakley J, Thomas N *et al.* (1989) Distinction of Becker from limb-girdle muscular dystrophy by means of dystrophin cDNA probes, *Lancet*, **1**, 466

Oesch B, Westaway D, Walchi M *et al.* (1985) A cellular gene encodes scrapie PrP 27-30 protein, *Cell*, **40**, 735

Parker WD, Oley CA, and Parks JK (1989) A defect in mitochondrial electron transport activity (NADH – coenzyme Q oxidoreductase) in Leber's hereditary optic neuropathy, *N Engl J Med*, **320**, 1331

Prusiner SB (1982) Novel proteinaceous infectious particles cause scrapie, *Science*, **216**, 36

Prusiner SB (1989) Scrapie prions, *Annu Rev Microbiol*, **43**, 345

Robbins C, Theilmann J, Youngman S *et al.* (1989) Evidence from family studies that the gene causing Huntington disease is telomeric to D4S95 and D4S90, *Am J Hum Genet*, **44**, 422

Schellenberg GD (1988) Absence of linkage of chromosomes 21q21 markers to familial Alzheimer's disease, *Science*, **241**, 1507

Scott M, Foster D, Mirenda C *et al.* (1989) Transgenic mice expressing hamster prion protein produce species-specific scrapie infectivity and amyloid plaques, *Cell*, **59**, 847

Singh G, Lott MT, and Wallace DC (1989) A mitochondrial DNA mutation as a cause of Leber's hereditary optic neuropathy, *N Engl J Med*, **320**, 1300

Snell RG *et al.* (1989) Linkage disequilibrium in Huntington's disease as improved localization for the gene, *J Med Genet*, **26**, 673

St. George-Hyslop PH, Tanzi RE, Polinsky RJ *et al.* (1987) The genetic defect causing familial Alzheimer's disease maps on chromosome 21, *Science*, **235**, 885

Theilmann J, Kanani S, Shiang R *et al.* (1989) Non-random association between alleles detected at D4S95 and D4S98 and the Huntington's disease gene, *J Med Genet*, **26**, 676

Vance JM, Pericak-Vance MA, Yamatha LH *et al.* (1989) Genetic linkage mapping of chromosome 17 markers and neurofibromatosis type I, *Am J Hum Genet*, **44**, 25

Wallace DC, Singh G, Lott MT *et al.* (1988) Mitochondrial DNA mutation associated with Leber's hereditary optic neuropathy, *Science*, **242**, 1427

Wasmuth JJ, Hewitt J, Smith D *et al.* (1988) A polymorphic DNA marker tightly linked to the Huntington disease gene, *Nature*, **332**, 734

Wexler NS, Conneally PM, Housman D *et al.* (1985) A DNA polymorphism for Huntington's disease marks the future, *Arch Neurol*, **42**, 20

Yankner BA, Dawes LR, Fisher S *et al.* (1989) Neurotoxicity of a fragment of the amyloid precursor associated with Alzheimer's disease, *Science*, **245**, 417

19

An approach to the genetic correction of defects and disorders of the central nervous system

T. Friedmann and Fred H. Gage

The development of the concepts and tools of molecular biology are revolutionizing approaches to the understanding, detection, and treatment of many kinds of human disease. Since Mendel's discovery of genetic mechanisms in the mid-19th century and the first scientific application of these principles by Sir Archibald Garrod to human illnesses at the beginning of this century, it has become possible to understand the mechanisms by which much of human disease reflects errors in our genetic material. Rapidly, we are identifying important genetic components in many diseases that most investigators would not previously have labeled 'genetic' in origin. Many of these disorders represent major illnesses of our society, including cardiovascular diseases such as coronary artery disease and atherosclerosis, most forms of human cancer, susceptibility to infections, auto-immune and degenerative diseases, and others. The major immediate effect of emerging molecular techniques has been in understanding mechanisms of pathogenesis, and in permitting more accurate and rapid diagnosis and detection of disease. Among the most stunning of all advances have been the emerging concepts of the biochemical and genetic components of normal and abnormal functions of neurological systems. However, advances in our understanding of the biochemistry of brain function and the very earliest beginnings of molecular genetic description of the CNS suggest that an understanding of some human CNS disorders may no longer be out of reach.

GENE THERAPY

The level of understanding of pathogenesis has led not only to improved detection and diagnosis, but also to a conceptually new approach to treatment of some kinds of genetic diseases, which is the concept of gene therapy. For the first time, it has become possible to imagine treating disease by restoring precisely the function that is defective, the mutant gene, to achieve a definitive correction of a disease phenotype. The concept underlying most current approaches to gene therapy relies on having available techniques to purify disease-related genes and then to deliver them in a functional, stable, and non-injurious way to genetically defective cells. The result of restored gene expression in such cells is to complement their genetic defect and correct the resulting disease phenotype. Both of these requirements are already being satisfied by rapidly improving methods of gene isolation and transfer. Methods of molecular genetics have made it possible, at least in principle, to isolate and purify the genes involved in the development of genetic disorders, whether or not the biochemical or metabolic nature of the disease is understood. The recent success in cloning the gene responsible for cystic fibrosis (Riordan *et al.*, 1989) is the first of what will certainly be a long list of genes isolated by 'reverse genetics', that is, without having any prior information of the biochemical nature of the disorder or any understanding of the function of the responsible gene or of its product. Progress in identifying some of the genes that specify quantitative traits has lent encouragement to the notion that even disorders resulting from complicated multigenic interactions will become amenable to molecular description (Paterson *et al.*, 1988).

Together with the techniques for efficient gene cloning have come efficient methods for transferring genes into human and other mammalian cells in a way that does not damage the cells but allows for long-term expression of the foreign gene (transgene). Particularly useful have been the viral vectors able to carry foreign genes into a very wide variety of target cells, to integrate their foreign genes into the genomes of the infected cells, and to have those foreign genes expressed stably and heritably in the cell and its progeny. A number of different viruses have been used for this purpose, but the most useful and versatile have been the vectors developed from murine and avian retroviruses (Temin, 1986). A large number of genes have been transferred safely and stably into mammalian cells with such vectors, and in a number of cases it has been shown that the newly expressed gene is able to complement a genetic defect in the cells and even to correct physiological consequences of the genetic deficiency, at least *in vitro*. Virus-mediated techniques of gene transfer have already been accepted for use in the relatively near future to correct genetic defects *in vivo* (Friedmann, 1989). There are many potential target diseases for these kinds of manipulation, including disorders of the hematopoietic system, forms of cancer, and systemic disorders resulting from metabolic enzymic deficiencies (inborn errors of metabolism). As important as many of these disease models have been for establishing concepts, it is now obvious that defects and diseases, even of the human central nervous system, offer some of the most attractive model disorders for early clinical intervention.

A GENETIC APPROACH TO THE CENTRAL NERVOUS SYSTEM

We have been developing approaches to CNS disorders that utilize genetic tools to replace functions that are defective as a result of genetic, degenerative, mechanical, or other causes. A genetic attack on CNS disease can be based on the presumption that gene products required for normal neurological function, such as neurotransmitters, trophic and tropic factors, and others, might be provided to a diseased or damaged CNS as a transgene, which can be introduced either directly into the CNS or, alternatively, in the form of a graft of cells expressing the desired new function. While it is very attractive to envision gene delivery directly to the CNS by means of a CNS-targeted vector, much less progress has been made with that approach than delivery into the CNS of a graft of genetically modified cells.

Several years ago, we proposed a conceptual scheme (Fig. 19.1) in which genetically modified cells grafted to the defective CNS were envisioned to correct abnormal CNS

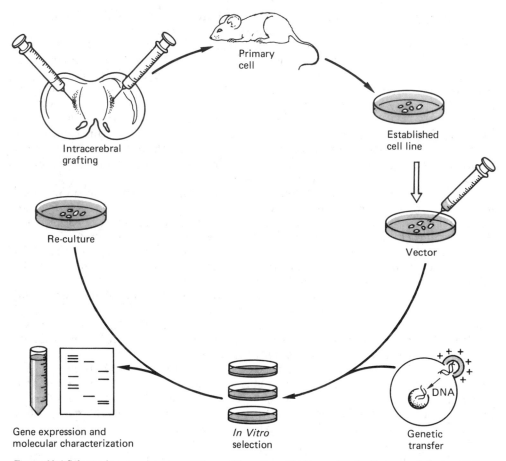

Figure 19.1 Schematic representation of the grafting of genetically modified cells into a defective CNS.

functions (Gage *et al.*, 1987). We have been able to present structural and functional evidence in several animal models that aberrant CNS functions can indeed be ameliorated by such manipulations. These studies have indicated that a genetic approach to the treatment of disease need not be restricted to classical genetic diseases. It may also be applicable to restore the function of CNS gene or metabolic products that become deficient because of pathological cell degeneration.

CHOLINERGIC NEURONS

While the precise role, if any, of nerve growth factor (NGF) in the pathogenesis of the degenerative human disorder Alzheimer's disease is not clear, many workers have suggested that at least some of the cognitive and memory deficits may result from the degeneration, death, or dysfunction of cholinergic neurons in the medial septum. Because these cells require a constant supply of the trophic factor NGF for their survival, it has been considered possible that restoration or augmentation of NGF supply to the diseased cholinergic neurons in patients with Alzheimer's disease may have beneficial clinical results (Hefti, 1983). Clinical studies are currently being designed to test the effectiveness of chronic infusions of NGF into patients. While most cases of Alzheimer's disease seem not to be genetic in etiology, a small subset of cases probably do result from the action of major genetic components (St. George-Hyslop *et al.*, 1987).

An animal model for the degeneration of cholinergic neurons that occurs in Alzheimer's disease is available in the rat. Degeneration of the cholinergic cells of the medial septum, analogous to those that degenerate in the human disease, can be induced through transection of the fimbria fornix, thereby interrupting the supply of NGF from the hippocampus. Under these conditions, the cells degenerate and die. Work in one of our laboratories and also by others has established that chronic infusion of NGF into fimbria fornix lesions prevents the degeneration of the cells (Williams *et al.*, 1986). Because of that knowledge, we anticipated that delivery of NGF to the lesion in the form of a cellular factory, consisting of a graft of rat fibroblasts genetically modified to produce and secrete NGF, might be equally effective.

For a number of technical reasons, we chose to use established lines of rat fibroblasts for our early grafting studies. Of course, it is obvious that the important and interdependent issues of graft survival, tumorigenicity, and continued transgene expression are related to the choice of cells for grafting (donor cells). The many factors contributing to these parameters must therefore all be understood before the most appropriate donor cells can be identified for each potential application. Nevertheless, we infected rat fibroblasts with a retroviral vector encoding and expressing a full length cDNA for mouse βNGF. Of the many infected cells, clones were chosen that expressed and secreted maximal amounts of NGF. Those cells were then grafted as a suspension into the lesion cavity of animals with fresh fimbria fornix lesions. The ability of the grafts to protect the cholinergic cells from degeneration was determined by staining sections of the medial septum for choline acetyl transferase to detect cholinergic cells.

Grafts containing cells that had not been infected with the NGF vector were ineffective in protecting the cholinergic neurons from degeneration. Less than 50% of the cells had survived, and many of those were pyknotic and otherwise morphologically abnormal. On the other hand, in animals that had received grafts of cells expressing and secreting NGF, the number and size of cholinergic neurons was similar to those found on the control, un-operated side of the brain, indicating a persistent trophic influence of NGF produced by the grafted cells. Furthermore, the grafts also induced a strong axonal sprouting response toward the functional grafts, indicating a tropic response to cells producing NGF.

Other animal models of cholinergic dysfunction and cognitive decline with aging that respond to chronic NGF will now be suitable for extending these observations. In particular we have shown that aged rats display a memory deficit that can be ameliorated by chronic NGF infusions into the lateral ventricle. The requirements of the infusion pumps and the relative instability of NGF suggest that the implantation of cells secreting NGF near the degenerating cholinergic neurons may be an ideal approach for long-term stable delivery of NGF. Furthermore, we have shown that chronic NGF is also effective in the non-human primate. This model will allow for further test of somatic cell therapy because it relates to the degenerating cholinergic neurons in Alzheimer's disease.

DOPAMINERGIC PATHWAYS

Parkinson's disease in the human results from degeneration of a specific set of neurons of the nigrostriatal pathway, a pathway whose integrity is required, among other things, for balanced voluntary muscle control. As in the case of Alzheimer's disease, the proximate cause of the cellular degeneration is not known, but in the vast majority of cases, genetic components have not been convincingly demonstrated. The symptoms of this disorder can be explained by a deficiency of the neurotransmitter, dopamine, the precursor for which, dopa, is synthesized from tyrosine through the action of the pterin-dependent enzyme, tyrosine hydroxylase (TH). Amino acid decarboxylase converts dopa to dopamine.

Systemic treatment with L-dopa can have striking, but often transient, effects on symptoms in some patients. It might be inferred from this empirical therapy that more precise regional and targeted delivery of dopamine or its precursor to the damaged caudate of a patient with Parkinson's disease might have more specific ameliorative effects without as many of the toxic side-effects that result from interference with normal CNS function caused by global delivery of the drug to the entire brain. One might imagine accomplishing this by introducing into the diseased caudate a graft of donor cells capable of synthesizing and secreting dopamine, or even L-dopa, into the extracellular space. Once secreted by the cell, the L-dopa could be decarboxylated by existing extracellular amino acid decarboxylase and converted to dopamine.

Such an approach has recently been taken in several neurosurgical centers. It has been shown that grafts of dopamine-rich human fetal substantia nigra may have dramatic ameliorative effects in patients with Parkinson's disease (Lindvall *et al.*, 1989). Earlier studies showing dramatic clinical improvement from grafting the patient's own adrenal medulla into the diseased caudate have not been substantiated by more recent studies. While the use of human fetal tissues may be clinically helpful in some instances, there are significant ethical and public policy difficulties associated with the need to harvest human fetal tissue following spontaneous and even elective abortions, and from anencephalic or otherwise non-viable newborns. In the current climate, with the debate on the question of abortion itself, it is unlikely that this therapeutic approach, as effective as it might be, will receive widespread public policy acceptance. It might be preferable, if possible, to design an autologous transplantation approach in which some readily accessible cells from the patient are modified genetically to produce dopa and then are grafted into the patient's brain.

To determine the feasibility of this approach, we have examined the effect of cell grafting in rats with unilateral destruction of the nigrostriatal pathway by the dopamine-analogue, 6-hydroxydopamine. Animals with unilateral lesions become susceptible to rotational behavior induced by a number of drugs, including apomorphine and amphetamine. The number of rotations, measured precisely in activity chambers, serves as a measure of the neurotransmitter dysfunction in those animals.

As in the case of the cholinergic neuronal degeneration discussed earlier, we have infected established or primary rat fibroblasts with a retroviral vector, in this case one expressing the cDNA for rat tyrosine hydroxylase. Infected cells express tyrosine hydroxylase enzyme activity and, in the presence of the pterin cofactor, synthesize and secrete dopa. These cells were grafted into the chemically-lesioned caudate in animals showing marked rotational activity. In animals with grafts successfully positioned in the more rostral portions of the caudate, the number of rotations was significantly reduced in animals grafted with TH-expressing cells but not in control animals (Wolff *et al.*, 1989).

APPLICATION TO HUMAN DISEASE

To demonstrate the feasibility of these kinds of combined genetic and grafting approaches for the therapy of human CNS disease, it is necessary to understand a number of features of the gene transfer and grafting technologies that are not yet fully characterized. Possibly the most important is the need to understand the pathophysiology of a disease sufficiently well to ensure that the replacement of a particular gene product or a metabolic product will in fact elicit an ameliorative effect for the patient. However, as in the case of the Parkinson's disease studies above, it may not be necessary always to understand the etiology of the disorder completely. Effective therapy with L-dopa and possibly with the grafted TH-producing cells does not approach questions of the mechanism for the degeneration of the nigrostriatal pathway in Parkinson's patients.

For long-term therapeutic effects for any disorder, it is important to ensure stable and, ideally, appropriately regulated gene expression from the transgene. Integrated viruses are indeed often, but not always, stable, and further studies of the parameters for most efficient and stable gene expression of the transferred foreign genes would be helpful. In many cases, it would be useful to be able to turn the level of foreign gene expression up, down, or even off, to satisfy variations in physiological needs. Future generations of virus vectors or other forms of the transferred genes will include portions of regulatory regions of the relevant genes to allow modulation of gene expression.

The genetic correction of some, or many, CNS disorders may require the establishment or re-establishment of faithful intercellular synaptic connections. Model systems to study these possibilities have not yet been developed and exploited because of the paucity of replicating non-transformed cell culture systems and the refractoriness of non-replicating neuronal cells to viral infection. As mentioned above, because vectors derived from neurotropic viruses, such as herpesviruses, continue to be developed as vehicles of gene transfer in non-replicating cells, modification of neurons for intracerebral transplantation will certainly become an import method. However, at present, technical difficulties of toxicity and latency must first be solved before such vectors become generally useful. On the other hand, studies, including those involving the immortalization of embryonic hippocampal neuronal cells (Frederiksen and McKay, 1988), suggest that replicating neuronal cell culture systems are now available for gene transfer *in vitro* and then for implantation *in vivo*. Such neurons might be susceptible to efficient transduction by retroviral or other viral vectors, and if they are also able to retain other neuronal characteristics, they may be able to establish synaptic connections with other cells after grafting into the brain. Alternatively, there are cells within the CNS that are late to develop, such as the ventral leaf of the dentate gyrus of the hippocampus, or continue to divide through adulthood, such as those in the olfactory mucosa and in the dentate gyrus. Such cells may be suitable targets for retroviral infection. The effects of possible neural connections established by such cells *in vivo* after grafting are impossible to predict, and will obviously be affected by any developmental and functional commitments made by the cells before implantation and synaptic connection. It is not immediately apparent whether hippocampal or olfactory area neurons, or neurons from any other specific area, will continue to function faithfully in other sites of the brain as they would have done in their area of origin, or if they will assume functions more characteristic of the implantation site.

Because of their accessibility and the presence of suitable replicating cell populations, bone marrow, skin, lymphocytes, endothelial cells, and hepatocytes have been studied most extensively as potential target organs for gene therapy. The use of non-neuronal cells for grafting, however, probably precludes the development of specific neural connections to resident target cells of the host. Therefore, the phenotypic effects of fibroblast or other non-neuronal donor cells or target cells *in vivo* would be through the diffusion of a required gene product or metabolite through tight junctions ('metabolic cooperation') or through specific uptake by target cells of secreted donor cell gene products or metabolites. Alternatively, the donor cell can act as a toxin 'sink' by expressing a new gene product and metabolizing and clearing a neurotoxin.

Advantages to the use of autologous cells as donor cells are that they need neither be CNS-derived nor have to express the desired function naturally. Instead, they may be selected solely on their ability to be grown and manipulated *in vivo* and to survive as grafts. In addition, by using cells derived from the donor, many immunological problems may be circumvented. Although they are not necessarily the most well suited cells for intracerebral grafting, skin fibroblasts have several advantageous features: they are easily obtained and grown from small biopsies with little discomfort to the patient; they can be genetically manipulated in culture by a number of methods, including retrovirus vectors; they can survive as intracerebral grafts in rats; and they are secretory cells and thus constituitively secrete many transgene products.

Certainly the human neurological diseases for which somatic gene therapy becomes relevant will dictate the type of cell and the requirements of the donor. Fibroblasts would be appropriate in the cases where a trophic factor or hormonal non-regulated release of a gene product would be sufficient for functional recovery. However, if the disease or disorder requires precise regulation of the secreted gene product or the establishment of accurate synaptic connections, more research will be needed to develop the appropriate cells and regulatory elements for the cells.

CONCLUSION

There is no longer any doubt that genetic approaches to the treatment of many kinds of human disease will soon become feasible and, indeed, necessary. The kinds of diseases amenable to genetic attack will include not only the conceptually straight forward enzymic deficiencies (inborn errors of metabolism), but also any disorders in which genetic factors play etiological or physiological roles. We know now that these include forms of cancer, cardiovascular diseases, and probably a number of neuro-psychiatric diseases. Certainly, the CNS presents some difficult barriers. The cells of the CNS are relatively inaccessible and therefore the biochemical basis for many CNS disorders have not been well understood. But the development of modern approaches to reverse genetic analysis will permit the identification of the mutant genes responsible for an increasing number of neuropsychiatric diseases, such as Alzheimer's disease, Huntington's disease, schizophrenia, and others. Our future ability to use the immense new powers of molecular genetics and neuroscience to modify the devastation caused by these and other CNS defects will be limited only by our imaginations.

References

Frederiksen K and McKay RDG (1988) Proliferation and differentiation of rat neuroepithelial precursor cells in vivo, *J Neurosci*, **8**(4), 1144–51

Friedmann T (1989) Progress toward human gene therapy, *Science*, **244**, 1275–81

Gage FH, Wolff JA, Rosenberg MB, Xu L, Yee J-K, Shults C *et al.* (1987) Grafting genetically modified cells to the brain: Possibilities for the future, *Neuroscience*, **23**, 795–807

Hefti F (1983) Is Alzheimer's disease caused by lack of nerve growth factor?, *Ann Neurol*, **13**, 109–10

Lindvall O, Brundin P, Widner H, Rehncrona S, Gustavii B, Frackowiak R *et al.* (1989) Grafts of fetal dopamine neurons survive and improve motor function in Parkinson's disease, *Science*, **247**, 574–7

Paterson AH, Lander ES, Hewitt JD, Peterson S, Lincoln SE, and Tanksley SD (1988) Resolution of quantitative traits into Mendelian factors by using a complete linkage map of restriction fragment length polymorphisms, *Nature*, **335**, 721–6

Riordan JR, Rommens JM, Kerem B-S, Alon N, Rozmahel R, Grzelczak Z *et al.* (1989) Identification of the cystic fibrosis gene: Cloning and characterization of complementary DNA, *Science*, **245**, 1066–73

St George-Hyslop PH, Tanzi RE, Polinsky RJ, Haines JL, Nee L, Watkins PC *et al.* (1987) The genetic defect causing familial Alzheimer's disease maps on chromosome 21, *Science*, **235**, 885–90

Temin HM (1986) Retrovirus vectors for gene transfer: Efficient integration into and expression of exogenous DNA in vertebrate cell genomes, In Kucherlapati R, ed, *Gene Transfer*, New York, Plenum, 149–87

Williams LR, Varon S, Peterson GM, Wictorin K, Fischer W, Björklund A *et al.* (1986) Continuous infusion of nerve growth factor prevents basal forebrain neuronal death after fimbria-fornix transection, *Proc Natl Acad Sci USA*, **83**, 9231–5

Wolff JA, Fisher LJ, Xu L, Jinnah HA, Langlais PJ, Iuovone PM *et al.* (1989) Grafting fibroblasts genetically modified to produce L-dopa in a rat model of Parkinson disease, *Proc Natl Acad Sci USA*, **86**, 9011–4

20
Summary and future needs

R. R. Young and P. J. Delwaide

This book has been published in an attempt to present restorative neurology in its larger biological, neurobiological, and rehabilitation engineering context. To understand more fully the pathophysiology of chronic neurologic disabilities, and to provide truly optimal therapy and management, we must become more successful in capturing the attention of our neuroscientist and engineering colleagues. Progress will not be sufficiently quick and comprehensive until many others outside the classical confines of rehabilitation and neurology become interested in specific problems of our patients; they can develop new methods to study neuropathophysiology. And before pathophysiology can really be understood, much more research must be done to explain normal function.

Classical neurology was based upon fundamentals of anatomy and neuropathology; modern imaging techniques (CT and MRI) are thus of immense clinical importance. Nevertheless, such anatomic approaches usually do not answer the questions posed by restorative neurology, especially not those concerned with function and disability. Unfortunately, probably because neurologic function is extremely complex, few reliable quantitative techniques have been developed to serve as imaging-equivalents of function. It also seems unlikely that future advances in molecular or cell biology, crucial as they have been and will be to progress toward our goals, will fully 'explain' the function of complex neural systems or provide needed insight into clinically relevant disabilities. We await the development of new, non-reductionist approaches to neuroscience, with quantitative and analytical, but integrative, approaches. Meanwhile, improved techniques are needed to measure function; and the tools used for evaluation, monitoring, and functional assessment must also be standardized. These advances are crucial if restorative neurology is to define normative values of motor and sensory function; to achieve more precise, functionally significant diagnostic categorizations (see Chapter 3); and to assess changes produced by therapy. The clinically pre-eminent question continues to be— which treatments really do work and to what extent? One naturally turns to clinical neurophysiology for help but, in addition, new concepts are needed from all levels of neurobiology, including neural systems and biomedical engineering. We asked the contributors to this volume to evaluate critically the available therapies. In almost every instance, lack of objective data in the literature prevented the achievement of that goal. A desperate need exists for the establishment of long-term efforts to assess quantitatively all rehabilitation therapies to prove which ones work and to what extent.

The 1990s, the decade of the brain, will be characterized by unprecedented options in neurology, particularly when therapy is taken to include restorative neurology or neurologic rehabilitation as well as pharmacotherapy and standard neurosurgical procedures. Molecular biology has provided DNA tests for carrier detection and diagnosis (including presymptomatic and prenatal diagnosis) of a variety of neurologic conditions, such as muscular dystrophies, familial polyneuropathies, Friedreich's ataxia, neurofibromatosis, retinoblastoma, tuberous sclerosis, and Wilson's disease. As many neurologic disorders become understood at a cellular or molecular level, new means are being discovered to prevent or repair damage to muscle or nervous tissue; for example, replacement of dystrophin in muscular dystrophy or transplanting glial cells into areas of demyelination (Blakemore, Crang, and Franklin, 1990). Prevention of functional deterioration is preferable to restoration, which takes place only after dysfunction has become clinically evident.

Methods are now being developed to minimize secondary neuronal damage by using drugs to downregulate cellular metabolism, so that neurons can survive longer after injury while they are receiving less glucose and oxygen than they ordinarily need; by using lazaroids to scavenge free radicals, which damage nervous tissue; and by blocking NMDA receptors to reduce excitotoxicity. Glutamate-related cell death may be mediated by nitric oxide, the first gas shown to be a normal neurotransmitter (Bredt *et al.*, 1991). How can this surprising development be used therapeutically?

Regeneration is being facilitated by antibodies against nerve growth inhibitors (Schnell and Schwab, 1990) and by using transplants or genetic modifications to increase neural growth factors and other neurotrophic substances. Brain-derived neurotrophic factor, for example, prolongs survival of midbrain dopaminergic neurons, which degenerate in Parkinson's disease (Hyman *et al.*, 1991). Gangliosides, which may modulate the action of endogenous trophic factors (see Sabel, Vantini, and Finklestein, in press, for review), have been reported to enhance recovery of motor function after spinal cord injury (Geisler, Dorsey, and Coleman, 1991). Aguayo has summarized recent developments in the field of neural regeneration in more detail (see Appendix, below).

We are beginning to understand stimulus-transcription coupling in nerve cells, intracellular molecular cascades underlying perception, cognition and learning (Dash, Hochner, and Kandel, 1990), and use-dependent synaptic plasticity even in mature cerebral cortex (Kaas, 1991). Long-term deafferentations of upper limbs in adult monkeys (C2-T4 dorsal roots) are associated with systematic, non-random reorganization of somatosensory cortical maps extending for 10 to 14 millimeters in a lateromedial direction, involving the entire deafferented area (Pons *et al.*, 1991). This is an order of magnitude greater than what had previously been considered possible and still may not represent the maximum reorganizational capability of the adult nervous system. Can this capability be used therapeutically? 'For example, inputs normally processed by regions of the sensory cortex damaged by stroke might be rechanneled for processing by undamaged regions of sensory cortex. If we know the mechanism and rules by which this is operating, there's the possibility that we can harness this type of reorganizational capacity for therapeutic purposes.' (Pons *et al.*, 1991.)

Monthly in neurological journals, papers relevant to restorative neurology appear describing, for example, functional anatomy of motor recovery after stroke in humans (Chollet *et al.*, 1991), results of intraspinal transplants (Tessler, 1991), and plasticity of sensory and motor maps in adult animals including reorganization of human motor cortex after spinal cord injury (Levy *et al.*, 1990). Plasticity is a much more widespread, ubiquitous, and powerful feature of CNS behavior than was once considered. Learning is, of course, its best known attribute but other examples exist, which suggest what may become possible once mechanisms underlying plasticity can be manipulated. For example, the deaf who use sign language often have remarkably enhanced powers of spatial perception (Poizner, Bellugill, and Klima, 1990) suggesting that areas of brain ordinarily devoted to hearing can be used for visual processing. As another example, more than half the corticospinal projections to spinal motorneurons and interneurons come from pre-motor and supplementary motor areas in the frontal lobe (Dum and Strick, 1991). This may have implications for restoration of function after lesions of the motor cortex or partial lesions of the corticospinal tract, particularly when whatever underlies plasticity can be manipulated appropriately.

New journals and national societies devoted entirely to restorative neurology or neurologic rehabilitation have sprung up in the past year or two (e.g. *Restorative Neurology and Neuroscience*, Elsevier; *Journal of Neurologic Rehabilitation*, Demos; American Society of Neurorehabilitation). We are at the threshold of exciting times for the mutually productive interaction of neurobiologists and clinicians. Not only has fundamental research provided the clinically useful (or potentially useful) techniques mentioned above, but careful clinical studies, interpreted critically, have begun to describe and define the operation of unknown neural mechanisms that need to be elucidated, thereby providing new and otherwise unsuspected problems for fundamental investigation. Clinical trials, if they have been performed carefully, may conceptualize mechanisms by which the therapy works as well as provide a rational basis for individualizing therapy. As therapeutic agents and techniques become more specific, they become more useful as tools for dissecting neural function.

Until this mutually supportive alliance between the bench and the clinic produces better ways to prevent secondary injury and to increase regeneration in the CNS, certain engineering solutions, which exist to restore function, must be implemented and new ones devised. Some of these efforts involve collaborations between engineering scientists and neurophysiologists to apply results obtained in the animal studies to human problems. High-tech solutions, such as those popularized in films, can be envisaged, but less complex ones may be more acceptable. For example, spinal cord injured patients whose knees are stabilized can be trained on a powered treadmill to produce bipedal stepping with weight bearing (Wernig and Mueller, 1991). Even simpler, and therefore more widely used, are custom fit boots that fix the ankles in 15° plantar flexion, which automatically lock the knees and hips in extension and permit patients with complete paraplegia to stand and walk using canes for balance (Lee *et al.*, 1991). It is surprising that it took so long for such a simple orthosis to be developed and reach clinical acceptance.

SUMMARY

This book is produced at an important turning point in the course of what has been called restorative neurology. Well-established techniques are now standards of practice and need to be critically evaluated; promises for the future, as outlined above, are exciting but still far removed from clinical reality. Dramatic changes are necessary in the way this field has been evolving. Empirical, and sometimes serendipitous, advances will continue slowly but clinical neuroscientists must be prepared to integrate new discoveries, coming from the application of first principles, into a clinical context. They must strike a balance between the pedestrian but clinically useful therapeutic trials, and the exciting but largely theoretical laboratory work. They must struggle to stay conversant in the many areas within neuroscience, such as genetic engineering, biomedical engineering, pharmacology, and rehabilitation medicine, and must plan for and undertake careful research projects to bridge the gap between theory and practice. These clinical neuroscientists will be known as Restorative Neurologists.

Appendix

A. J. Aguayo

Functional deficits engendered by injury and diseases of the nervous system tend to be permanent, largely as a result of the death of cells, neurons, and glia, and the interruption of the cellular appendages that make synaptic contacts possible.

Clinical and experimental studies have provided greater insight into the progressive nature of many CNS injuries where only a proportion of the damaged cells may be destroyed by the trauma-inducing forces but many others die as a result of subsequent changes at the injury site, altered patterns of neuronal and non-neuronal activity, and the loss of critical sources of trophic support. In this regard, there have been important advances in understanding the role played by the release of calcium, free radicals, excitatory aminoacids, and genes whose expression can result in cell death (Choi, 1988; Martin *et al.*, 1988). Moreover, studies have resulted in the identification of several new trophic factors and their genes, as well as major advances in understanding the way these proteins are synthesized, released, and interact with their receptors (Barde, 1989). The availability of expression systems, which permit the synthesis and production of many of the molecules that are critical to the survival of injured neurons, suggest the possibility that some may soon be ready for clinical trials aimed at mitigating progressive neuronal damage and cell death.

There is also a continuing interest in the possibility of replacing lost or damaged nerve cells and glia by means of transplants of immature or genetically engineered cells (Björklund, 1991). Work based on a thoughtful and scientific approach to neural grafting continues to move forward towards its use in patients afflicted by specific disorders of the nervous system.

While it has long been accepted dogma that nerve cells in the mature mammalian CNS are incapable of restoring lost connections, recent *in vivo* animal studies have shown that such injured neurons have the capacity to initiate and sustain extensive fiber regrowth, which can lead to the formation of new functional synapses with distant targets. This capacity is made apparent when the glial substrate of CNS axons is changed by grafting peripheral nerve segments into the brain or spinal cord (Aguayo *et al.*, 1991). Furthermore, the formation of novel connections after axonal regeneration does not appear to be totally random, a finding that suggests regrowing axons may continue to exhibit specific post-synaptic preferences in the adult (Carter *et al.*, 1989). Additional, indirect evidence for the persistence of such recognition cues also arises from the observation that transplants containing immature neurons, selectively innervate and functionally influence appropriate targets in the vicinity of the graft (Björklund, 1991).

The overall significance of many of the studies, in which non-neuronal and neural grafts have been used to investigate regenerative capacities, suggests that while injured neurons in adult mammals may be intrinsically capable of replicating many of the developmental steps that led to the establishment of functional neural circuits, their innate responses are strongly influenced by components of their immediate environment. Investigators in several laboratories have begun to unravel the complex extrinsic mechanisms that curtail such an axonal regrowth in the CNS. Studies by Schwab (1990) suggest that two proteins in central myelin, with a molecular mass of 35 and 250 kd, block neurite extensions both *in vitro* and *in vivo*. Antibodies generated against these proteins, when administered to laboratory animals with spinal cord injury, result in a greater regrowth of interrupted corticospinal tract axons, presumably as a result of a specific perturbation of the axon-blocking action of these myelin components. It is of additional interest that these two inhibitory proteins have not been identified in peripheral nerves or in the CNS of fish and amphibians, where severed axons can regenerate spontaneously.

Advances in understanding the role of nerve cells and their cellular and extracellular environment in regeneration, and the possibility that some of the critical molecular mechanisms involved in axonal growth and target recognition may be unravelled, have generated increasing study of cues used by extending axons to appropriately select and reach their remote targets. Observations in vertebrates and invertebrates (see Rutishauser and Jessell, 1988, for review) suggest that specific substrate molecules guide axons along complex pathways in the developing nervous system to establish the circuits that make neural behavior possible.

It will be important to determine if the suppression of the molecules that inhibit growth in the mammalian CNS lead not only to a more extensive regrowth of the cut axons but also to re-expression of the substratum conditions responsible for their guidance. The remarkable precision and order with which many axotomized nerve cells in the CNS of amphibian and fish re-establish damaged axonal projections provide an encouraging argument for continuation of studies in the injured mammalian brain and spinal cord.

References

Aguayo AJ, Rasminsky M, Bray GM, Carbonetto S, McKerracher L, Villegas-Perez MP *et al.* (1991) Degenerative and regenerative responses of injured neurons in the central nervous system of adult mammals, *Philos Trans R Soc Lond [Biol]* **331**, 337–43

Barde Y-A (1989) Trophic factors and neuronal survival, *Neuron*, **2**, 1525–34

Björklund A (1991) Neural transplantation – an experimental tool with clinical possibilities, TINS, **14**, 319–21

Blakemore WR, Crang AF, and Franklin FJM (1990) Transplantation of glial cell cultures into areas of demyelination of the adult CNS, *Prog Brain Res*, **82**, 225–32

Bredt DS, Hwang PM, Glatt CE, Lowenstein C, Reed RR, and Snyder SH (1991) Cloned and expressed nitric oxide synthase structurally resembles cytochrome P-450 reductase, *Nature*, **351**, 714–8

Carter DA, Bray GM, and Aguayo AJ (1989) Regenerated retinal ganglion cell axons can form well-differentiated synapses in the superior colliculus of adult hamsters, *J Neurosci*, **9**, 4042–50

Choi DW (1988) Glutamate neurotoxicity and diseases of the nervous system, *Neuron*, **1**, 623–34

Chollet, F, DiPiero V, Wise RJS, Brooks DJ, Dolan RJ, and Frackowiak RSJ (1991) The functional anatomy of motor recovery after stroke in humans, *Ann Neurol*, **29**, 63–71

Dash PK, Hochner B, and Kandel ER (1990) Injection of cAMP-responsive element into the nucleus of *Aplysia* sensory neurons blocks long-term facilitation, *Nature*, **345**, 718–21

Dum RP and Strick PL (1991) The origin of corticospinal projections from the premotor areas in the frontal lobe, *J Neurosci*, **11**, 667–89

Geisler FH, Dorsey FC, and Coleman WP (1991) Recovery of motor function after spinal-cord injury – a randomized, placebo-controlled trial with GM-1 ganglioside, *N Engl J Med*, **324**, 1829–38

Hyman C, Hofer M, Barde Y-A, Juhasz M, Yancopoulos GD, Squinto SP *et al.* (1991) BDNF is a neurotrophic factor for dopaminergic neurons of the substantia nigra, *Nature*, **350**, 230–2

Kaas JH (1991) Plasticity of sensory and motor maps in adult mammals, *Annu Rev Neurosci*, **14**, 137–67

Lee IY, Craffey E, Davidson D, Durso V, Tun CG, Walsh N *et al.* (1991) Complete paraplegics can walk using a below-the-knee boot orthosis, *Neurology*, **41**, 221

Levy WJ, Amassian VE, Traad M, and Cadwell J (1990) Focal magnetic coil stimulation reveals motor cortical system reorganized in humans after traumatic quadriplegia, *Brain Res*, **510**, 130–4

Martin DP, Schmidt RE, DiStefano PS, Lowry OH, Carter JG, and Johnson EM (1988) Inhibitors of protein synthesis prevent neuronal death caused by nerve growth factor deprivation, *J Cell Biol*, **106**, 829–44

Poizner H, Bellugill, and Klima ES (1990) Biological foundations of language: clues from sign language, *Ann Rev Neurosci*, **13**, 283–301

Pons TM, Garraghty PE, Ommaya AK, Kaas JH, Taub E, and Mishkin M (1991) Massive cortical reorganization after sensory deafferentation in adult macaques, *Science*, **252**, 1857–60

Rutishauser U and Jessell TM (1988) Cell adhesion molecules in vertebrate neural development, *Physiol Rev*, **68**, 819–57

Sabel BA, Vantini G, and Finklestein SP (1992) The role of neurotrophic factors in the treatment of neurological disorders, In Vecsei L, ed, *Neurological Disorders: Novel Experimental and Therapeutic Strategies*, New York, Simon and Schuster

Schnell L and Schwab ME (1990) Axonal regeneration in the rat spinal cord produced by an antibody against myelin-associated neurite growth inhibitors, *Nature*, **343**, 269–72

Schwab ME (1990) Myelin-associated inhibitors of neurite growth, *Exp Neurol*, **109**, 2–5

Tessler A (1991) Intraspinal transplants, *Ann Neurol*, **29**, 115–23

Wernig A and Mueller S (1991) Improvement of locomotion by laufband training in patients with severe spinal cord lesions, *Pfluegers Arch*, **418**, 52

Index